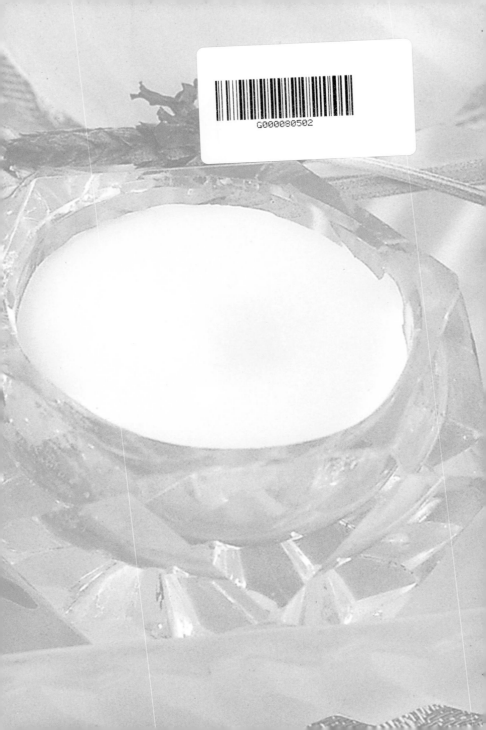

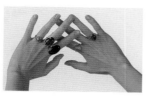

THE HANDBOOK OF
ALTERNATIVE
HEALING

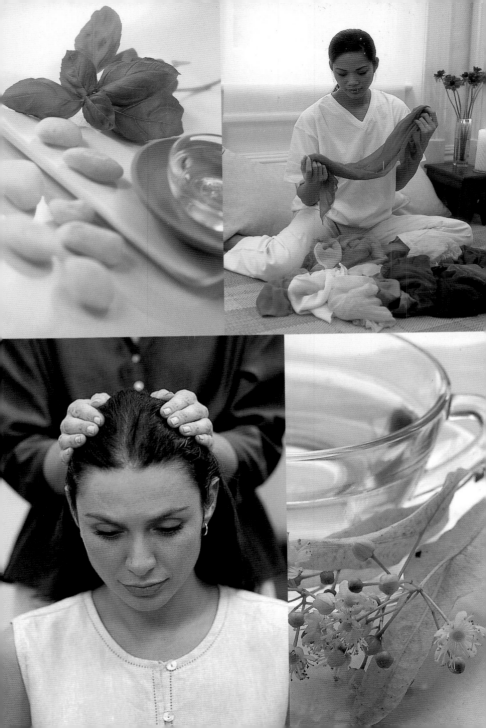

THE HANDBOOK OF
ALTERNATIVE HEALING

A safe and comprehensive guide to using nature's remedies for healing mind, body and spirit, including flower healing • herbal remedies • aromatherapy • healing foods • ayurveda • energies • crystals • colour therapy • therapeutic touch • yoga • meditation

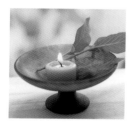

LORENZ BOOKS

This edition is published by Lorenz Books

Lorenz Books is an imprint of Anness Publishing Ltd Hermes House, 88–89 Blackfriars Road, London SE1 8HA; tel. 020 7401 2077; fax 020 7633 9499 www.lorenzbooks.com; info@anness.com

© Anness Publishing Ltd 2004

UK agent: The Manning Partnership Ltd, 6 The Old Dairy, Melcombe Road, Bath BA2 3LR; tel. 01225 478444; fax 01225 478440; sales@manning-partnership.co.uk

UK distributor: Grantham Book Services Ltd, Isaac Newton Way, Alma Park Industrial Estate, Grantham, Lincs NG31 9SD; tel. 01476 541080; fax 01476 541061; orders@gbs.tbs-ltd.co.uk

North American agent/distributor: National Book Network, 4501 Forbes Boulevard, Suite 200, Lanham, MD 20706; tel. 301 459 3366; fax 301 429 5746; www.nbnbooks.com

Australian agent/distributor: Pan Macmillan Australia, Level 18, St Martins Tower, 31 Market St, Sydney, NSW 2000; tel. 1300 135 113; fax 1300 135 103; customer.service@macmillan.com.au

New Zealand agent/distributor: David Bateman Ltd, 30 Tarndale Grove, Off Bush Road, Albany, Auckland; tel. (09) 415 7664; fax (09) 415 8892

A CIP catalogue record for this book is available from the British Library.

Publisher: Joanna Lorenz
Editorial Director: Helen Sudell
Project Editors: Caroline Davidson, Emma Grey, Melanie Halton, Simona Hill, Debra Mayhew, Catherine Stuart
Contributors: Raje Airey, Mark Evans, Jenni Fleetwood, Doriel Hall, Jessica Houdret, John Hudson, Tracey Kelly, Simon Lilly, Rosalind Oxenford, Lilian Vernier-Bonds
Designers: Ann Cannings, Jane Coney, Lilian Lindblom, Nigel Partridge, Ian Sandom
Production Controller: Claire Rae
Editorial Reader: Jay Thundercliffe

Previously published in twelve separate volumes as *Healing with Flowers, Healing with Herbs, Healing with Aromatherapy, Healing with Food, Healing with Ayurveda, Healing Energies, Healing with Crystals, Healing with Colour, Healing Hands, Healing with Reflexology, Healing with Yoga* and *Healing with Meditation.*

10 9 8 7 6 5 4 3 2 1

Disclaimer
The author and publishers have made every effort to ensure that all instructions within this book are accurate and safe, and cannot accept liability for any resulting injury, damage or loss to persons or property, however it may arise. If you do have any special needs or problems, consult your doctor or a physiotherapist. This book cannot replace medical consultation and should be used in conjunction with professional advice.

Contents

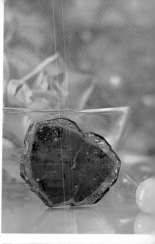

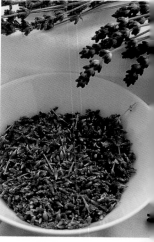

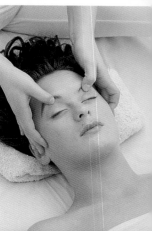

Introduction

Alternative healing is a term given to a range of practices that aim to promote well-being by considering body, mind and spirit, and by using natural, organic ingredients. Although increasingly popular in today's society, many remedies in this book draw from the wisdom of ancient practices.

POWERFUL PLANTS

Flowers and herbs have formed the basis of medicine since the dawn of human history. Even today, it is estimated that about three-quarters of all medicines are derived from living plants. The chapters on HEALING WITH FLOWERS and HERBS show how to harvest, dry, prepare and store your own healing plants, and subsequently unleash their potent curative powers in floral and herbal teas, tisanes, infusions, inhalations and compresses. Treatments for particular ailments are outlined – such as soothing stomach upset with chamomile

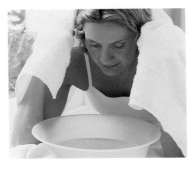

▲ A BOWL OF SCENTED, HOT WATER WILL LIFT THE SPIRITS OR SOOTHE A COLD.

and cramp bark, or alleviating winter blues with rosemary tonic wine – and an alphabetical directory of the most effective healing plants offers further advice on their properties and safe self-administration.

A section on HEALING WITH AROMATHERAPY explores ways in which to use the essential oils of flowers, herbs, shrubs, vines, fruits, spices and trees to lift the spirits and stimulate the senses. These potent oils can be added to restorative massages, soothing baths and cleansing inhalations.

▼ PLANTS CAN BE USED IN A VARIETY OF WAYS TO STIMULATE THE SENSES.

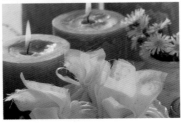

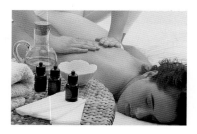

▲ AROMATHERAPY MASSAGE CAN EASE TENSE MUSCLES AND HELP US FEEL RELAXED.

Moreover, their natural perfume and protective properties make them a perfect organic addition to luxurious skin creams, hair rinses and soaps.

FORTIFYING FOODS

"You are what you eat" – never has this old adage seemed so appropriate. Scientific research is proving time and time again the therapeutic and preventive benefits of eating a nutritious selection of foods. Cruciferous vegetables and fruits, such as carrots, for example, are rich in antioxidants, which are now known to help guard the body against cancer. The fatty acids present in oily fish, nuts and seeds supply wide and varied benefits ranging from healthy brain function to great-looking skin. Brimming over with suggestions for healthy snacks, storage tips, advice on

where to source essential vitamins and minerals, plus recipes for common ailments, HEALING WITH FOOD offers constructive and delicious advice on how to eat your way towards good health.

A chapter on HEALING WITH AYURVEDA harnesses the wealth of knowledge contained in this ancient medicinal system, which originated in India some 5,000 years ago. You'll learn about the

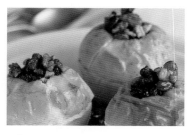

▲ HEALTHY SNACKS NEED NOT BE BORING: MANY FRUITS ARE NATURALLY SWEET.

Tridosha – the three universal energies – plus the ways in which to balance them. Complete a questionnaire on personality and physical traits to reveal your ayurvedic "dosha", or type, and use this knowledge to make lifestyle choices on diet, exercise, work and relaxation, to take your daily routine in a new direction entirely suited to you.

Harnessing energies

Natural phenomena such as colour, light and sound hold a wealth of vitality for those who know how to channel their subtle vibrations. HEALING WITH ENERGIES illustrates the effect of biorhythms and cosmic influences on stamina, and how the body's energy field can be accessed using simple diagnostic methods such as kinesiology, dowsing, homeopathy and water therapy.

The properties of gemstones have long been known to promote health and harmony, and an eye-

▼ THE COLOUR OF ANY CRYSTAL DETERMINES ITS MAIN HEALING FUNCTION.

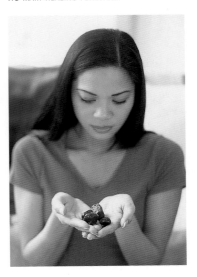

opening chapter on the dynamics of HEALING WITH CRYSTALS explores practical ways to harness the power of these precious stones. Did you know, for example, that placing quartz near to your computer helps to combat the effects of electro-magnetism, or that headaches can be soothed by contact with healing amethysts?

Both this and a subsequent chapter on using COLOUR to heal explain the links between the seven chakras – which materalize as seven layers of coloured light – and natural energy flow. By applying the principles of full-body chakra healing to your choice, and usage, of crystals and colour, you can balance, energize or soothe through adjustments to your home and work environment.

Therapeutic touch

The HANDS have long been used as instruments of healing, and a number of hands-on therapies have evolved to combat pain, boost immunity and increase stamina. Shiatsu is a holistic method of healing whereby finger pressure is applied to key points on the body to bring the female yin and male

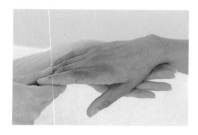

▲ THE POWER OF TOUCH IS EVIDENT IN
THERAPIES SUCH AS MASSAGE AND SHIATSU.

yang energies into balance. Reiki healing – which has roots in Tibetan Buddhism – works by harnessing the invisible energies of the cosmos and directing them towards the body as a force for well-being. Like shiatsu, reflexology works with finger pressure, by stimulating the body's reflexes through contact with the hands and feet.

MIND OVER MATTER

Health practitioners are learning that so many ailments begin with prolonged and negative stress on the mind, which, if left unchecked, can weaken the body and open it to a whole host of ailments. It is vitally important to regain control of our emotional being. To this end, a chapter on HEALING WITH YOGA unites body and mind through dynamic yet easily-perfomed postures and breathing exercises, to promote balance, resolve and flexibility. HEALING WITH MEDITATION reveals how the power of the mind can be channelled using mantra, memory, even day-dreaming, to enable you to fulfil ambitions, work with greater clarity, and simply relax.

With such a wealth of methods to choose from, use this guide to see for yourself how alternative healing can turn your life around by dissolving tension, restoring energy and promoting a healthy mind and body.

▼ MEDITATING WITH CRYSTALS CLEARS THE
MIND AND HELPS TO REKINDLE RESOLVE.

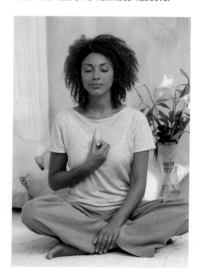

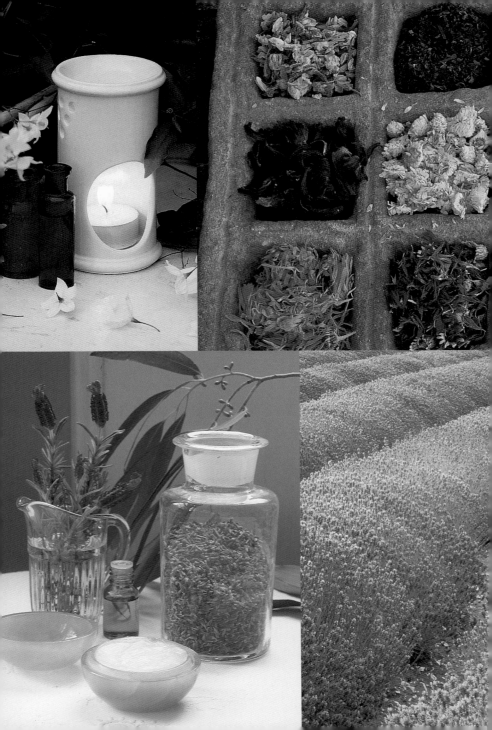

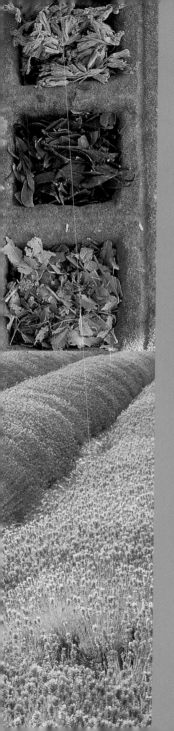

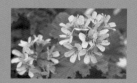

HEALING WITH
FLOWERS

Healing with flowers and herbs is as ancient as humankind, and, for much of our history, was the only medical option available. Even today, it is estimated that three-quarters of our pharmaceutical drugs are plant-based, and medical research continues to prove the healing powers of natural flower remedies.

The following section describes how to cultivate, harvest, dry, prepare and store healing flowers. It also explains how to use the various parts of a flower in therapeutic teas, tinctures, oils, infusions, compresses and inhalants. A directory of healing plants introduces some of the most useful flowers, with tips on how to recognize them and harness their healing properties.

History of healing with flowers

Until the advent of pharmaceutically based medicine at the beginning of the 19th century, healing systems in all cultures relied upon plants. Indeed, many of today's manufactured pills were originally made from plants.

EARLY HEALING SYSTEMS

Many ancient civilizations had well-developed medicinal plant healing systems. The earliest recorded natural healing methods were in China nearly 5,000 years ago, but because China remained closed to the West for many centuries, it is the texts recorded on tablets and papyri from the early civilizations of Sumeria and Egypt which are the antecedents of the later European healers. The great physicians of ancient Greece – Hippocrates, Galen, Theophrastus and Dioscorides – drew on these earlier cultures when writing their own works.

The name of Paracelsus (1493–1541), a 16th-century Swiss physician and alchemist, stands out in particular. He declared that he had not taken his knowledge from the Greek

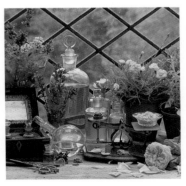

▲ FLOWERS HAVE BEEN USED FOR HEALING PURPOSES THROUGHOUT HISTORY.

"father of medicine" Hippocrates, the influential Roman physician Galen or anyone else, but "from the best teachers: experience and hard work". Paracelsus believed that disease originated from a departure with essential spirituality, and that by balancing the four elements, a substance called a "quintessence" was created, which healed the soul. The right essence, whether of a flower or mineral, would renew the connection with the spirit within, which was the true healer.

THE RENAISSANCE

From earliest times there has been a belief in the power of flower fragrance to protect from disease. This led to the 15th-century production of pomanders, the use of posies, strewing herbs and herbal fumigation. Diet was also considered integral to healing – herbs and flowers were added to food for their medicinal action as much as for their nutritional or flavouring capabilities.

THE MODERN ERA

In the early 19th century, the medical establishment moved away from remedies made with plants to laboratory-produced chemical drugs. This was a great step forward for civilization as general health improved and cures were found for many diseases, but a side-effect was that much of the responsibility for their own minor health problems was taken out of the hands of ordinary people and home remedies began to be forgotten.

During the last century Edward Bach (1886–1936), the founder of modern flower essence therapy, pioneered the treatment

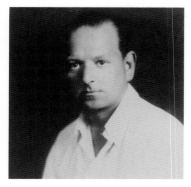

▲ EDWARD BACH, PIONEER OF MODERN FLOWER REMEDIES.

of the whole person by using safe and natural remedies. Of Welsh origin, Bach was born in Birmingham and trained as a bacteriologist. Later, in 1919, he joined the staff of the London Homeopathic Hospital.

Bach believed that for healing to succeed, the emotions, particularly fear, uncertainty and shock had to be addressed in depth. By 1928, he was experimenting with flowers, finding that impatiens, clematis and mimulus worked well to calm certain mental states.

Much ancient plant lore has recently been revived in the use of flowers in both internal and external forms of self-healing.

Using flowers to heal

The ways in which you can use flowers to heal include inhaling uplifting flower scents, drinking soothing teas, unwinding with a relaxing flower oil massage, or allowing the subtle energy of a flower essence to work on your deepest emotions.

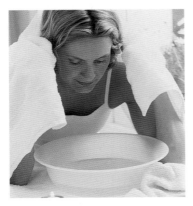

▲ An essential oil steam inhalation is an excellent way to relieve the congestion of a cold or blocked sinuses.

Flower oils

Essential oils extracted from flowers have a powerful effect on mental and emotional states. Breathing in their vapours can be relaxing, restorative or uplifting. One way to inhale the scent is simply to put a few drops on a handkerchief and keep it on your pillow overnight. But for a more controlled and concentrated method, which is also longer lasting, an essential oil burner is ideal. Other ways of benefiting from oils include adding a few drops to a warm bath, or diluting and massaging into the skin.

Flower teas

Also known as tisanes, flower teas have been used for medicinal purposes for many centuries. Lavender, hyssop and thyme were taken to alleviate cold symptoms, while chamomile and lime flower were used against insomnia. Whatever the virtues, the scent of these tisanes alone is a tonic and they can be enjoyed simply for this reason.

Flower tonics

Plants that affect the nervous system interact powerfully with the body. These are known as nervines, and invigorate and nourish the whole nervous system. Restorative nervine tonics include St John's wort, sage and mugwort. Relaxing tonics include skullcap, vervain and wood betony.

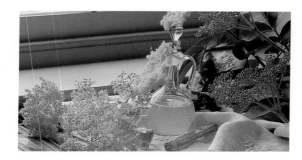

◀ YOU CAN STORE YOUR HOME-MADE FLOWER REMEDIES IN ORNATE BOTTLES.

FLOWER ESSENCES

Natural flower remedies do not address the organs of our bodies, like our heart, liver and lungs, and their ailments. Rather, the remedies work on basic mental and emotional states.

Recent research suggests that water has a "memory" and can hold the imprint of a flower's properties, passing these on to us. Bach himself made sun-potentized flower essences in pure water.

Just as beautiful music can inspire us and help us feel whole, so can flower essences, Bach said. Some people now use the term "vibrational medicine" to make the analogy between music and the flowers clearer.

▶ THE SEPARATE COMPARTMENTS OF THIS SPECIALLY DESIGNED ESSENCE BOX KEEP THEIR INDIVIDUAL HEALING PROPERTIES CLEAR.

So, if our particular challenge is the anger or jealousy aspect of oversensitivity, holly essence will encourage acceptance of the emotion and bring out our love and tolerance. If the struggle is with the discouragement aspect of uncertainty, gentian essence can revive our courage and faith.

There is no harm in taking flower essences along with herbal tonics or essential oils, herb teas, aromas or inhalants. Each of these are healing expressions of the positive power of herbs and plants.

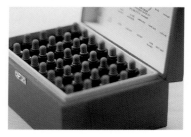

Flower cultivation

The process of cultivating, harvesting, drying and storing flowers can be a healing experience in itself. It is also the best way to learn the qualities of many remarkable healing plants, although buying flowers also gives good results.

GROWING

It is relatively easy to grow healing flowers, partly because many of these plants are wild in origin and do not suffer much from pests and diseases. Their aromatic smells often keep away harmful insects.

Cultivating your own healing flowers means you know exactly what has been put on them, and you can choose to go organic, using compost or mulches if you wish. Since many healing flowers are considered to be weeds — including red clover, horehound,

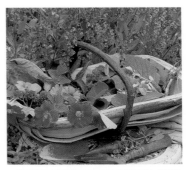

▲ GATHER FLOWERS IN THE MORNING, WHEN THE SUN HAS CAUSED THE DEW TO EVAPORATE AND ENCOURAGED THE FRAGRANCE TO DEVELOP.

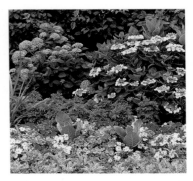

▲ MANY OF THE PLANTS FOUND IN GARDENS TODAY HAVE BEEN USED FOR THEIR HEALING PROPERTIES FOR 2,000 YEARS.

elder, selfheal and yarrow of those listed in the healing plants directory — they actually thrive on neglect and can colonize otherwise unused land.

HARVESTING

Reaping the flowers is a continuous rather than a one-off process. Most plants will be vigorous enough to allow repeated picking in small amounts, which encourages their further growth. It is best to gather flowers, stems and leaves when they are at their peak, which for flowers means on a sunny morning and for leaves before flowering begins. Roots should be dug up in the autumn, cleaned and chopped into small pieces.

If gathering wild flowers, be sure you have identified the plant correctly. Use a wild flower book, and pick them away from busy roads. Many wild plants are protected by law and should be left alone.

Drying

In order to dry flowers and herbs successfully, the moisture needs to be removed without losing the plant's volatile oils. Natural drying in an airing cupboard that is well ventilated is good. Loosely

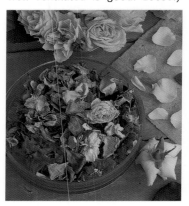

sealed brown paper bags can be used for drying small quantities. Using an oven even at a low setting is usually too hot for flowers and leaves, although it may be needed for roots.

Storing

Keep dried flowers and herbs in separate airtight containers in the dark, and label and date them. If hanging bundles, keep them in a dry, airy place out of the sunlight. If you prefer, store freshly gathered plants in the freezer. This method works well for lemon balm and parsley, which lose their flavour when dried. Tinctures are used to preserve selected herbs in alcohol.

Buying

If buying flowers is your preference, choose ones that seem fresh, and which have retained their colour and aroma.

◀ Dried rose petals make a colourful and fragrant potpourri which can help to promote a feeling of well-being.

Flower preparation

Flowers should be gathered on a warm dry morning, before the sun has become too strong and drawn out the essential oils. They are best picked in bud or freshly opened, when their scent and flavour are at their most enticing.

GATHERING FLOWERS

Those who are allergic to pollen should not eat flowers. In any case, it is still best to cut out the central reproductive areas, where the stamens and pollen are to be found, if you can. Individual flowers vary greatly but some, such as lilies and hibiscus, are particularly heavy with pollen and it is obvious which parts should be removed. With smaller flowers such as primroses, cowslips, violas and marjoram this would be difficult in the extreme, so if anyone is susceptible to allergy it is best to avoid all flowers.

Separate the petals from the green parts surrounding them – it is easier in some plants, such as marigolds, than others, for example violets or hollyhocks. Plants that flower in umbels, such as fennel, are best used whole.

▼ MAKE SURE THAT YOU IDENTIFY WILD FLOWERS CORRECTLY BEFORE PICKING THEM.

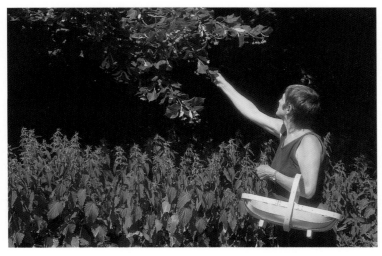

The body can benefit from the healing properties of flowers by using treatments both internally and externally.

INTERNAL USES

Flowers can be taken internally in infusions, inhalations, tinctures, teas, as capsules and powders, and in the many different types of preparations used to flavour and enhance cooking.

EXTERNAL USES

Flowers can be used externally in compresses, poultices, ointments, potpourris, skin creams, infused oils, massage and bath oils.

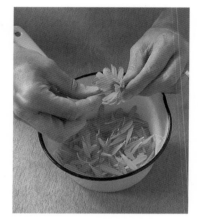

▲ CREAMS MADE FROM POT MARIGOLD PETALS ARE IDEAL FOR SOOTHING ALL MANNER OF SKIN IRRITATIONS.

▼ DRINKING SOOTHING HERBAL TEAS IS A GENTLE WAY TO RELAX BOTH BODY AND MIND.

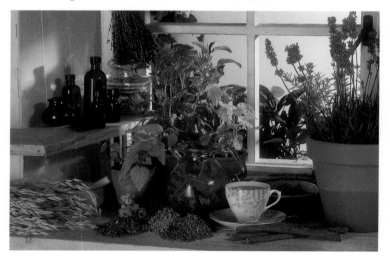

Infused oils and syrups

Active flower ingredients can be extracted in oil and used externally as a massage oil or added to creams and ointments. The two methods of extraction are hot infusion, using simmering heat, and cold infusion, using sunlight.

INFUSED OILS

Hot infusion is preferred for spicy herbs, including ginger or cayenne, and leafy herbs, such as comfrey, chickweed or mullein. The cold method is often used for fresh plants with delicate flowers, such as St John's wort, marigold, chamomile and melilot.

MAKING COLD INFUSED OILS

Pack a glass storage jar with the flowers or leaves of the herb. Pour in a light vegetable oil to cover the herbs, close the jar and shake well. Sunflower and grape

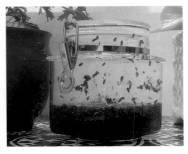

▲ PLACE THE FLOWERS AND THE OIL IN A GLASS JAR AND ALLOW THE CONTENTS TO STEEP FOR ONE MONTH IN A SUNNY LOCATION.

seed oil are good but olive oil is probably the best oil since it will not go rancid.

Allow the jar to stand on a sunny windowsill or in a greenhouse for a month, shaking it every day. The more sunlight there is and the longer the mixture is allowed to steep, the stronger it will be.

Strain the flowers or leaves, using a sieve or muslin bag. For a stronger infusion, renew the flowers in the oil every two weeks and infuse again. Pour the liquid into airtight bottles, label, and store in a cool dark place for up to a year.

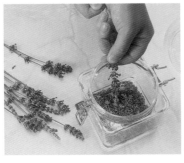

▲ FILL A GLASS STORAGE JAR WITH YOUR CHOSEN FLOWERS OR LEAVES.

Hot-syrup infusions

Since they use honey or unrefined sugar as a sweet preservative, syrups can disguise the taste of bitter plants such as motherwort or vervain. They are thus a good choice of remedy for children. Syrups are soothing in conditions such as sore throats and coughs.

Making syrups

Place 500g/1¼lb sugar or honey into a pan and add 1 litre/1¾ pints/4 cups water.

Heat gently and stir until the honey or sugar dissolves fully. Add 130g/4½oz flowers. Heat the ingredients gently for 5 minutes. Turn off the heat and allow the mixture to steep overnight.

Strain and store the syrup in an airtight container in the refrigerator or a cold cupboard. The sugar acts as a preservative so it should keep for up to 18 months.

▼ KEEP PREPARED SYRUPS AND INFUSED OILS IN AIRTIGHT GLASS STORAGE BOTTLES IN A COOL DARK PLACE.

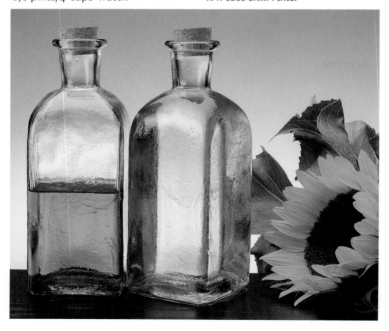

Flower essential oils

Aromatic flowers are so-called because they contain essential oils that carry specific and often therapeutic scents. The use of such oils and aromas to relax, sedate or stimulate has been known for millennia.

Flower therapy

Aromas have the power to produce emotional reactions within us. A distinctive smell can evoke a long-forgotten memory of a pleasurable or perhaps disturbing experience; it can be an instinctive reaction of attraction or repulsion, or a learned response. We quickly realize that hydrogen sulphide smells bad, like rotten eggs, while a rose is sweet. Some essential oils such as chamomile and lavender are sedating, others such as rosemary and geranium uplifting, but such general qualities can also be modified by our moods.

What are essential oils?

These are natural, volatile substances, which possess medicinal properties and a distinctive aroma. Essential oils evaporate easily, releasing their scent into the air, as demonstrated when someone brushes against an aromatic plant.

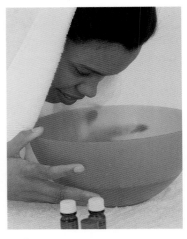

▲ STEAM INHALATION IS A QUICK AND EASY WAY TO ABSORB ESSENTIAL OILS.

Aromatherapy largely grew out of the perfumery industry, at first with the distillation of essential oils and later with the blending of aromatic oils to yield pleasurable scents. Combining oils is important to aromatherapy, as the effects of individual oils can be magnified in combination. A balanced scent from a blend is likely to be more enjoyable and have a greater therapeutic effect.

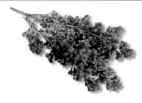

◀ AROMATIC PLANTS CONTAIN ESSENTIAL OILS THAT CAN BE USED TO RELAX, SEDATE, REFRESH OR STIMULATE.

In the early 20th century, the French chemist René-Maurice Gattefosse was working in the family perfumery laboratory, when he badly burned his hand. Plunging it into the nearest liquid, Gattefosse found that the jar of lavender oil he had accidentally used eased the pain, prevented scarring and promoted healing.

Gattefosse then began to examine the therapeutic properties of essential oils, and in 1928 coined the term "aromatherapy" to describe the use of aromatic oils for treating physical and emotional problems.

MASSAGE WITH ESSENTIAL OILS

Essential oils are very concentrated and can damage the skin. Before using them in massage, dilute them with a vegetable carrier oil, such as wheatgerm or almond oil. In general, mix one drop of essential oil with 10ml/ 2 tsp of carrier oil, but use less essential oil if there is any sign of a reaction.

Once diluted, essential oils have a short life, so prepare fresh mixtures in small quantities as needed. Use dry, clean utensils, measuring out about 10ml/2 tsp of vegetable oil into a blending bowl and adding the essential oil one drop at a time. Mix gently.

Body massage is a skill that takes some experience and knowledge of physiology, but essential oils can easily be self-administered for conditions such as chest colds or painful joints. Massage the spot gently with the diluted oils, then rest.

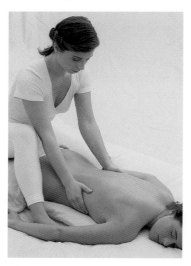

▲ THE NURTURING TOUCH OF MASSAGE IS ENHANCED BY THE AROMA OF ESSENTIAL OILS.

Flower essences

Although people have known of the medicinal benefits of flowers for centuries, modern flower essence therapy began with the work of Edward Bach in 1928. Flower essences are easy-to-use liquid herbal preparations.

A HOLISTIC APPROACH

As people's awareness and healing methods become more holistic, the flower essence philosophy of restoring our health by non-invasive treatment of mental-emotional conditions is gaining ground.

The essences are chosen according to how a person feels about their difficulty, a treatment process that is non-invasive. The compactness of the Bach set makes it a good starting point for people who are beginning their journey into flower essences.

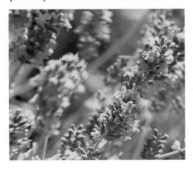

▲ "FLOWERS ARE CONSCIOUS, INTELLIGENT FORCES. THEY HAVE BEEN GIVEN TO US FOR OUR HAPPINESS AND HEALING." LILA DEVI

THE SEVEN HELPERS

Gorse	Heather
Oak	Olive
Rock Water	Vine
Wild Oat	

THE 38 BACH REMEDIES

The Seven Helpers are sun-potentized essences for deep, chronic conditions. They are used to support the Twelve Healers.

The Twelve Healers are sun-potentized essences, which correspond to the positive and negative states of 12 basic personality types. These "type essences" support us as we try to find balance and growth, and as we explore inner being throughout our lives.

The second half of the Bach 38 remedy set are essences prepared by the boiling method, and are known as the "New Nineteen Essences". These extend the work of the sun-potentized essences in developing positive spiritual qualities.

The Twelve Healers

Negative	Essence	Positive
Restraint	Chicory	Love
Fear	Mimulus	Sympathy
Restlessness	Agrimony	Peace
Indecision	Scleranthus	Steadfastness
Indifference	Clematis	Gentleness
Weakness	Centaury	Strength
Doubt	Gentian	Understanding
Over-enthusiasm	Vervain	Tolerance
Ignorance	Cerato	Wisdom
Impatience	Impatiens	Forgiveness
Terror	Rock Rose	Courage
Grief	Water Violet	Joy

Travelling scents

Flower essences do "travel" quite well beyond their place of production, but some users insist on using essences prepared in their own country. In Australia, the bush essences are well known, while in the USA, Alaskan, Californian and Hawaiian essences are popular. In Europe there are French, Dutch and German essence makers, but the UK still has the largest number of makers and suppliers, including the Bach Centre in Sotwell and Findhorn and Harebell Remedies, Scotland.

The New Nineteen Essences

Aspen	Elm	Mustard	Walnut
Beech	Holly	Pine	White Chestnut
Cherry Plum	Honeysuckle	Red Chestnut	Wild Rose
Chestnut Bud	Hornbeam	Star of Bethlehem	Willow
Crab Apple	Larch	Sweet Chestnut	

Nature's role in preparing essences

Flower essences are prepared using either of two classical methods: sun potentizing or boiling. In both methods, flowers should be picked from plants growing in a clean, unspoiled environment.

THE DOCTRINE OF SIGNATURES

A belief popularized by Paracelsus nearly 500 years ago, is the doctrine of signatures. It holds that the appearance of a plant relates to its qualities and conveys a message to the healer.

Colour, shape, size and other features all offered insights to the flower healer. The dandelion's yellow colour, for example, suggested a role in healing liver complaints. The patches on lungwort leaves resemble diseased lungs, and the plant was used for bronchitis and tuberculosis.

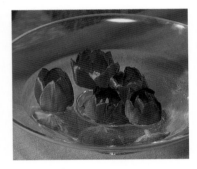

▲ A FLOWER'S ESSENCE ENTERS THE WATER.

This theory was very useful in the development of physical healing, while the Bach tradition has added the vital element of emotional healing.

THE "MEMORY" OF WATER

Edward Bach suggested in the 1930s that the sun is the catalyst which fuses water molecules with the imprint of the flowers used. His claims for potentization were supported by the French scientist Jacques Benveniste, whose experiments showed that water retains the imprint of a substance dissolved in it.

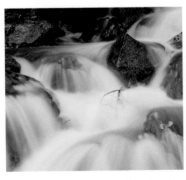

▲ WATER HAS THE POWER TO "MEMORIZE" THE IMPRINT OF FLOWERS.

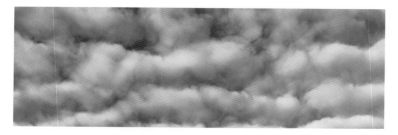

▲ IF CLOUDS APPEAR DURING THE SUN-POTENTIZING PROCESS, CONSIDER STARTING AGAIN ON ANOTHER DAY.

SUN-POTENTIZING METHOD

Start early in the morning. Fill a thin glass bowl with pure water. Pick your chosen flowers and float them on the water.

Leave the bowl close to where the flowers were growing, in clear sunshine for up to four hours or until the petals fade. The life force of the flowers will pass into the water, which may have changed colour, acquired flavour and feel "zingy" if held. Remove the flowers.

Pour the essence into a clean, clearly labelled bottle. Add an equal amount of brandy. This tincture now forms the "mother essence", which is diluted later to produce the dosage essence.

▶ FLOAT YOUR FRESHLY PICKED FLOWERS IN A BOWL OF PURE WATER FOR UP TO 4 HOURS.

BOILING METHOD

This is used for flowering trees, such as walnut, which need fire energy to bring out their essence, especially when the blooms are in spring, before the sun is hot.

Instead of picking only blossoms, add twigs too. Place the ingredients in a pan and cover with pure water. Bring to the boil and simmer for 30 minutes. When cool, filter the essence into a bottle with an equal amount of brandy. This tincture is diluted to create flower essence "stock", which can then be diluted for individual use.

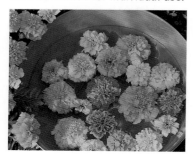

Using flower essences internally

Flower essences can be taken internally at any time of day, using a small dropper bottle. A few drops are taken several times a day, depending on the chosen brand, and treatment can be fitted easily into the daily routine.

TAKING ESSENCES

The best times to take the essences are morning and night, when the system is clear, and also before meals. A rhythmical approach like this will give the best results. No advantage is gained by taking a double dose if the previous dose has been forgotten, as taking more than the suggested number of drops is a waste.

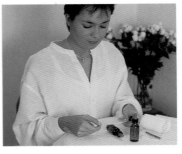

▲ CLEARLY LABEL EACH DOSAGE BOTTLE WITH THE DATE AND CONTENTS LIST.

PREPARING A DOSAGE BOTTLE

1 Almost fill a 30ml/1fl oz dropper bottle with spring water. Add 5ml/1tsp brandy or vodka as a preservative. Use cider vinegar or glycerine if you prefer to avoid alcohol. For babies and animals, omit the preservative, but keep the bottle in the fridge.

2 Add 2 drops of each of your chosen mother essences to the water and brandy mixture. Bang the bottle on your palm to mix.

3 Carry the bottle with you, or prepare several dropper bottles of the essence and have these to hand for different situations.

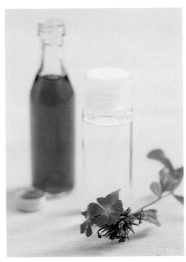

▲ STILL SPRING WATER AND BRANDY FORM THE LIQUID BASE IN DOSAGE BOTTLES.

Dosage is usually 4 drops, four times a day for 3 weeks. Then stop and allow a week to assess the results and decide what to put in a new bottle. Each treatment is based on a four-week cycle.

Alternatively, you may prefer to take essences internally by diluting in a glass of water, adding 2 drops per glass and stirring well. Sip four times a day, and make a fresh batch daily.

The essences can also be taken in pill form. To make the pills, weigh 25g/1oz sugar or lactose pilules in a small jar, add 2 drops of each chosen essence and shake well. Dry the pills on a plate. Chew two a day, with water.

There is no limit on the number of essences that can be taken together. Some herbalists like to use combinations of ten essences, while others will address a core issue using only one essence. Four essences in a treatment bottle is probably a good guideline.

▾ ONCE THE DROPS ARE DISPERSED IN A LARGE GLASS OF WATER, IT IS VIRTUALLY IMPOSSIBLE TO TASTE THE BRANDY.

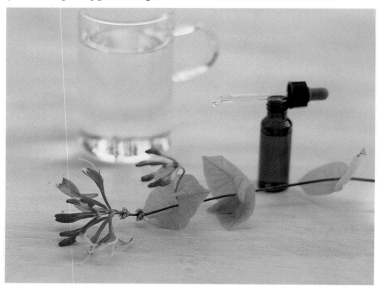

Using flower essences externally

The wide use of flower essences in oils and creams confirms their powerful effect when used externally. Many therapists believe that such usage greatly enhances the effect of the flowers.

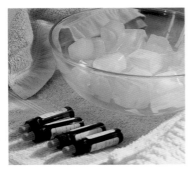

▲ ADD ICE TO A FLOWER COMPRESS TO EASE ACHES CAUSED BY SPRAINS AND SWELLINGS.

SOOTHING COMPRESSES

Lay the compress on any sprain, burn, bite or swelling, and repeat until relief is felt. Seek medical help if appropriate. Fill a bowl with hot or cold water, adding four drops of each chosen essence and four drops of essential oil. Soak a flannel or cotton wool in the water and apply to the affected area.

RELAXING ESSENCE BATHS

Add 12–20 drops of your current dosage essence in a warm bath, or four drops of each chosen mother essence, and swirl the water in a figure of eight pattern to activate the essences. Soak in the bath for 20 minutes and then rest for a further 20 minutes.

HEALING CREAMS

Use a hypoallergenic, non-perfumed cream as a base. Fill a jar with 50g/2oz cream, add four drops of each chosen essence and four drops of an essential oil. Mix with a wooden stick, screw on the jar lid. Apply the finished cream twice daily or as needed.

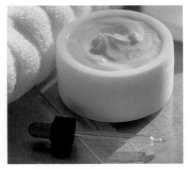

▲ ADD A FEW DROPS OF ESSENTIAL OIL TO YOUR FLOWER ESSENCE CREAM TO ENHANCE ITS HEALING PROPERTIES.

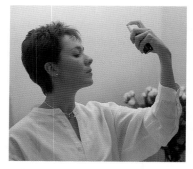

▲ USE FLOWER ESSENCE SPRAYS TO REFRESH YOUR MIND AND UPLIFT YOUR SPIRITS.

FLOWER ESSENCE SPRAYS

Sprays help to cleanse a room of negative energy and refresh stale air. Adding essential oils to flower essences gives an uplifting smell and heightens the healing benefits. Lighter oils such as lavender, geranium and lemon grass work best. Fill a plastic or glass spray bottle with 50ml/2fl oz spring water. Add 10 drops of essential oil and four drops of each chosen flower essence. Shake the bottle and spray as needed.

FLOWER ESSENCE MASSAGES

Put four drops of an essential oil and four drops of chosen flower essences into a bottle. Pour in 50ml/2fl oz of cold-pressed almond oil. Shake the bottle to mix and pour the contents into a bowl.

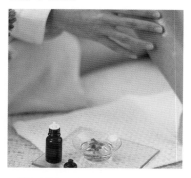

▲ ADD FLOWER ESSENCE TO MASSAGE OILS.

A FLOWER ESSENCE MASSAGE MIXTURE

- dandelion, for relaxing muscles
- comfrey, also to relax muscles
- chamomile, to relax involuntary muscle spasms
- rock water, to relax the whole body
- valerian, to release stress and tension
- orange hawkweed, to release trauma and energy blocks

Emergency essences

Most people's first introduction to flower essence therapy, and the most well-known of the Bach remedies, is Rescue Remedy. This emergency formula has proved to be helpful for all kinds of stressful situations.

RESCUE REMEDIES

The five classic components in Rescue Remedy are:

- rock rose, for fear
- impatiens, for mental agitation and tension
- cherry plum, for panic and fear of losing control
- clematis, for "faraway" feelings, and unwillingness to face up to a crisis
- star of Bethlehem, for treating panic and shock

Other composite remedies have names such as Five Flower Formula, Emergency Essence, Recovery Remedy, and Calming Essence. All work to restore our emotional and mental balance after shock or trauma, and in "heavy" situations, such as accidents, arguments, bad news, stress at work, or bereavement.

In a crisis, take four drops in a glass of water, sipping slowly. If no water is available,

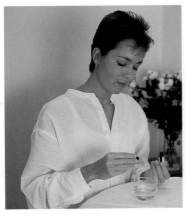

▲ IN A CRISIS ADD FOUR DROPS OF RESCUE REMEDY TO WATER.

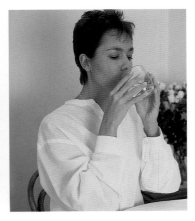

▲ THE QUANTITY OF WATER IS NOT IMPORTANT, BUT SIP SLOWLY.

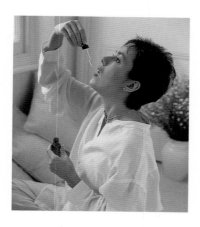

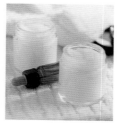

◀ IF NO LIQUID IS AVAILABLE, TAKE DROPS DIRECTLY ON THE TONGUE.

▶ TRY MAKING YOUR OWN RESCUE CREAM.

take directly on the tongue. Take the remedy every few minutes, as the effect is cumulative.

If a crisis is approaching, make up a dosage bottle: add four drops of Rescue Remedy to a 30ml/1fl oz dropper bottle of spring water. Add 5ml/1 tsp brandy and shake well. Take four times a day or up to 10 times if in need.

Carry a bottle of emergency essence with you at all times, and keep a bottle in the family first aid kit and in the office.

EMERGENCY SPRAYS AND CREAMS

The remedy can also be used as a spray or in cream form. To prepare the cream, add 10 drops of the remedy to 50g/2oz of a hypoallergenic base cream and mix. Useful healing additions are up to four drops of lavender or tea tree essential oil.

The cream should be applied at once if bruises, stings, cuts or blisters occur. Apply every two minutes or so for 15 minutes, as the skin absorbs the cream quickly. The liquid remedy should also be taken, or if no cream is to hand, the liquid can even be applied direct to the injury.

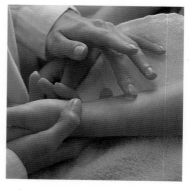

▲ APPLY CREAM IMMEDIATELY IF POSSIBLE.

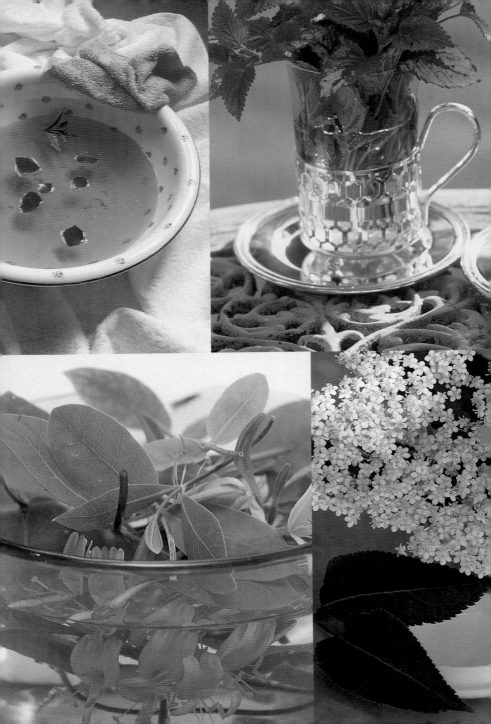

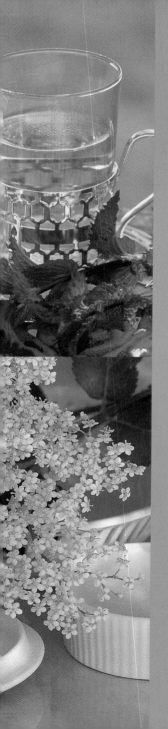

FLOWER
TREATMENTS

The flower remedies introduced in the following section will help you to deal with some of the difficult situations that we all experience from time to time. The recipes are designed to treat some of the most common health problems, from calming anxiety to relieving a painful abscess.

These natural treatments, which include the use of flower essential oils and essences, can be safely self-administered in the home, but do not exceed the doses stated, and seek further advice if you are pregnant or over 70 years of age. You can refer to the healing plants directory for further information, but always be sure to seek professional help if a problem persists or if you are uncertain.

Calming anxiety

Anxiety often involves over-excitement and frustration. In such states the body produces adrenaline but in the office or in traffic there is no safe outlet for all this negative energy. Flower remedies can help to calm you down.

ALLEVIATING SYMPTOMS OF ANXIETY
Flower essences and herbal treatments can help tackle symptoms of anxiety such as palpitations, sweating, irritability and sleeplessness.

Use Rescue Remedy in emergencies. If you can, take a hot bath, add lavender essential

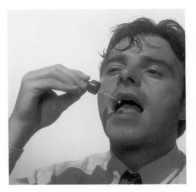

▲ TAKE A FEW DROPS OF RESCUE REMEDY WHEN SUFFERING FROM PANIC ATTACKS.

oil and relax. Passionflower, cut and dried when fruiting, is a good sedative and can relieve nervous conditions such as palpitations.

A TEA FOR ANXIETY
Try combining the nerve tonics and specific remedies listed. Put 5ml/1 tsp of three plants in a tea pot (use only 2.5ml/½ tsp passion flower). Add 600ml/ 1 pint/2½ cups boiling water, leave to steep for 10 minutes. Strain and drink. Take two cups a day for up to 2 weeks.

REMEDIES FOR ANXIETY
• To help calm your nervous system choose: oats; vervain; skullcap; or wood betony. These are all nervine tonics. Choose whichever one suits you best and combine it with a specific remedy for the symptom that troubles you most. Caution: these are powerful herbs, do not exceed the recommended doses (not more than 5ml/1 tsp a day of skullcap and betony, or 2.5ml/½ tsp if in combination).
• To ease palpitations: motherwort or passionflower.
• To reduce sweating: valerian or motherwort.
• To help you sleep: passionflower or valerian.

Fighting nervous exhaustion

We are more susceptible to illness or depression when hard pressed at work or when we face heavy emotional demands. Drinking flower teas is a safe and cheap way to support our nervous systems when stressed.

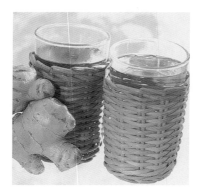

▲ A CUP OF GINGER TEA IS A TASTY TONIC FOR BOOSTING THE NERVOUS SYSTEM.

NERVOUS SYSTEM BOOSTERS

There are a number of flower and herb tonics that can strengthen the nervous system and prevent it running down to the point where nervous exhaustion occurs. Try ginseng, ginger, echinacea or hawthorn.

REVITALIZING TEAS

Mix equal amounts of the following six dried plants that work for nervous exhaustion: oats, licorice, skullcap, borage flowers, rosemary and wood betony.

Put 15ml/1 tbsp of the mixture into a tea pot, and add 600ml/1 pint/2½ cups of boiling water. Steep for 10 minutes and strain. Take one to two cups daily for up to 2 weeks or until the exhaustion passes.

Vervain is another traditional healing plant with a reputation for restoring the nervous system following periods of tension. Vervain's aerial parts, including its stiff, thin stems and small lilac flowers, can be made into a bitter but stimulating tea. It has been used for centuries as an ideal tonic for convalescence from chronic illness.

A well-known restorative tea, for whenever you are tired or stressed, is Earl Grey, which acquires its distinctive flavour from the addition of bergamot oil. Note that the pure essential oil should not be taken internally.

▸ WOOD BETONY RESTORES THE NERVOUS SYSTEM.

Relieving PMS

Many plants have been found to have beneficial effects on the reproductive system, especially in women. Menstrual problems, including cramps, pre-menstrual syndrome and heavy bleeding, can be alleviated by self-treatment.

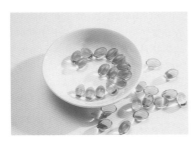

▲ CAPSULES OF EVENING PRIMROSE PROVIDE THE BODY WITH ESSENTIAL FATTY ACIDS, OFTEN LACKING WITH PMS.

Breast tenderness, sore nipples, and fluid retention can often accompany PMS. Lifestyle changes, such as eating extra fresh fruit and vegetables, stopping smoking, taking more exercise, cutting down on salt and processed foods, and relaxing by baths or meditation are all helpful in easing the symptoms.

Good remedies to try are evening primrose capsules or chaste tree (*Agnus castus*) tincture – 12 drops every morning for 3 months, are recommended. Vervain, valerian, lady's mantle and rosemary are also beneficial.

Vervain and rosemary are often taken in infusion form, while valerian is given as tablets or tincture. The name of lady's mantle refers to this plant's traditional value in healing women's conditions, especially in reducing heavy bleeding; it is best avoided during pregnancy.

VERVAIN AND LADY'S MANTLE TEA
Put 5ml/1 tsp each dried vervain and lady's mantle in a pot, and add 300ml/½ pint/1¼ cups boiling water. Steep for 10 minutes, strain and sweeten to taste. Take one cup twice a day from day 14 of the cycle, or from 2 weeks after your period begins.

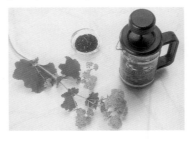

▲ LADY'S MANTLE AND VERVAIN TEA.

Easing periods

Pain during or before periods arises from contraction of the muscles of the womb, which reduces blood flow and causes the muscles to ache. Tisanes and hot compresses can help to ease these menstrual cramps.

Cramp bark (guelder rose) is well-known for reducing spasm, and rosemary is a circulatory stimulant and relaxant.

The leaves of feverfew, lady's mantle, peppermint and valerian have all been used in tisane form to relieve period pain. Among garden flowers, marigold petals in a tisane are known to normalize the menstrual process, and pasque flowers (use only the dried form in tisanes) are a noted relaxant. In each case, infuse 5–10ml/1–2 tsp of the leaves or flowers for up to 10 minutes in boiling water.

A hot-water bottle on the abdomen gives relief, as does a soothing hot herbal compress.

▲ ROSEMARY STIMULATES CIRCULATION.

HOT COMPRESS

Boil 10ml/2 tsp cramp bark in 600ml/1 pint/2½ cups water for 10–15 minutes. Add 10ml/2 tsp dried rosemary. Steep for 15 minutes and strain into a bowl.

Soak a clean cotton cloth or bandage in the liquid. When cool, wring out the cloth. Place the hot compress on the abdomen and relax until it cools.

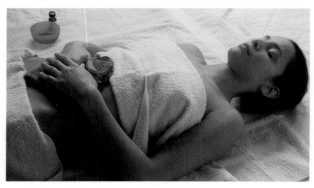

◀ PLACE A HOT COMPRESS ON YOUR ABDOMEN, LIE BACK AND RELAX.

Helping with the menopause

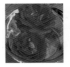

Menopause causes levels of the hormones progesterone and oestrogen to decline. This leads to reduced bone density and adds to the risk of osteoporosis. It is therefore important to support both hormones at this time.

Hormonal changes often lead to unpleasant hot flushes and night sweats. Using plant parts like the berries of chaste tree (*Agnus castus*), lime blossom and sage leaves will help maintain hormone levels, but general vitalizers or tonics are also useful in pepping up a run-down system.

Drinking rose water made by immersing damask rose petals in distilled water is a traditional remedy in the Middle East for alleviating the worst of menopausal symptoms.

TEA FOR HOT FLUSHES

Put 5ml/1 tsp each of motherwort flowers and sage leaves into a cup. Pour on 600ml/1 pint/ 2½ cups of boiling water. Sweeten

with licorice (unless you have high blood pressure). Allow to cool, and sip throughout the day.

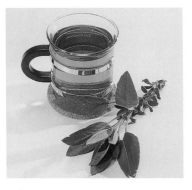

▲ TAKING REGULAR SIPS OF MOTHERWORT AND SAGE TEA THROUGHOUT THE DAY MAY HELP TO EASE MENOPAUSAL HOT FLUSHES.

LIME BLOSSOM TEA

The flowers should be gathered immediately after flowering in midsummer. Collect on a dry day and leave them to dry slowly in the shade. Use as a tincture or make a tisane by mixing a cup of boiling water with 5ml/1 tsp blossom. Leave to steep for up to 10 minutes, then allow to cool. Drink a cup three times a day.

CAUTION

Sage is a powerful herb and should only be taken for up to 3 weeks at a time. Allow a break of at least a week before taking again.

Lifting depression

Prolonged conditions of stress, anxiety and tension can lead to depression. Physical and mental energy leach away, leaving us vulnerable and unable to recover our equilibrium. There are, however, natural means of helping ourselves.

If external circumstances don't seem to be changing, sometimes all we can do is hang on to our routine until we feel able to cope again. Try to avoid taking pharmaceutical drugs or stimulants at this time. Cooking food may be hard to manage, so this could be the opportunity to buy fresh fruit and vegetables. Keep busy, walk more or do some grounding exercises. Give yourself extra time to relax. Helping others even when we feel depressed is very healing. Flower essences such as mustard, sweet chestnut and gentian, can address our depression, and wild rose and gorse can be used for hopelessness and despair.

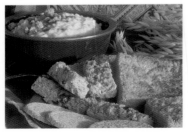

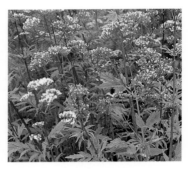

▲ THE ROOT OF WHITE-FLOWERED VALERIAN IS USED TO PROMOTE CALM AND SLEEP.

VALERIAN INFUSION

Use the dried and shredded root of valerian to make a remedy to calm the nerves. Using 10ml/ 2 tsp to a 250ml/8fl oz/1 cup of water, simmer the ingredients gently for 20 minutes in a covered, non-aluminium pan. Leave the concoction to cool, then strain. Re-heat and drink just before you go to bed to reduce the nervous tension and anxiety that hinder sleep.

◀ THERE ARE MANY TASTY WAYS IN WHICH YOU CAN INCREASE YOUR INTAKE OF OATS AS AN ANTIDOTE TO DEPRESSION.

Skin treatments

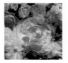

The skin needs regular cleansing and nourishment to remain healthy. Its condition reflects the general state of your body's health, but many minor skin problems can be improved by the external use of flower remedies.

ABSCESSES

A localized inflamed swelling containing pus is called an abscess. External abscesses on the skin can be treated with hot compresses, but internal abscesses in the mouth or other mucous membranes need qualified medical treatment.

To soothe an external abscess, make a compress by adding no more than 5–6 drops of an essential oil, such as bergamot, chamomile, lavender or tea tree, either separately or combined, to a bowl of boiling water and soak your compress in it. Keep this on the abscess for up to 30 minutes and renew when the compress cools.

ACNE

A common skin condition in adolescence, acne can affect people in later life

◄ WITCH HAZEL

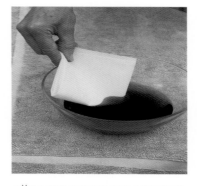

▲ USE A SOFT CLOTH TO MAKE A COMPRESS.

too. It is a sign that the sebaceous glands are producing excess sebum, and the glands and hair follicles are becoming blocked and infected.

Treat with the antiseptic and skin-growth-promoting essential oils tea tree, geranium, lavender or palmarosa, mixing a few drops into a bland carrier oil. Herbal treatments for external use include infusions of elderflower, lavender, marigold or witch hazel. Internally, a decoction of either red clover, burdock or echinacea can tone up the system.

Athlete's foot

This is a fungal infection that causes inflammation and itching between and under the toes, or in the groin. Preventive and controlling measures include scrupulously keeping the feet dry and clean, avoiding synthetic socks and tight-fitting shoes.

Use tea tree or lavender essential oil, or a clove of garlic, rubbed onto the skin twice or more a day. The Indian spice turmeric mixed with a tincture of marigold or myrrh can be applied between the toes.

Skin tonics

Stress and tension cause our muscles to contract, leaving the skin deprived of blood, and often resulting in dryness.

Make up a skin tonic by mixing essential oils into an unperfumed skin cream. Add either 3 drops rose and 3 drops sandalwood, or 4 drops neroli and 2 drops rose to a 25g/1oz pot of skin cream. Arnica, marigold, tea tree and witch hazel can also be applied in paste or cream form.

▸ ROSE WATER IS MILD AND SOOTHING ON THE SKIN AND ALSO BENEFITS THE EYES.

A rose and chamomile facial

Hot water facials open up the pores and leave the skin refreshed and relaxed. Fill a wide bowl with hot water, add 3 drops rose and 4 drops chamomile essential oil. Cover your head with a towel and stay over the bowl for 5 minutes.

Relax for a further 15 minutes. Then apply a toning lotion: for dry skin, mix 75ml/5 tbsp rose water and 30ml/2 tbsp orange flower water; for oily skin, mix 90ml/6 tbsp rose water and 30ml/2 tbsp witch hazel.

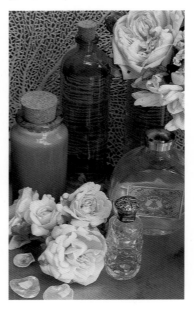

Respiratory ailments

The respiratory tract extends from inside the eyes and nose through the sinuses, throat and airways to the lungs. Flower treatments can combat infection, clear congestion, soothe the membranes and alleviate inflammation.

Avoidance of mucus-forming foods, such as dairy products and refined starches, is advised. So cut out morning cereals and milk, replacing with fruit or fruit juice. Also start taking raw garlic.

CATARRH

When the membranes of nose and throat are irritated, excess mucus may be formed, for example, after a cold. Nasal catarrh occurs higher up in the airways and bronchial catarrh lower down.

A steam inhalation of essential oils, with peppermint, alone or combined with eucalyptus, or tea tree oil helps to loosen mucus and fight infections. For longer-term catarrh, try oil of pine and lavender.

Infusions of peppermint or eucalyptus leaves or chamomile flowers help to ease nasal congestion, as can infusions of the herbs elderflower, golden rod and hyssop.

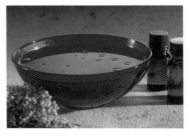

▲ STEAM INHALATIONS HELP TO CLEAR CONGESTION IN THE SINUSES AND CAN AID RECOVERY FROM COLDS AND SORE THROATS.

COLDS

It is difficult to stop a cold virus once it takes hold, and it will usually run its course. Flower treatments, though, can help to relieve symptoms and prevent catarrh or a worse infection taking over. Take plenty of fruit and vitamin C along with other treatments, and cut out mucus-forming foods.

Aromatherapy remedies include baths and steam inhalations. For night-time baths add 10 drops of lavender and 5 drops of cinnamon oil; earlier in the day, use tea tree or eucalyptus (10 drops of each).

A hot infusion of equal parts elderflower, peppermint and yarrow, taken before bedtime will raise the temperature and may sweat out the cold.

Coughs

A cough is a reflex response to irritations or blockages in the airways, so it is better to help the cough rather than suppress it with drugs. Essential oils, such as lavender, thyme and eucalyptus, in a steam inhalation, will do this.

Among many good infusions are marshmallow, thyme, coltsfoot, echinacea and hyssop. For dry coughs, thyme and licorice are recommended, and for mucusy coughs, eucalyptus and licorice.

Sinusitis

The sinus cavities are air spaces in the bones of the skull, around the eyes. Lined with mucous membranes, they are quickly infected by coughs or colds.

Steam inhalations using pine, peppermint, eucalyptus, tea tree, chamomile and lavender essential oils, singly or combined, are all

▶ Aromatic plants such as eucalyptus are ideal for treating nasal congestion.

▶ Peppermint 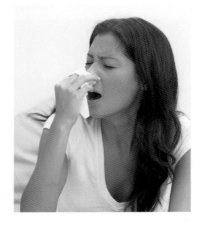 effective at loosening mucus. Catmint, elderflower and golden seal all make strong infusions.

Sore throats

A strong and effective treatment for sore throats and colds is a garlic, ginger and lemon mix: crush a clove of fresh garlic and a similar-sized piece of fresh ginger, adding the juice of a squeezed lemon. Add honey as a sweetener, and mix in hot water. Take up to three times a day.

Steam inhalations of oils such as lavender and thyme help to soothe a swollen throat, as will infusions or gargled tinctures of these herbs, or agrimony and sage.

Digestive settlers

If we are what we eat, we owe it to ourselves to keep our digestive system in good health. The two main roles of plants and flowers in maintaining digestive peace are as stimulants and relaxants.

FOR STOMACH ACHE AND NAUSEA
A cramping stomach pain may be caused by poor digestion or food poisoning, nervous tension or infection. Stomach ache may lead to diarrhoea (see opposite). In general, marigold and garlic are good for fighting digestive infection, while relaxing herbs such as chamomile and cramp bark (guelder rose) will relieve stomach spasms. Nausea can be alleviated by taking frequent sips of a ginger infusion, or by diluting 10 drops of tincture in a glass of water. Lemon is a good cleanser.

FOR A NERVOUS STOMACH
You can make a soothing infusion from chamomile, lemon balm and hops, using them either together or separately.

Place 5ml/1 tsp each of chamomile

▲ MARIGOLD

flowers, peppermint and lemon balm into a small tea pot. Fill with boiling water and allow the tea to steep for 10 minutes before straining. Drink the tea three times a day or following meals. Hops can be added to the mixture in the evening to settle the stomach.

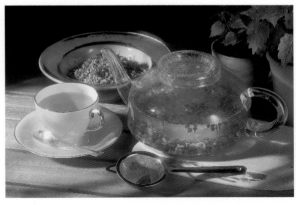

◀ CHAMOMILE TEA IS HIGHLY EFFECTIVE IN TREATING MANY DIGESTIVE DISORDERS AND FOR SETTLING THE STOMACH IN MOMENTS OF NERVOUS TENSION.

A soothing compress

One of the easiest ways to settle an excited stomach is to use an aromatherapy compress, taking the time to relax and allow the soothing essential oils to ease your abdomen.

Measure out 2 drops orange and 3 drops peppermint or 3 drops chamomile and 2 drops orange into a bowl of hot water. Soak a flannel or a bandage in the mixture and place the compress onto the stomach. Lie back and relax for 10 minutes, or longer.

For wind, bloating and colic

Drinking hot teas of catmint, chamomile, ginger or peppermint will help to ease the symptoms. Alternatively, gently massage the abdomen in a clockwise direction with essential oils of chamomile, lemon verbena or peppermint. Dilute the oils at the ratio of 1 drop per 10ml/2 tsp of base oil.

For constipation

One of the most effective methods of self-help is daily clockwise massage of the lower

▶ Lemon balm makes a soothing and delicious tea that calms the stomach.

abdomen, and this can be performed using 2 drops of oils of lavender, marjoram or rosemary in 5ml/1 tsp of base oil. Alternatively, try chewing on a stick of licorice.

For diarrhoea

An infusion of agrimony or chamomile may help to reduce the impact of tension on the digestive tract. An infusion of meadowsweet may help to settle an acidic stomach. Thyme fights infections and improves digestion generally by settling churning, loose bowels and killing off harmful bacteria.

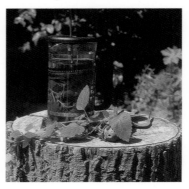

Enhancing sleep and relaxation

Flowers and herbs are unsurpassed in their ability to help us sleep and to relax. Sedative herbs aid in relaxation when taken at night, and stimulating herbs are used when we are overstimulated and there is nervous exhaustion.

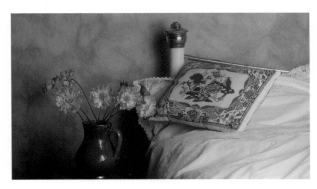

◀ A SOFT FLOWER PILLOW, WHETHER MADE OR BOUGHT, IS A GOOD FIRST STEP IN IMPROVING YOUR SLEEP ENVIRONMENT.

Sedative flowers often used in infusions are, in ascending order of strength, chamomile, lime, lavender and passion flower. Infusions in the evenings are relaxing, as are baths (see opposite). A hop or herbal pillow works for some people. The important thing is to take some time to relax and unwind, doing something peaceful after a day's work, such as gentle exercise, meditation, reading, yoga or tai chi.

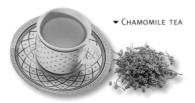

▼ CHAMOMILE TEA

SLEEPY-TIME TEA

Put 5ml/1 tsp each of dried chamomile, lemon balm and vervain in a pot, and pour on 600ml/ 1 pint/2½ cups boiling water. Steep for 10 minutes. Strain and drink a cup after supper and another before going to bed.

For a stronger blend, add a decoction of 5ml/1 tsp valerian root or 2.5ml/½ tsp dried hops or Californian poppy. Never take more than 2.5ml/½ tsp hops per day.

Bath therapy

A hot bath, with the aroma of exotic flowers, and perhaps a candle and soothing music is an inexpensive, easily arranged yet unsurpassed relaxation therapy we can enjoy in our own homes.

In addition to quick baths or showers to get clean, we should often award ourselves the time for a relaxing bath, using essential oils to make our bathtimes particularly healing experiences. Pour 5 drops of an oil into the bath water just before you are ready to enter. This will form a thin film on the surface of the water, and the oil will be easily absorbed by the skin, whose pores are being opened up by the heat. Breathing in the aroma is also therapeutic for both the mind and body.

A refreshing morning bath is produced by adding 3 drops bergamot and 2 drops geranium oil. For an unwinding evening bath, blend 3 drops lavender and 2 drops ylang ylang. For aching muscles at any time, use 3 drops marjoram and 2 drops chamomile essential oils.

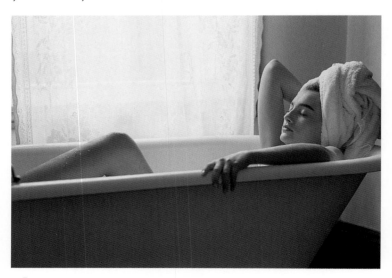

▲ Treat yourself to a long bath with essential oils.

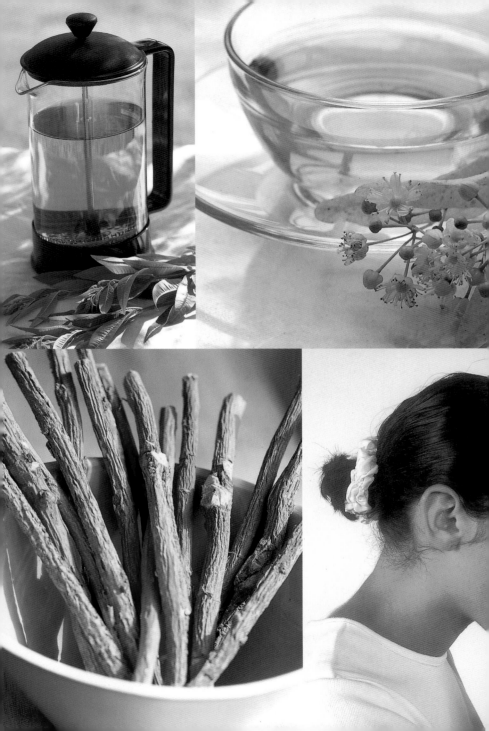

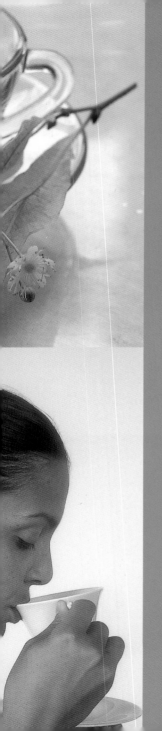

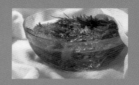

HEALING WITH
HERBS

Herbs have always played a key role in physical and emotional health, and many widely available herbs have a direct medicinal action, thanks to their antiseptic, antibacterial qualities. Cultivating healing herbs is easy – as shown in this section, they are prolific growers and require little effort in order to thrive. Taken as a regular part of the diet, sprinkled over food or used in a range of herbal teas and decoctions, herbs can help to ward off illness and cure minor ailments.

Other herbs have uplifting scents that promote a feeling of renewed energy when used externally in ointments, inhalations, essential oils, compresses and poultices. Refer to the healing plants directory for more information on the most useful herbs and their properties.

The benefits of herbs

The definition of what constitutes a herb has broadened over the centuries. Nowadays the term "herb" includes any plant whose roots, stem, leaves, flowers or fruit is used to flavour food, as medicine or for scent.

Most people are familiar with herbs that are commonly used in cooking, such as basil, bay, chives, mint, oregano, parsley, sage and thyme. But taking into account the broader definition of the term "herb", one can include plants such as aloe vera, spices such as ginger, flowers such as marigolds and roses, and fruits such as lemons and rose-hips.

As well as adding aroma and delicious flavour to food, culinary herbs have some nutritional value, often containing appreciable amounts of vitamins, minerals and trace elements. Adding herbs to your food on a daily basis actively promotes good health. Many herbs have excellent digestive qualities, helping the body to process and eliminate oily, fatty or gas-producing foods. But adding a generous sprinkling of fresh or dried herbs to your food is not the only way to benefit from these versatile plants.

▼ HERBS WILL GROW IN THE SMALLEST OF SPACES, SO LONG AS THEY ARE NURTURED.

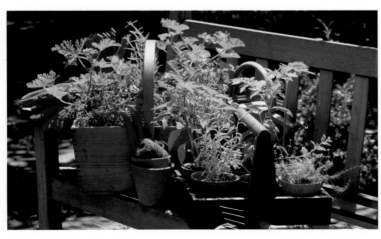

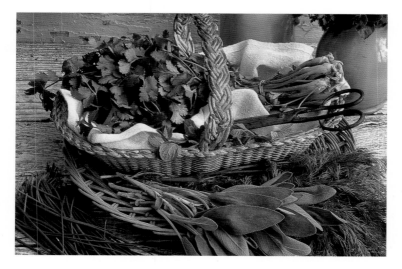

HERBAL MEDICINE

Many herbs have a therapeutic and medicinal value and can be taken in a variety of forms to prevent and cure illness and to promote health. Taken internally they can be made into herbal teas, decoctions, tinctures and inhalations. Externally they can be applied as compresses, poultices, ointments, creams or infused oils. Herbs add their aroma to bath water for a therapeutic soak and essential oils distilled from the flowers can be used for a massage.

Best of all, herbs are widely available and grow in the smallest of spaces ensuring a continual year-round supply for everyone.

▲ FRESH HERBS AID DIGESTION AS WELL AS ADDING VITAL FLAVOUR TO FOOD.

▼ WARMING SPICES SUCH AS GINGER AND CINNAMON ADD HEAT TO FOOD AND DRINKS, HELPING TO WARD OFF COLDS AND CHILLS.

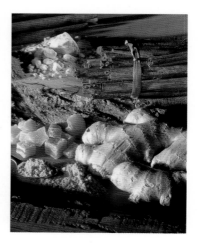

Growing herbs for healing

If you are new to growing herbs, take heart, they are not very difficult to grow and reward you over and over again for very little effort. The easiest way to start is to buy pot-grown herbs and plant them out.

SOIL

On the whole, herbs are undemanding and easy to grow. A free-draining lightish soil will suit the majority. Many herbs prefer light, sandy soils, similar to that provided by their Mediterranean homeland, and most will not stand heavy clay soils or waterlogged conditions. You can lighten soil by digging in sand, grit and organic matter, or you could consider growing your herbs in containers. The rule tends to be: silvery, needle-like leaves or tough foliage require sunny, well-drained conditions; soft green leaves tolerate partial shade; golden-leaved herbs will need sun.

▼ HERBS OFFER GLORIOUS SCENTS AND ADD STUNNING COLOUR TO A GARDEN.

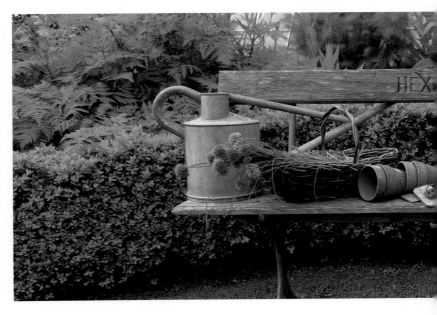

Site

A sunny, sheltered position protected from bitter winds will suit many herbs best. Some will need winter protection and a few, such as basil, will not survive and will need replanting every year. Aloe vera must be treated as a houseplant in colder regions.

Maintenance

Many herbs are prolific growers. Harvesting them helps to keep them under control, but do not be afraid to cut them back ruthlessly from time to time and root out those that are overpowering their neighbours. Herbs kept on a kitchen windowsill should be rotated with other container herbs to ensure that they do not become so bereft of foliage that they die.

Weeding

Remove weeds regularly to prevent them from competing with your herbs for moisture and nutrients. A light mulch of compost, applied in spring or autumn, can help to keep the herbs at their best.

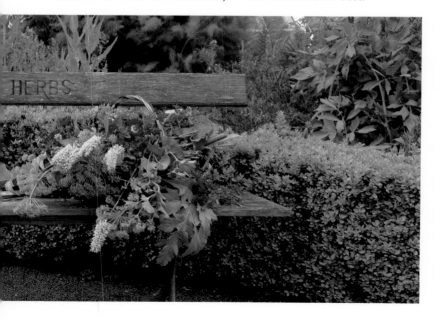

Growing herbs in containers

Herbs grow well in containers if you follow a few simple tips. Choose from a small pot, hanging basket, old clay sink, window box, large wooden tub or trough, old chimneystack or even an old barrel.

Make sure your container can give the roots room to spread out and that it has holes in the base. Put a layer of broken shards of terracotta pots in the base, then add a layer of sand or grit before filling with potting compost (soil mix). Never use garden soil, no matter what condition it is in – it may harbour weeds, pests and diseases. Add water-retaining gel if you like, since this helps with watering later on.

Extra fertilizer must be added after two weeks, with subsequent weekly feeds throughout the summer growing season to ensure you get the best from your plant.

Water frequently during the growing season. During the winter months water just enough to avoid drying out completely.

▼ A GROUP OF HERBS PLANTED IN DECORATIVE CONTAINERS CAN MAKE AN ATTRACTIVE FEATURE IN THE GARDEN.

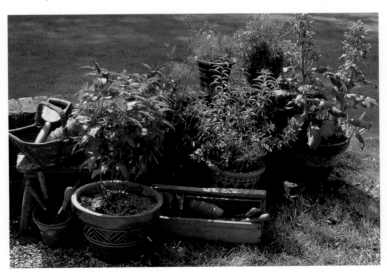

A trough for winter colds

Most of the herbs used here keep their leaves through the winter. However it is best to harvest them while they are growing vigorously and dry them for later use since they do not have the same potency while dormant in the winter.

YOU WILL NEED
  trough
  broken terracotta pots
  gravel or horticultural grit
  potting compost (soil mix)
  watering can

HERBS – black peppermint, hyssop,
  horehound, sage, purple sage,
  golden sage, thyme

▼ THIS TROUGH WILL KEEP YOU SUPPLIED WELL THROUGHOUT THE YEAR WITH HERBS FOR TEAS AND COUGH REMEDIES.

1 Put a layer of broken terracotta at the bottom of the trough. Add a layer of gravel or horticultural grit. Almost fill with a good quality potting compost.

2 Tap the plants out of their pots and plant, firming around each one with extra compost. Put the tallest plants at the back and the thymes at the front. Top up with extra compost as necessary and water the plants in well.

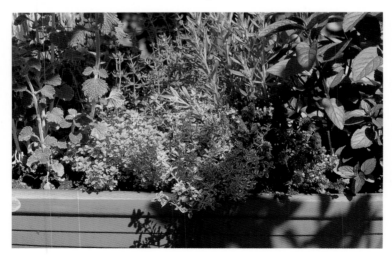

Pots for headache remedies

Fresh or dried herbs made into teas and compresses can help to relieve the tension brought on by headaches and migraines. Feverfew will relieve a migraine, but it is bitter, so eat the leaves sandwiched between bread slices.

YOU WILL NEED
  half-barrel with drainage holes
  heavy-duty black plastic
  staples
  broken terracotta pots
  horticultural grit
  soilless compost (growing medium)
  sharp sand
  watering can

HERBS – feverfew, lavender, borage, marjoram, rosemary

▼ TAKING HERBS AS TEAS WILL HELP RELIEVE THE SYMPTOMS OF A HEADACHE.

1 Insert the plastic liner into the tub and staple it to the side, overlapping the plastic where necessary.

2 Put in a layer of broken terracotta pots at the bottom, and top up with grit. Add soilless compost (growing medium), mixed with sand, to come a third of the way up the tub.

3 Fill with a gritty, open-textured potting compost (growing medium). Arrange the herbs in the tub. Plant up and water in well.

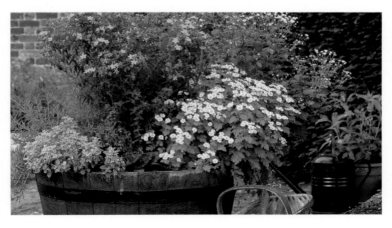

Pots for bites and bruises

The plants used here make good salves and ointments to counteract the effects of bites and bruises. If you are susceptible to bruising or live in areas infested with insects having herbs to hand will make life easier.

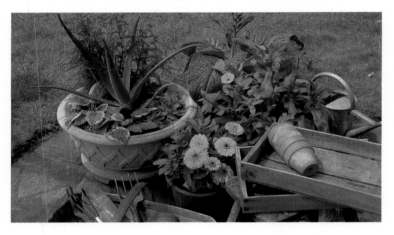

▲ Herbs with structure make striking features in pots.

You will need
  stone urn
  broken terracotta pots
  horticultural grit
  loam-based potting compost
  (soil mix) mixed in equal parts
  with soilless potting compost
  (growing medium)
  trowel
  watering can

Herbs − *aloe vera, comfrey, house-leek, pot marigold, yarrow*

1 Put a layer of broken terracotta pots in the base of the urn, then add a layer of grit.

2 Two-thirds fill the urn with the compost (soil mix).

3 Plant the aloe vera in the middle in its own pot so that it can be removed before the first frosts. Plant the yarrow and comfrey near the middle of the pot. Put the houseleeks around the outside, filling in with extra compost as necessary. Water the plants in well.

Harvesting herbs

 The best time to harvest the aerial parts of herbs is after their flower buds have formed but before they are in full bloom. Roots should be dug up in the autumn, cleaned and chopped into small pieces.

Never pick herbs without being able to correctly identify them, or pick so many that you reduce next year's growth.

Spread the herbs out to dry in an airy position out of direct sunlight – an airing cupboard is an ideal place. Leafy bunches can be tied into little bundles and hung up. Spread flower heads on tissue or newspaper and dry them flat. It can take a week for them to dry.

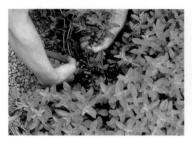

1 Cut bunches of healthy material at mid-morning on a dry day.

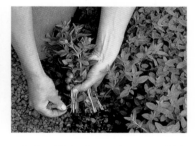

2 Strip off the lower leaves, which may otherwise become damaged.

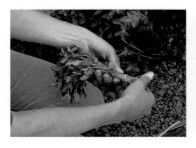

3 Bind the lower stems tightly with a rubber band.

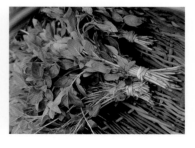

4 Gather as many bunches as you need, then hang them up to dry.

Storing herbs

The volatile oils in herbs start to deteriorate quickly once the herbs are put in the light. Store dried herbs in separate, airtight containers away from the light and they will keep for up to six months.

Although many herbs retain an aromatic scent for several years, for medicinal purposes it is best to replace stocks every year since their potency declines with age.

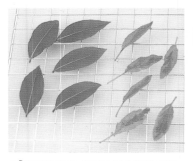

▲ DRY INDIVIDUAL LEAVES ON A WIRE RACK, BEFORE STORING THEM.

▼ SOME HERBS CAN BE LAYERED IN SALT TO PRESERVE THEM. THIS ALSO FLAVOURS SALT.

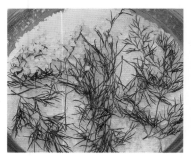

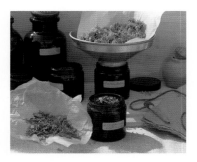

▲ DARK BOTTLES CAN BE USED TO STORE DRIED HERBS, OILS AND CREAMS.

Many shops stock dried herbs. Buy these only if they seem fresh – brightly coloured and strongly aromatic. Some herbal remedies are now available over the counter in the form of capsules, tablets or tinctures. Choose the simpler types that tell you exactly the type and quantity of herb involved.

FREEZING HERBS
Instead of drying your herbs, you can store them in the freezer. This is especially useful for herbs such as parsley or lemon balm, which lose their flavour when dried.

Herbal teas

One of the easiest ways to benefit from the properties of a herb is to drink it as a tea. Taken regularly, herbal teas can make a significant contribution to well-being with their soothing, refreshing, and invigorating qualities.

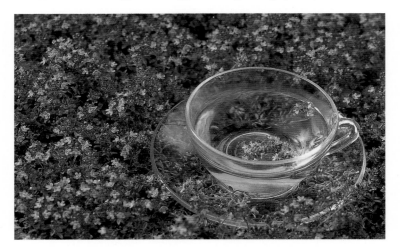

▲ THYME TEA IS GOOD FOR STOMACH CHILLS AND CHEST INFECTIONS.

Herbal infusions make wonderfully refreshing drinks and can be drunk as caffeine-free alternatives to ordinary tea and coffee. Herb teas, or tisanes, as they are sometimes known, are an acquired taste, so if you are unsure whether or not you like them, persist a little longer. The flavour of most can be sweetened with honey, a licorice stick, slices of fresh ginger or a squeeze of fresh lemon.

Herbal tisanes contain general health-giving properties and act as a refreshing tonic when taken regularly. Many commercial brands are available, but the taste is inferior to those made from fresh or

CAUTION

Herbs are powerful and can be harmful if taken in excess. Do not make teas stronger or drink them more frequently than recommended. Seek medical advice before taking herbal remedies when pregnant.

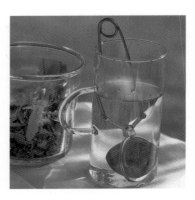

▸ A TEA INFUSER IS USEFUL FOR MAKING A SINGLE CUP OF TEA FROM DRIED HERBS.

home-dried garden herbs. Using herbs from your garden also ensures that the maximum benefit will be extracted. Since many herbs have a specific medicinal quality, you could grow those that suit your needs for a year-round supply.

Herbal teas can be taken to help ward off colds and flu, to aid digestion, promote sleep, to relieve headaches, anxiety and stress, even to promote energy. Drink a cupful of the appropriate tea no more than three times a day. Teas can be stored for up to 24 hours in the refrigerator.

1 Allow either 30ml/2 tbsp fresh or 15ml/1 tbsp dried herbs to each 600ml/1 pint/2½ cups water. For a single cup (250ml/8fl oz), use two small sprigs of fresh or 5ml/1 tsp dried herb. Wash fresh herbs first.

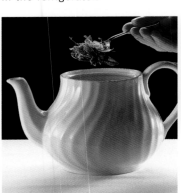

2 Put the herbs into a warmed pot. Pour on boiling water. Replace the lid to prevent vapour dissipation.

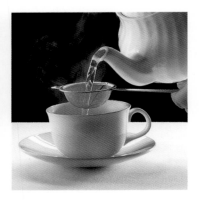

3 Leave to brew for three or four minutes, then strain the tea into a cup for a refreshing drink.

herbal teas **63**

Herbal tea remedies

 You don't necessarily have to feel ill to enjoy the benefits of a herbal brew, since many can be taken as a refreshing drink at any time of day. However, if you do have specific symptoms, the combinations below will certainly help.

Coughs and colds

PURPLE SAGE AND THYME	USE 5ML/1 TSP OF EACH FRESH PER CUP. ADD 1.5ML/ ¼ TSP CAYENNE PEPPER FOR A MORE POWERFUL EFFECT.
PEPPERMINT, ELDERFLOWER; CHAMOMILE AND LAVENDER	USE 2.5ML/½ TSP OF THE FIRST THREE, WITH A PINCH OF LAVENDER, PER CUPFUL OF WATER.
HOREHOUND	USE FRESH OR DRIED, AND SWEETEN WITH HONEY.
HYSSOP	USE FRESH OR DRIED, AND SWEETEN WITH HONEY OR MIX WITH ORANGE JUICE.
THYME	USE 5ML/1 TSP DRIED OR 10ML/2 TSP FRESH PER CUP.

Digestive troubles

CHAMOMILE	USE 5ML/1 TSP OF DRIED FLOWERS PER CUP.
PEPPERMINT AND LEMON BALM	USE FRESH HERBS IN EQUAL MEASURE AFTER A MEAL.
DILL	CAN BE GIVEN TO BABIES AND YOUNG CHILDREN. ALLOW 2.5ML/½ TSP LIGHTLY CRUSHED DILL SEED TO A CUP OF WATER AND BOIL FOR TEN MINUTES. STRAIN AND LEAVE TO COOL.
FENNEL SEED	CRUSH THE SEEDS AND SIMMER IN AN ENAMEL PAN FOR 10 MINUTES BEFORE STRAINING. CARAWAY SEEDS CAN BE PREPARED IN THE SAME WAY.
CINNAMON	INFUSE A CINNAMON STICK IN BOILING WATER FOR THREE OR FOUR MINUTES. LEAVE TO COOL, THEN CHILL.

Tonics and pick-me-ups

STINGING NETTLES	CHOP A SMALL HANDFUL OF YOUNG, FRESH LEAVES AND INFUSE IN 600ML/1 PINT/2½ CUPS BOILING WATER BEFORE STRAINING.
SPEARMINT	USE 15ML/1 TBSP CHOPPED FRESH LEAVES PER CUP AND SWEETEN TO TASTE.
GINGER	INFUSE FRESHLY GRATED ROOT GINGER IN TONIC WATER FOR A NATURAL ENERGY BOOST.

Early morning wakeners

LEMON VERBENA	USE FRESH OR DRIED LEAVES TO WAKE UP YOUR SYSTEM.
PEPPERMINT	USE ONE SPRIG OF FRESH HERBS PER CUPFUL.
BERGAMOT	USE FRESH FLOWERS FOR AN "EARL GREY" TASTE.

Disturbed sleep

CHAMOMILE	MAKE WITH 5ML/1 TSP DRIED CHAMOMILE TO A CUP AND ADD A PINCH OF LAVENDER FOR EXTRA RELAXATION.
LIMEFLOWER AND ELDERFLOWER	ADD A DASH OF GRATED NUTMEG AND SWEETEN WITH HONEY OR FLAVOUR WITH LEMON JUICE.
VALERIAN	USE 10ML/2 TSP DRIED AND SHREDDED ROOT TO A CUP OF WATER AND SIMMER FOR 20 MINUTES IN AN ENAMEL PAN WITH A LID. LET IT COOL, THEN STRAIN AND REHEAT IT.

Headaches, anxiety and depression

ROSEMARY	USE ONE OR TWO SMALL SPRIGS PER PERSON.
LEMON BALM	USE FRESH LEAVES.
BORAGE	USE FRESH OR DRIED FLOWERS.
PASSIONFLOWER, VALERIAN AND MOTHERWORT	USE 5ML/1 TSP DRIED VALERIAN AND MOTHERWORT AND ADD TO IT 2.5ML/½TSP OF PASSIONFLOWER.

▼ CHAMOMILE TEA IS SOOTHING AND CALMING.

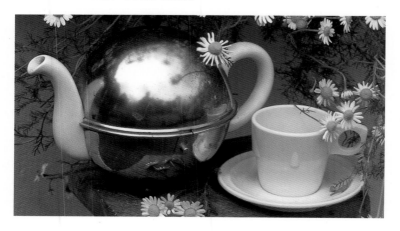

Herbal decoctions

Infusing herbs in boiling water is not enough to extract the constituents from roots or bark, such as valerian or licorice. Harder plant material needs to be boiled, and the resulting liquid is called a decoction.

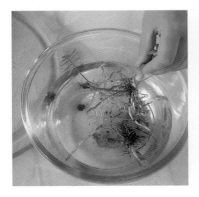

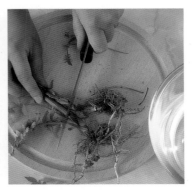

1 To make a decoction, wash the roots thoroughly.

2 Chop the root into small pieces.

3 Add 5ml/1 tsp of the root or bark to a pan of cold water. Leave it to soak for at least ten minutes, then bring it to the boil. Let it simmer for 10–15 minutes. Strain off the liquid and allow to cool before drinking. Decoctions can be kept for 24 hours in the refrigerator. They can be drunk hot or cold.

TIP
Always use a stainless-steel, glass or enamel pan when preparing herbal remedies.

Herbal decoction recipes

CHILBLAINS SIMMER 15G/½OZ CHOPPED GINGER ROOT IN 750ML/1¼PT/3 CUPS OF WATER UNTIL THE LIQUID REDUCES TO 600ML/ 1 PINT/2½ CUPS. STRAIN AND STORE IN THE REFRIGERATOR. TAKE 5–20ML/ 1–4 TSP THREE TIMES A DAY.

GALL BLADDER PROBLEMS SIMMER 50G/2OZ CLEAN, CHOPPED DANDELION ROOT IN WATER. STRAIN THROUGH A SIEVE AND STORE IN THE REFRIGERATOR FOR UP TO THREE DAYS. TAKE IN DOSES OF 5–20ML/1–4 TSP THREE TIMES A DAY.

Herbal tinctures

A tincture is a medicinal extract in a solution of alcohol and water. Take it diluted in a little water or fruit juice, but do not exceed 5ml/1 tsp, three or four times a day. Alternatively, use it externally, by adding it to liniments and compresses.

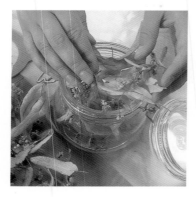

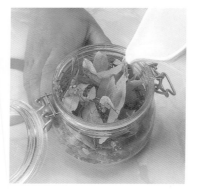

1 Place 115g/4oz dried herbs or 300g/11oz fresh herbs in a jar.

2 Add 250ml/8fl oz/1 cup vodka and 250ml/8fl oz/1 cup water.

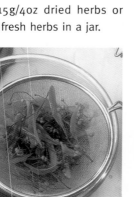

3 Leave to steep for two weeks, in a sunny place. Strain. Store in a dark, cool place for up to 18 months.

Herbal tincture remedies

HEADACHES AND DEPRESSION
USE LAVENDER IN THE QUANTITIES GIVEN ABOVE. TAKE DILUTED, OR ADD TO A COMPRESS.

MOUTH ULCERS AND INFLAMED GUMS
USE RASPBERRY LEAF IN THE QUANTITIES GIVEN ABOVE. DILUTE IN AN EQUAL QUANTITY OF WARM WATER AND USE AS A MOUTHWASH.

RHEUMATISM USE JUNIPER IN THE QUANTITIES GIVEN ABOVE AND ADD IT TO A LINIMENT FOR ACHING JOINTS.

COLDS AND HAYFEVER USE DRIED ELDERFLOWER IN THE QUANTITIES GIVEN.

Herbal ointments

An ointment contains oils or fats, but not water, and helps to form a protective layer over the skin. For a natural method use a vegetable oil such as sweet almond or sunflower, with beeswax. This is easy to make at home.

BASIC RECIPE

25g/1oz beeswax
120ml/4fl oz/½ cup vegetable oil, such as almond, safflower, sesame, or grapeseed oil blended with almond oil.
20–30 drops essential oil, or 10 drops if the ointment is for sensitive skin

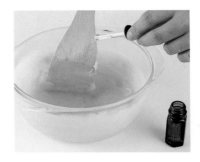

1 Place the beeswax and the oil in a glass bowl over a pan of water. Bring the water to the boil and simmer until the wax has melted into the oil. Remove from the heat.

2 Stir continually as the oil/wax mixture cools and stiffens. Add your choice of essential oils and stir into the mixture.

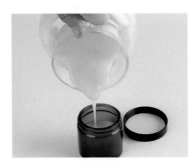

3 Pour or spoon into small, clean ointment jars, seal and store. Make small quantities and use it as soon as it is made.

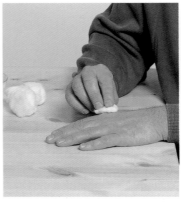

▲ APPLY OINTMENTS SPARINGLY AND COVER THE TREATED AREA TO PROTECT FROM DIRT.

Herbal creams

Making an organic cream is very similar to making an ointment, again using beeswax. Keep the cream in a cool place away from direct sunlight, and preferably in a dark glass or china pot. It should not be kept indefinitely.

BASIC RECIPE

25g/1oz beeswax
25ml/1½ tbsp water
120ml/4fl oz/½ cup vegetable
   oil such as almond, safflower,
   sesame or grapeseed oil
20–30 drops essential oil, or
   10 drops if the ointment is
   for sensitive skin

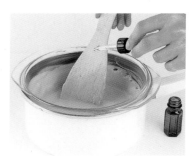

1 Melt the oil and beeswax, as for the herbal ointment. Add water to the melted wax/oil mixture, drop by drop, stirring all the time until the cream thickens and cools.

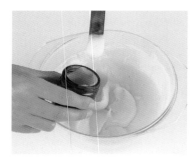

3 Carefully pour or spoon the cream into small, clean dark-coloured ointment jars. Seal and then store in the refrigerator.

2 Add the essential oils and gently stir them into the cream.

Herbal cream recipes

PROBLEM SKIN ADD ROSE OIL.

MATURE SKIN ADD JASMINE OIL.

FOR HEALING CUTS AND GRAZES ADD MARIGOLD OIL.

FOR HEALING ACNE ADD SANDALWOOD OIL TO THE CREAM.

TO NOURISH, CLEANSE AND SOOTHE THE SKIN MELT 50G/2OZ WHITE BEESWAX WITH 115G/4OZ ALMOND OIL. IN A SEPARATE BOWL DISSOLVE 2.5ML/½TSP BORAX IN 50ML/2FL OZ/¼ CUP OF ROSEWATER. SLOWLY POUR THE BORAX MIXTURE INTO THE OIL AND WAX, WHISKING UNTIL IT COOLS. WHEN IT THICKENS POUR INTO GLASS POTS.

Herbal poultices

Mashed herbs form the basis of a poultice. Its main purpose is to aid the healing of bruises, sprains and sores. Poultices are applied direct to the skin, either hot or cold. Hot poultices help sprains, while cold help inflammations.

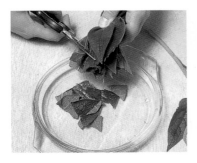

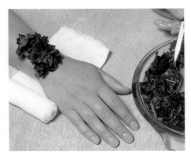

1 Snip a handful of herb leaves into a dish. Cover with boiling water and mash to a pulp with a spoon.

▼ A POULTICE IS AN INSTANT METHOD OF USING HERBS.

2 Leave to cool slightly, then spread the pulp directly on to the affected area. Cover with a piece of gauze and a bandage. Leave in place for several hours.

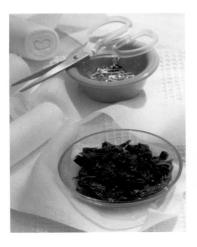

Herbal poultice recipes

SUNBURN LIGHTLY CRUSH THE LEAVES AND STEMS OF ANGELICA AND APPLY DIRECT TO THE SKIN.

GRAZES AND SCRAPES MASH SAGE LEAVES. APPLY DIRECT TO THE SKIN.

ACHING JOINTS AND MUSCLES MIX EQUAL AMOUNTS OF THE FRESH OR DRIED LEAVES OF MARJORAM AND ANGELICA AND APPLY TO THE SKIN.

STINGS AND BITES MIX OATMEAL TO A PASTE WITH AN INFUSION OF COMFREY OR MARIGOLD. LEAVE TO COOL. APPLY TO THE SKIN.

Herbal compresses

A compress is a length of fabric that is applied to the skin after it has been dipped into a herbal infusion. Compresses are gentle remedies that can be used for many different complaints from headaches to period pains.

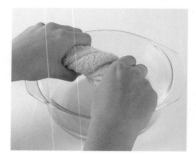

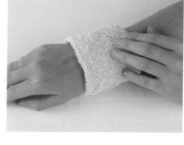

1 Put fresh or dried herbs into a clean bowl. Pour over boiling water. Leave to stand for one hour, then strain the liquid. Allow to cool and mix in any essential oil. Soak a length of cotton in the infusion and wring out lightly.

2 Position on the affected area and hold in place with a bandage.

▾ COMPRESSES CAN BE USED EFFECTIVELY ON ANY PART OF THE BODY.

Herbal compress recipes

TIRED EYES USE A SMALL HANDFUL OF CHAMOMILE FLOWERS TO MAKE AN INFUSION. DIP MUSLIN IN THE COOLED LIQUID AND APPLY TO THE CLOSED EYELIDS FOR 20 MINUTES.

BRUISES MAKE AN INFUSION USING 25G/1OZ FRESH WORMWOOD OR 15G/½OZ DRIED WITH 500ML/17FL OZ/2¼ CUPS BOILING WATER. LEAVE FOR 30 MINUTES THEN STRAIN. APPLY COOL.

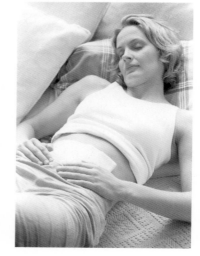

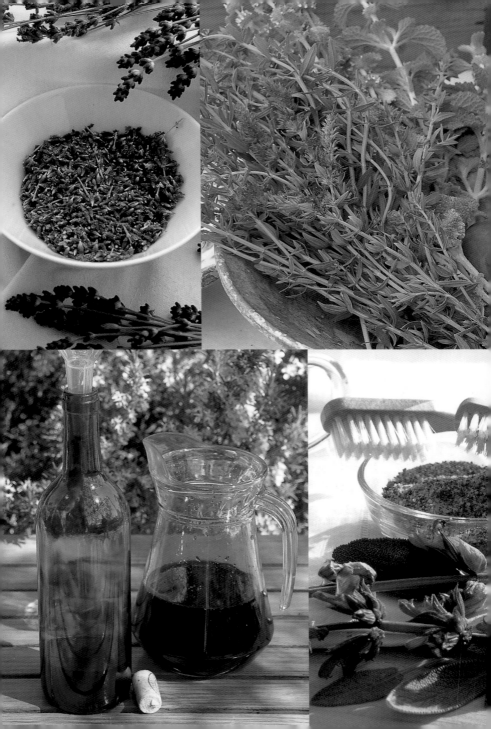

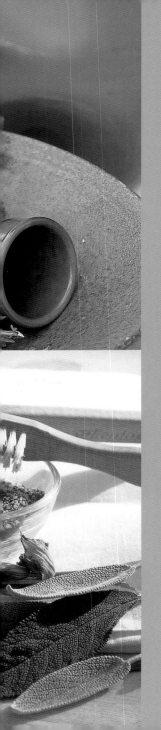

HERBAL
TREATMENTS

The recipes that follow use the roots, bark, leaves, stems and flowers of many kinds of herbs in healing remedies for everyday complaints such as cuts, bruises, aches and winter blues. Be aware that, while herbs are therapeutic if used in the correct quantity and manner, they are also a potent source of medicine, containing essential oils which can become toxic if dosage is exceeded.

Pregnant women should avoid any herbal remedies unless under professional supervision. Always use herbs from a reliable source, and if you are unsure of what the herb is, do not use it. Consult the healing plants directory for more information on key herbs and their properties, but always seek further advice if unsure.

Coughs and colds

The common cold affects most people at some point in the year. And since there are over 200 strains of cold virus, it is not surprising that a cure has not been found. Herbal treatments can help to relieve many of the symptoms.

GARLIC COLD AND FLU SYRUP

With antiseptic and antibacterial qualities, garlic is ideal for a cold.

INGREDIENTS

1 head garlic, crushed
300ml/½ pint/1¼ cups water
juice of ½ lemon
30ml/2 tbsp honey

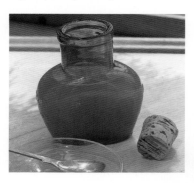

1 Bring the garlic and water to the boil. Simmer gently for 20 minutes.

2 Add the lemon juice and honey and simmer for two minutes. Allow to cool, then strain into a clean, dark bottle with an airtight lid. Take 10–15ml/2–3 tsp three times a day. Keep chilled for up to three weeks.

EVERYDAY ROSE-HIP TEA

Rose-hips are high in vitamin C and help to ward off colds.

INGREDIENTS – MAKES ABOUT 6 CUPS

45ml/3 tbsp rose-hips
1.5 litres/2½ pints/6¼ cups filtered or bottled still water

1 Top and tail the rose-hips. Cover them in tap water for 24 hours. Strain and discard the water.

2 Bring the filtered water to the boil. Add the rose-hips. Simmer for about 30 minutes. Strain and serve, sweetening to taste with honey.

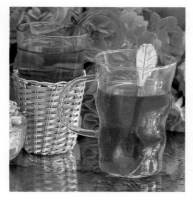

LAVENDER AND EUCALYPTUS VAPOUR
The fresh and uplifting scents of lavender and eucalyptus clear the bronchial and nasal passages. Rub on the chest before bedtime.

INGREDIENTS

50g/2oz petroleum jelly
15ml/1 tbsp dried lavender
6 drops eucalyptus essential oil
4 drops lavender essential oil

1 Melt the jelly in a bowl over a pan of simmering water. Stir in the lavender and heat for 30 minutes.

2 Strain the liquid through muslin. Cool, then add the oils. Pour into a clean jar and leave until set.

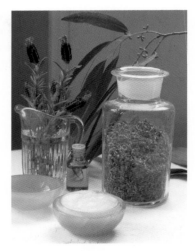

▲ THIS VAPOUR RUB CAN ALSO BE INHALED. MELT A SMALL QUANTITY IN A BOWL OF STEAMING WATER. LEAN OVER THE BOWL, WITH A TOWEL OVER YOUR HEAD AND INHALE. KEEP THE CREAM REFRIGERATED.

Herbal cough remedies

TRY A WARM INFUSION OF ONE OR A MIXTURE OF THE FOLLOWING:
COLTSFOOT – PARTICULARLY GOOD FOR IRRITATING, SPASMODIC COUGHS
HYSSOP – A CALMING AND RELAXING EXPECTORANT
MARSHMALLOW – FOR A HARSH, DRY, PAINFUL COUGH
THYME – POWERFULLY ANTISEPTIC, THIS RELIEVES A HARSH, DRY AND PAINFUL COUGH
HOREHOUND – AN EXPECTORANT, FREEING UP MUCUS AND HELPING IT TO BE REMOVED.

Herbal cold remedies

TAKE AN INFUSION OF EQUAL AMOUNTS OF PEPPERMINT, ELDERFLOWER AND YARROW JUST BEFORE BED TO INDUCE A SWEAT. YOU CAN ALSO ADD:
CAYENNE PEPPER – USE 1.5ML/¼ TSP OF THE POWDER TO STIMULATE THE SYSTEM. CAYENNE ADDS INSTANT HEAT AND WILL MAKE YOU SWEAT.
CINNAMON – BREAK A CINNAMON STICK INTO THE HERBS FOR A GENTLE, WARMING AND SWEAT-INDUCING EFFECT.
GINGER – GRATE A SMALL PIECE OF FRESH ROOT GINGER INTO THE MIXTURE FOR EXTRA HEAT.

Sore throats

Often a sore throat goes hand-in-hand with the symptoms of a cough or cold. Sometimes sore throats can be caused by air conditioning in office buildings. Discomfort can be eased by gargling with herbs or sipping herbal teas.

ALLIUM STEAM INHALATION
Garlic has antiseptic properties that will ease a sore throat.

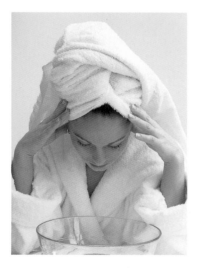

1 Put two unpeeled garlic cloves in a heatproof bowl containing 1 litre/ 1¾ pints/4 cups of steaming water.

2 Lean over the bowl, cover your head with a towel and inhale the garlic steam for several minutes.

▸ HYSSOP YIELDS BOTH FLOWERS AND LEAVES WITH MEDICINAL BENEFITS.

HYSSOP TISANE
Originally from Asia, hyssop is a widely-used medicinal plant with beautiful aquamarine flowers and aromatic leaves with expectorant properties. When used alone, it makes an excellent tisane for coughs and sore throats, but it is quite bitter, so it's worth adding a little honey, or a splash of orange juice for vitamin C, to sweeten the taste.

To prepare, simply infuse a few fresh or 5ml/1 tsp dried leaves and flowers in 250ml/8fl oz/1 cup boiling water.

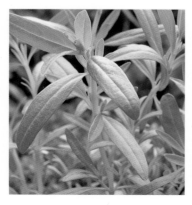

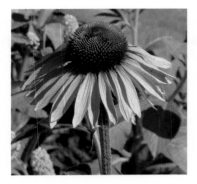

▲ The coneflower, *Echinacea angustifolia* or *E. purpurea*, boosts the immune system and may be taken in tablet form or as a tincture.

Soothing laryngitis

Laryngitis is an acute inflammation of the larynx or vocal chords, leading to a sore throat, hoarseness and even loss of voice. Local treatment is by gargle or cold infusions. The best herbs to use are sage, thyme, agrimony or raspberry leaf. Leave a small handful of leaves to infuse in boiling water, then strain and allow to cool. For a soothing effect, add marshmallow.

Tonsillitis remedies

Make an infusion of agrimony, licorice, sage, or thyme to gargle with. A tincture of myrrh is also good.

Thyme and sage gargle

This recipe will relieve sore throats, mouth ulcers, gum disease, laryngitis and tonsillitis.

Ingredients

> 15g/½oz fresh sage and thyme, or horehound
> 600ml/1 pint/2½ cups boiling water
> 30ml/2 tbsp cider vinegar
> 10ml/2 tsp honey
> 5ml/1 tsp cayenne pepper

1 Put your choice of herbs into a bowl, pour in the boiling water, cover and leave for 30 minutes. Strain the liquid.

2 Stir in the vinegar, honey and cayenne. Gargle or swallow 10ml/ 2 tsp at a time, twice a day.

▼ Sage and thyme are both antiseptic.

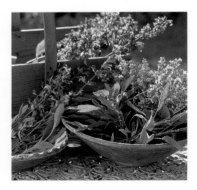

Blocked sinuses

Inhaling steam scented with aromatic herbs relieves the congestion of a cold or blocked sinuses, and can remove headaches which are often a symptom of the problem. You could put essential oils on your pillow and in your bath too.

ESSENTIAL OIL INHALANT
Add 5 drops of eucalyptus, 2 drops of camphor and 1 drop of citronella essential oils to 600ml/1 pint/ 2½ cups of boiling water and inhale.

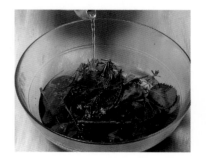

FRESH HERB INHALANT
To relieve blocked sinuses, immerse fresh herbs and spices in steaming water and breathe in the vapours. Choose from: eucalyptus leaves, basil, cayenne pepper, cinnamon stick, hyssop, juniper berries and foliage, lavender, lemon balm, mint, rosemary, sage, thyme.

1 Put a large handful of your chosen herbs in a bowl and pour in about 1 litre/1¾ pints/4 cups of boiling water. Lean over the bowl, covering both it and your head with a towel. Inhale deeply.

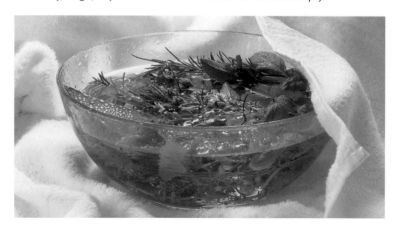

Earache

Earaches most often develop through an infection, often following a cold or sinusitis. They should not be neglected – infections can spread through into the middle or even inner ear with potentially serious complications.

If earache is associated with catarrh, this should be treated too. Earache in children needs to be treated quickly as an infection in the middle ear can be both painful and damaging. Seek medical help if earache worsens or persists.

Do not put anything into the ear, unless it has been examined by a doctor to check that the eardrum has not been perforated.

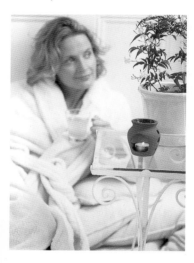

▲ Burning lavender and chamomile oil will bring relief to earache sufferers.

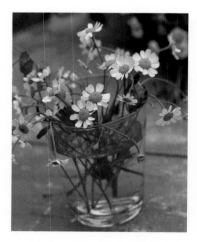

▲ Chamomile contains the anti-inflammatory chemical azulene which is useful for treating conditions such as earache, acne, insect bites and allergies.

Earache remedies

Chamomile – make a hot compress, or an infusion. Apply to the outside of the ear with cotton wool (swab).

Garlic – eaten with food, or if the eardrum is not perforated, crush 1 clove of garlic into 5ml/1 tsp of olive oil; warm it to blood temperature and gently insert a few drops into the ear. This is an excellent antibiotic.

Winter blues

The transition from autumn to winter is not always easy, particularly when the nights draw in and the warm weather disappears. To help you to adapt to this changing time, there are plenty of uplifting herbal remedies.

ROSEMARY TONIC WINE

This pungent and aromatic herb has a long tradition of use as a tonic herb with a reputation for lifting the spirits.

INGREDIENTS

handful of fresh rosemary
*   leaves*
2 small cinnamon sticks
5 cloves
5ml/1 tsp ground ginger
grating of nutmeg
bottle of claret or other good
*   quality red wine*

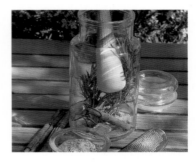

1 Put the rosemary, cinnamon and cloves into a jar and crush using a pestle to release their essential oils. Add the ginger and nutmeg to the mixture.

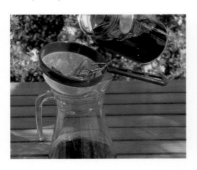

2 Add the wine, seal the jar and leave in a cool place for ten days. Strain into a sterilized bottle and seal with an airtight stopper.

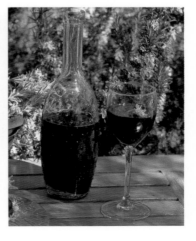

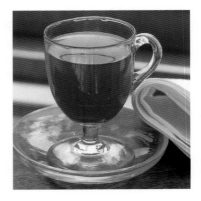

WINTER WARMER

Ginger is one of the oldest and most popular herbal medicines, and makes an excellent, warming addition to a cup of tea on a cold day. This uplifting drink helps to ward off low blood sugar, headaches, nausea and fatigue.

To make the tea, pour boiling water over a teaspoon of freshly grated ginger root. Add the juice of half a lemon and sweeten with 1 tsp of honey. Drink warm in winter as an uplifting tonic or allow to cool thoroughly, and add ice, for a deliciously chilled tea in summer.

▶ FRESH OR HOME-DRIED HERBS MAKE THE BEST HERBAL TEAS, BUT IF YOU DON'T HAVE ACCESS TO A SUPPLY, THERE ARE SOME GOOD SHOP-BOUGHT VARIETIES.

ALCOHOL-FREE TONIC

This excellent tonic should be drunk warm twice a day for a total of three weeks to thoroughly cleanse the system. Add 600ml/ 1 pint/2½ cups of boiling water to 2.5ml/½ tsp each of oats, vervain and borage. Flavour with peppermint or licorice. Allow to steep for ten minutes and strain.

AROMATIC BOOSTER

Pulsating with freshness and the promise of spring, this delicate infusion is perfect for reawakening the senses at a dark time of year. Simply add three or four fresh leaves of basil to a 250ml/ 8fl oz/1 cup boiling water and allow to steep for 10 minutes. Strain while still warm.

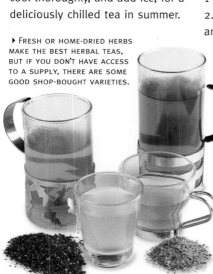

Headaches

The majority of headaches are caused by nasal congestion or sinusitis, eyestrain, fatigue or tension. They can also be caused by stress or worries, with muscle spasms in the neck and upper back leading to head pains.

WOOD BETONY AND LAVENDER TEA
These herbs soothe the nerves and are helpful for tension headaches. You could try chamomile, or lime blossom tea to relieve a headache.
INGREDIENTS
> *2.5ml/½ tsp dried wood betony*
> *2.5ml/½ tsp dried lavender*
> *200ml/7fl oz/scant cup boiling water*

1 Put the herbs into a cup and leave to steep in the boiling water for up to ten minutes.

2 Strain and drink twice a day.

Caution: Do not take more than 5ml/1 tsp betony per day.

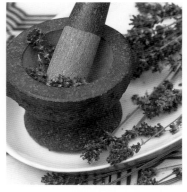

▲ LAVENDER HAS A DELICIOUS, UPLIFTING SCENT. USE IT TO PERFUME A BATH.

▼ RUB LAVENDER OR ROSEMARY OIL INTO YOUR TEMPLES TO RELIEVE A HEADACHE.

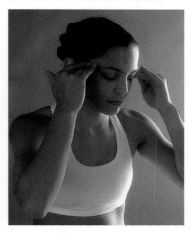

Herbal headache remedies
HANG A MUSLIN (CHEESECLOTH) BAG OF FRESH OR DRIED HERBS UNDER THE TAP WHEN YOU RUN A BATH.
MAKE A LAVENDER COMPRESS BY SOAKING SOFT COTTON FABRIC IN A LAVENDER INFUSION AND WRINGING IT OUT SLIGHTLY.

Hangovers

Most hangover symptoms – headache, nausea, fuzzy head and depression – are connected with the liver being unable to perform many of its functions. Bitter herbs can stimulate the liver, but avoid vervain if you suffer from liver disease.

MORNING-AFTER TEA

Vervain is bitter and lavender aids digestion; both lift the spirits.

INGREDIENTS

5ml/1 tsp dried vervain
2.5ml/½ tsp lavender flowers
600ml/1 pint/2½ cups water

1 Bring the water to the boil and add the herbs. Cover the pan of boiling water to retain the volatile oils, and remove from the heat.

2 Allow to steep for ten minutes. Strain and sweeten with a little honey. Sip a cup of this tea slowly.

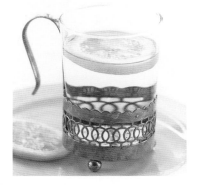

▲ IF YOU HAVE A HANGOVER, DRINK PLENTY OF WATER TO FLUSH THROUGH YOUR BODY, AND TAKE EXTRA VITAMIN C. A CUP OF BOILING WATER WITH A SLICE OF LEMON IN IT, OR FRESHLY SQUEEZED LEMON JUICE, WILL GIVE THE LIVER A BOOST.

▼ HERBAL TEAS ARE EXCELLENT CLEANSERS.

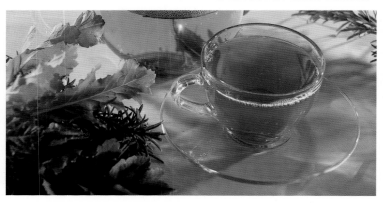

Migraines

These are more than a severe headache. They generally involve acute pains, often over one eye, and perhaps distorted vision or flashing lights. There may also cause nausea or vomiting and sensitivity to bright lights.

NECK MASSAGE FOR MIGRAINE
Use rosemary essential oil to massage your neck with. Keep your arms relaxed while massaging.

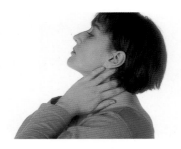

1 For stiff, aching neck muscles massage the neck with firm circular movements.

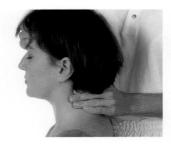

2 Ideally have someone else massage your neck for you. They can support your head while massaging.

Herbal tea remedies to relieve migraines

CHOOSE FROM CHAMOMILE OR ROSEMARY, ACCORDING TO YOUR TYPE OF MIGRAINE. MAKE AN INFUSION OR TEA WITH THE CHOSEN HERB AND SIP IT THROUGHOUT THE DAY.

CHAMOMILE IS GOOD FOR A DULL, THROBBING HEADACHE WITH A FEELING OF QUEASINESS – ADD A LITTLE GINGER TO RELIEVE MORE SEVERE NAUSEA.

FEVERFEW RELIEVES THE FEELING OF A TIGHT BAND AROUND THE HEAD. IT IS ALSO AVAILABLE IN TABLET FORM.

ROSEMARY HELPS WHERE STRESS IS A TRIGGER FOR MIGRAINES AND WHERE LOCAL WARMTH GIVES RELIEF.

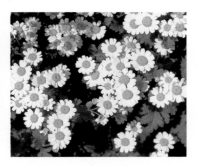

▲ FEVERFEW LEAVES ARE VERY BITTER. THE BEST WAY TO TAKE THEM IS SANDWICHED BETWEEN TWO SLICES OF BREAD.

Tense muscles

When we are anxious, we raise our shoulders and contract our back muscles. The effort of maintaining our muscles in this way is tiring. Tight neck muscles can also partially restrict blood flow to the head and so bring on a headache.

COLD-INFUSED LAVENDER OIL
This recipe is easy to make and very versatile. You could make marjoram or rosemary oils in the same way.
INGREDIENTS
dried lavender heads
clear vegetable oil

1 Fill a jar with lavender heads and cover completely with oil. Replace the lid. Allow to steep in a sunny place for a month. Shake daily.

2 Strain and bottle. Massage into stiff muscles or add to your bath to encourage relaxation.

CAUTION
• Do not use concentrated essential oil on your skin, dilute it by adding 2 drops of oil to 20ml/4 tsp of grapeseed or almond oil.

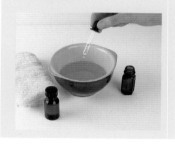

▼ IF YOU SPEND A LOT OF TIME STANDING OR SITTING IN THE SAME POSITION YOU NEED TO KEEP STRETCHING AND RELAXING YOUR LIMBS.

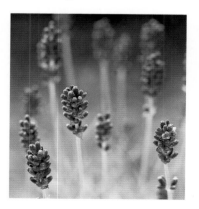

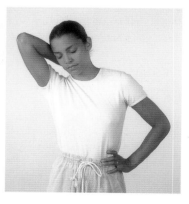

Insomnia

It is important to distinguish between habitual sleeplessness and temporary insomnia caused by worry. Do not become obsessed with trying to get a certain amount of sleep; not everyone needs eight hours.

LAVENDER TINCTURE
Store tinctures in dark bottles in a cool place for best results.

INGREDIENTS
   15g/½oz dried lavender
   250ml/8fl oz/1 cup vodka, made
   up to 300ml/½ pint/1¼ cups
   with water

1 Put the lavender into a glass jar and pour in the vodka and water. Put a lid on the jar and leave in a cool, dark place for ten days (no longer), shaking occasionally. The tincture turns dark purple.

2 Strain off the lavender through a muslin before pouring into a sterilized glass bottle. Seal with a cork.

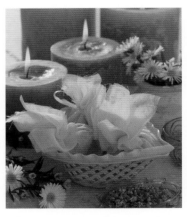

▲ TRY FILLING A MUSLIN (CHEESECLOTH) BAG WITH LAVENDER AND HOLD IT UNDER THE WATER FLOWING FROM THE BATH TAP. ADD LIGHTED CANDLES TO HELP CREATE MOOD.

▼ TAKE TIME TO UNWIND BEFORE YOU GO TO BED. LISTEN TO SOOTHING MUSIC AND TREAT THE EYES TO A CUCUMBER FACIAL.

Herbal insomnia remedies
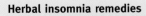
MAKE THE HERBS LISTED BELOW INTO TINCTURES OR USE THE DRIED HERB TUCKED UNDER YOUR PILLOW.

CHAMOMILE	LAVENDER
HYSSOP	LEMON BALM
LIME BLOSSOM	VIOLET
PASSIONFLOWER	

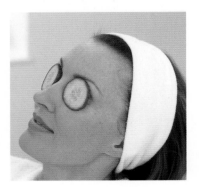

Stress

Stress in itself is not harmful and can in fact be motivating. But when the amount of stress is too much for our system to cope with, then it can cause other more harmful medical conditions.

STRESS-BUSTER TEA

Choose relaxing infusions from herbs such as lavender, lime blossom, lemon balm and valerian. A mixture of vervain, rosemary and betony (no more than 2.5ml/½tsp per cup) are a tonic for exhaustion.

INGREDIENTS

30ml/2 tbsp fresh or 15ml/
1 tbsp dried herb
600ml/1 pint/2½ cups boiling
water

1 Put the herbs and water in a teapot. Steep for ten minutes.

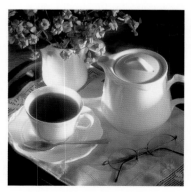

▲ AVOID CAFFEINE WHEN YOU ARE STRESSED. CHOOSE HEALTHY HERBAL TEAS INSTEAD.

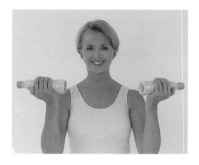

▲ EXERCISE HELPS TO REMOVE TENSION AND CHANGES THE FOCUS OF YOUR ATTENTION.

SYMPTOMS OF STRESS
• Constantly on edge and on the verge of tears.
• Difficulty in concentrating.
• Always tired, even after a night's sleep, and unable to relax or unwind – even if not working.
• Feelings of being unable to cope with life.
• Poor appetite or else nibbling without hunger.
• No sense of fun or enjoyment.
• Mistrustful of everybody.
• Problems in relationships, no interest in sex.
• Always fidgeting or biting nails or chewing hair.

Acidity and heartburn

Bouts of acidity and heartburn may occur after consuming rich foods or eating too quickly, and can be a symptom of indigestion. If the condition is temporary, make teas from the suggested herbs. Seek help if the problem persists.

MEADOWSWEET TINCTURE

This herb is a traditional remedy for heartburn, gastric ulcers and excess acidity.

INGREDIENTS

   *115g/4oz dried, or 300g/11oz
      freshly picked meadowsweet
      flowers
   250ml/8fl oz/1 cup vodka
   250ml/8fl oz/1 cup water*

1 Place the herb flowers in a jar. Pour in the vodka and water.

2 Put a tight-fitting lid on the jar and leave to steep for a month, preferably on a sunny windowsill. Gently shake the jar.

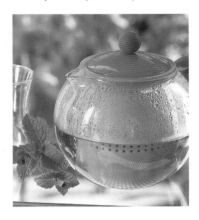

▲ PEPPERMINT TEA IS A GOOD TEA TO TAKE FOR INDIGESTION AND ACIDITY.

3 Strain and store the tincture in a dark glass bottle (it will keep for up to 18 months).

4 Take 5ml/1 tsp, three times a day, diluted in a little water or fruit juice.

◄ GROW MEADOWSWEET IN YOUR GARDEN AND ADD THE LEAVES TO STEWS OR SOUPS IF YOU ARE PRONE TO HEARTBURN.

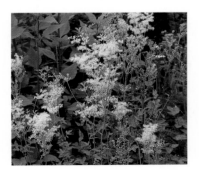

Herbal teas for acidity and heartburn

CHAMOMILE	LEMON BALM
MEADOWSWEET	SLIPPERY ELM

Abscesses

An abscess is a localized, inflamed swelling containing pus which can develop externally on the skin or internally in the mouth or other mucous membranes – the latter should be treated by a medical professional.

HOT MARSHMALLOW POULTICE

A poultice made of marshmallow to heal an inflammation is one of the earliest recorded uses for a herb.

INGREDIENTS

2 handfuls fresh marshmallow leaves or 15ml/1 tbsp powdered marshmallow root
250ml/8fl oz/1 cup of boiling water or about 45ml/3 tbsp of hot water
olive or almond oil

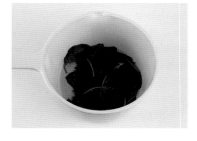

1 Pour the boiling water over the leaves in a bowl. If you are using powdered root, mix it with a little hot water to make a paste.

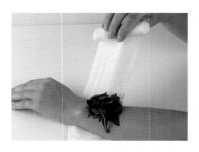

2 Apply a little oil to the skin in the affected area first, so that the poultice does not stick and burn the skin. Place the leaves or the paste on the abscess and cover with clean gauze or strips of cotton, lint or muslin.

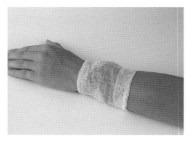

3 Hold in position with tape or a safety pin. You can keep the poultice on for several hours but may need to replace the contents of it every couple of hours. It may feel a little damp and uncomfortable to begin with.

Bites and stings

Summer brings a host of insects such as bees, wasps and hornets that can sting. In any situation where a bite or sting affects the mouth or throat, or if there are signs of an allergic reaction, get medical help immediately.

MARIGOLD INFUSION

Only the pot marigold *Calendula officinalis* has a medicinal value, so make sure you choose the right one when picking your flowers.

INGREDIENTS

> heatproof bowl
> 1 litre/1³⁄₄ pints/4 cups boiling
>   water
> 20 marigold flower-heads

1 Warm the bowl. Place the flowers in the bowl and pour over the just-boiled water. Cover with a tea towel and leave to stand for ten minutes.

2 Strain the liquid into a bottle. Apply the infusion as a skin lotion or on a cold compress to ease the pain of a bite or sting.

REMOVING A STING

Some stings, for instance those of bees, result in the sting being left behind in the skin. This should be carefully removed before applying any ointments or herbal treatments to the affected area. Try using a pair of tweezers if you cannot steady your hand. Take care, though, not to burst the poison sac when removing the sting, and thereby send more toxin into the puncture, causing further irritation.

Bite and sting remedies

COMPRESS – WORMWOOD, WITCH HAZEL, CHAMOMILE, ELDERFLOWER, RED CLOVER, MARIGOLD, LAVENDER, LEMON BALM, PLANTAIN, YELLOW DOCK.
FRESH HERBS – ALOE VERA, HOUSELEEK, LEMON BALM, BASIL, DOCK LEAF, ONION.
OINTMENT – CHICKWEED, MARIGOLD.
POULTICE – CARROT (FOR SUNBURN), OATMEAL.
TINCTURE – ST JOHN'S WORT.

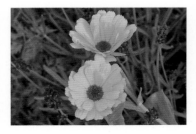

◀ MARIGOLD IS USED IN SKIN CREAMS TO SOOTHE AND HEAL.

Cuts, grazes and bruises

Before treating any cuts, grazes and bruises, make sure that the affected area is properly cleaned with water and a clean cloth to remove any dirt. An ointment will help to draw out dirt that is deeply embedded in the skin.

COMFREY BRUISE OINTMENT
Apply this ointment to varicose veins, bruises and inflamed muscles.

INGREDIENTS
200g/7oz petroleum jelly or
*   paraffin wax*
25g/1oz fresh comfrey leaves

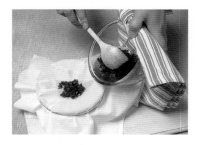

1 Put the petroleum jelly in a bowl. Set it over a pan of boiling water, add the chopped comfrey leaves and stir well. Heat over gently simmering water for about one hour.

2 Strain the mixture through muslin secured to the rim of a bowl with a rubber band. Gradually pour the liquid into a clean glass jar, before it has chance to set.

Herbal remedies for cuts and grazes

COMPRESS – WITCH HAZEL (THOUGH NOT ON BROKEN SKIN).
OINTMENT – MARIGOLD, COMFREY.
POULTICE – SAGE.
TINCTURE – MARIGOLD, MYRRH, YARROW.

Herbal remedies for bruises

COMPRESS – WITCH HAZEL, COMFREY, WORMWOOD.
ESSENTIAL OILS – LAVENDER.
OINTMENT – HOUSELEEK, YARROW.
POULTICE – COMFREY.

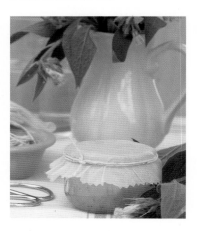

▲ USE COMFREY SPARINGLY AND NEVER TAKE IT INTERNALLY.

Burns and sunburn

Severe burns require medical assistance. The immediate treatment is to apply cold water for up to ten minutes to reduce the heat. With sunburn, be sure to avoid further exposure to the sun until all the symptoms have cleared.

AFTER SUN SOOTHING OIL

A cooling oil for burnt skin.

INGREDIENTS

> 5 drops rose essential oil
> 5 drops chamomile essential oil
> 45ml/3 tbsp grapeseed oil
> 45ml/3 tbsp virgin olive oil
> 15ml/1 tbsp wheatgerm oil

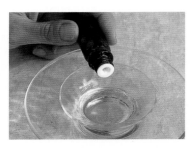

1 Combine the oils in a small bowl. Massage gently into the burn.

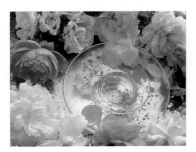

MARIGOLD OINTMENT FOR BURNS

This ointment moisturizes and soothes the skin.

INGREDIENTS

> 200g/7oz petroleum jelly
> about 25g/1oz marigold flower
>   heads, roughly chopped

1 Put the petroleum jelly in a bowl. Set it over a pan of boiling water, add the marigolds and stir. Heat over simmering water for one hour.

2 Strain the mixture through muslin secured to the rim of a jug with a rubber band. Pour the liquid immediately into a clean glass jar, before it has a chance to set. Leave to cool then refrigerate.

TIPS

• Aloe vera gel is an excellent first-aid treatment for burns. Break open a leaf and spread the gel directly on to the burn.
• You could also try infusions of elderflower, rose, chamomile, lavender, and tea tree.

Halitosis and mouth ulcers

Bad breath can result from several things such as an upset stomach, or teeth that need cleaning. For an instant breath freshener chew fresh parsley after a meal. Mouth ulcers are an indication of being run down. Herbs can help both.

SAGE AND SALT TOOTHPOWDER
This toothpaste replacement will clean your teeth and keep your breath fresh.

INGREDIENTS
  25g/1oz sage leaves
  60ml/4 tbsp sea salt

1 Shred the sage leaves into an ovenproof dish using scissors.

2 Mix in the salt, grinding it into the leaves with a pestle. Bake in a very low oven for about one hour until crisp.

3 Pound the baked ingredients until reduced to powder. Use in place of toothpaste on a damp toothbrush.

Herbal mouth ulcer tinctures

MYRHH	MARIGOLD
RASPBERRY LEAF	SAGE
THYME	

Herbal teeth cleansers
RUB TEETH WITH FRESH SAGE LEAVES.

MYRRH AND SAGE MOUTH ULCER RINSE
Sage has antiseptic qualities and is a good herb for mouth complaints.
INGREDIENTS
  15ml/1tbsp dried sage
  100ml/½ pint/1¼ cups boiling water
  10ml/2 tsp tincture of myrrh

1 Put the sage leaves in a bowl. Pour the boiling water over. Leave to stand for 20 minutes, strain and mix in the myrrh. Allow to cool. Use to rinse your mouth.

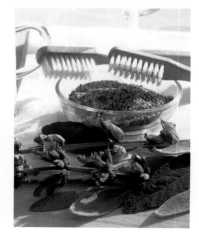

Acne and spots

Acne is caused by increasing levels of hormones, which, during the teens, cause the skin's glands to overproduce sebum (the natural oily skin lubricant), blocking the pores. Regular cleansing will help to remove this oily excess.

FEVERFEW COMPLEXION MILK
Feverfew is easy to grow in the garden and self-seeds prodigiously. When the leaves are heated with milk, they produce an excellent tonic which, once applied to the skin, helps to clear blemishes, discourage blackheads and moisturize dry skin.

INGREDIENTS
1 large handful of feverfew
leaves
600ml/1 pint /2½ cups milk
A saucepan, strainer and bottle

1 Place the feverfew leaves and milk into a small pan, bring to the boil, then reduce the heat and simmer for 20 minutes.

2 Remove the pan from the heat and allow the mixture to cool. Strain into a bottle and store in the refrigerator until needed.

3 Apply cold to the skin, taking care to massage in thoroughly.

▼ FEVERFEW LEAVES CAN BE USED BOTH TO CLEANSE AND MOISTURIZE FACIAL SKIN.

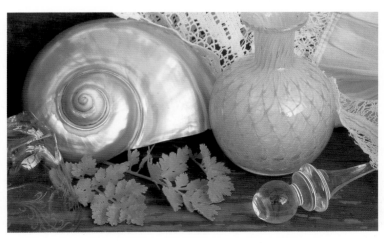

Dry and sore lips

It is quite simple to make your own soothing cream for lips chapped by sun, wind, weather or illness. You can also apply a simple mixture of honey and rosewater as a salve for sore or chapped lips.

LAVENDER LIP BALM

Beeswax and cocoa butter are rich emollients; lavender oil is well known for its healing ability.

INGREDIENTS

5ml/1 tsp beeswax
5ml/1 tsp cocoa butter
5ml/1 tsp wheatgerm oil
5ml/1 tsp almond oil
3 drops lavender essential oil

1 Put all but the last ingredient, into a bowl and set over a pan of simmering water. Stir until melted.

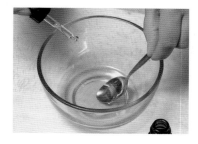

2 Remove from the heat and allow to cool for a few minutes before mixing in the lavender oil. Pour into a small jar and leave to set.

▼ BEESWAX HAS A HIGH MELTING POINT, SO BE PATIENT.

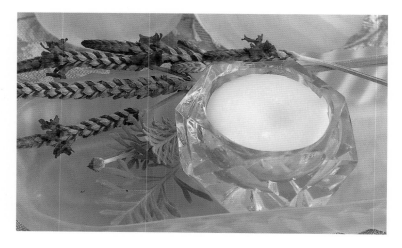

Dry and oily skin

Moisturizing cream prevents dryness of the skin, keeps wrinkles at bay and protects your skin from the weather. If you like, substitute pot marigolds for the elderflowers. Splash a little tonic on to your face first to feel refreshed.

DRY SKIN MOISTURIZER

Elderflowers have a reputation for lightening dry skin. Store this face cream in the refrigerator. It keeps for several months.

INGREDIENTS

> *120ml/4fl oz/½ cup water*
> *10ml/2 tsps dried elderflowers*
> *30ml/2 tbsp emulsifying*
>   *ointment*
> *5ml/1 tsp beeswax*
> *30ml/2 tbsp almond oil*
> *2.5ml/½ tsp borax*

1 Boil the water and pour over the dried elderflowers in a jar. Leave to stand for 30 minutes then strain.

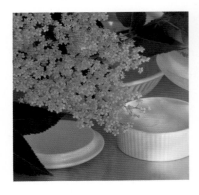

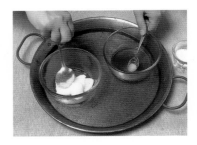

2 Put the emulsifying ointment, beeswax and almond oil into one bowl and the elderflower infusion and borax into another. Set both over hot water and stir until the oils melt and the borax dissolves.

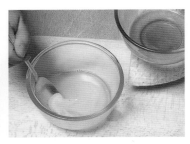

3 Remove from the heat and pour the elderflower mixture into the oils. Stir gently until incorporated. Leave to cool, stirring at intervals. Pour into a jar before it sets.

Elderflower skin tonic

This refreshing skin tonic can be made to suit your skin type and should be applied to your face direct from the refrigerator. It keeps for a few days, or can be frozen in small quantities and thawed as required.

Ingredients

10 dried elderflower heads
300ml/½ pint/1¼ cups still bottled water, boiled
15ml/1 tbsp either cider vinegar for normal skin, or witch hazel for slightly oily skin, or vodka for very oily skin

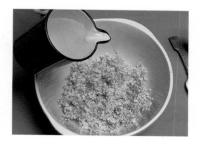

1 Strip the elderflowers from the stems and place in a bowl. Pour the boiling water over the flowers. Cover with a tea towel and leave for 20 minutes. Add either the cider vinegar, witch hazel or vodka, cover and leave overnight to infuse.

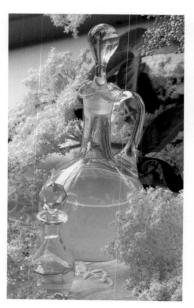

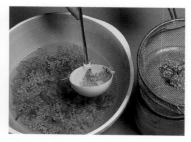

2 Strain into a sterilized jar, cover and allow to cool. Store chilled.

Mint and marigold moisturizer for oily skin

USE 25G/1OZ FRESH MINT LEAVES WITH 15G/½ OZ FRESH MARIGOLD PETALS AND 600ML/1 PINT/2½ CUPS BOILING WATER WITH 30ML/2 TBSP VODKA.

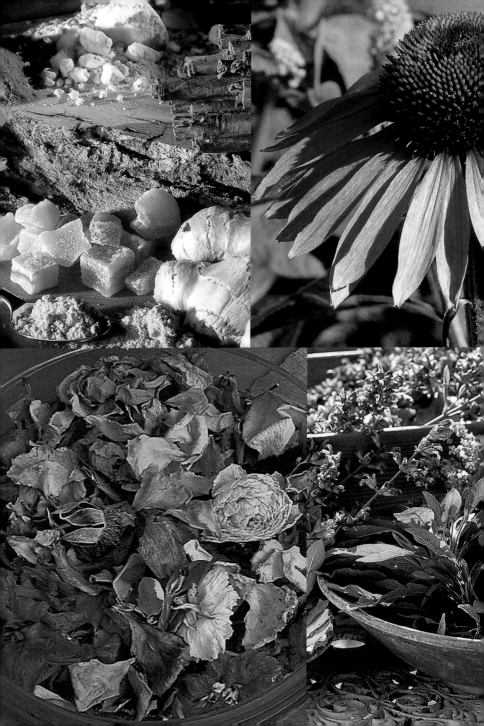

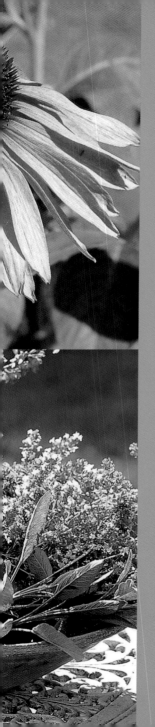

HEALING PLANTS
DIRECTORY

This directory features up to 80 of the best-known healing flowers and herbs, many of which can be grown easily at home. There is information on characteristics such as height and leaf shape, to help you to identify them, plus advice on how to use the various parts of each plant to heal safely and effectively.

Special care should be taken when using flowers or herbs as part of internal remedies. It is essential that you use the correct dosage as prescribed by a qualified herbalist, and, if pregnant or taking other medicines, discuss usage with a medical professional. Remember that plant remedies do not work instantly, so give them time to take effect. Seek further medical advice if symptoms persist.

The directory

Achillea millefolium,
YARROW
Pungent perennial herb with flat, whitish or pink flowerheads and feathery leaves. The essential oil can treat catarrh; the bitter-tasting infusion sweats out colds and fevers. Yarrow is also used externally to treat wounds, nose-bleeds and as a skin toner.

Agrimonia eupatoria,
AGRIMONY
Perennial herb with yellow flower spikes which, when dried, can be used in anti-inflammatory, anti-bacterial infusions. Used internally to treat sore throats, catarrh, diarrhoea, cystitis and urinary infections. Forms the basis of lotions used to treat skin wounds and stem external bleeding.

Allium sativum,
GARLIC
This versatile herb has many medicinal properties and can be taken orally in a variety of forms. It helps to lower blood pressure and reduce blood cholesterol, and is thought to inhibit blood clotting which leads to circulatory diseases. Garlic is also used as a decongestant, and has strong antiseptic properties.

Aloe vera,
ALOE VERA
The fleshy, spiny-toothed leaves of this famous plant ooze a thick gel which is used in a whole host of health and beauty treatments. Aloe vera contains various anti-inflammatory agents, minerals, anti-oxidant vitamins C, E, B12 and beta carotene. The gel from the leaves is applied to burns, bites, bruises and skin irritations.

Althaea officinalis,
MARSHMALLOW
Hardy perennial with pale pink flowers. Flowers and roots are famed for soothing, sweet mucilage, and as lozenges relieve inflamed gums, mouth and gastric ulcers, and bronchial infections. Used externally, the flowers help to soothe inflamed skin. The modern confectionery of the same name no longer contains the herb.

Anemone pulsatilla,
PASQUE FLOWER
A hardy perennial with bell-shaped purplish-blue flowers, followed by silky seedheads. Pasque is used for treating menstrual cramps, PMS, and in remedies for male reproductive problems. The flowers are usually prescribed in homeopathic rather than fresh form, as the plant can be toxic. **Caution:** Avoid usage during pregnancy.

 Anethum graveolens,
DILL
An aromatic annual with a soft, feathery texture. Dill is a cooling, soothing herb which, taken orally, aids digestion and constipation, and is also used to treat inflammation. Poultices made from the leaves soothe boils and ease swellings and joint pains. The seeds are chewed to cure bad breath.

 Arnica montana,
ARNICA
An alpine perennial with cheerful, yellow, daisy-like flowers. Used internally to relieve shock and pain, and to prevent colds, but should only be taken in prescribed, homeopathic doses as can be toxic in excess. Arnica is also used externally as part of a soothing lotion for bruises and sprains.

 Artemisia absinthium,
WORMWOOD
Perennial shrub with hairy stems and aromatic, downy, grey-green leaves. To taste, wormwood is extremely bitter (*absinthium* means "without sweetness"). It is a strong tonic for the digestive system but can be toxic if used in excess. It is useful for curing anaemia, easing wind and during periods of recuperation.

 Borago officinalis,
BORAGE
Hairy annual plant with bristly leaves and mauve, star-shaped flowers. As a herbal infusion it can be applied to inflamed skin, and flowers produce a safe, essential oil used to treat hormonal problems and PMS. The flowers can be taken as tea to dispel depression and nervous anxiety.

Calamintha nepeta,
CALAMINT
A bushy perennial mint with tubular, pink-mauve flowers. Leaves and flower tops are used as a stimulating tea or as a tonic or infusion for settling wind and indigestion. **Caution:** Avoid usage during pregnancy.

Calendula officinalis,
MARIGOLD
The marigold, or pot marigold, is a low-growing annual with cheerful orange-yellow petals. Herb is antiseptic, anti-inflammatory, anti-bacterial and anti-fungal. Added to soothing ointments for burns, eczema, sunburn, stings and bites. Has many benefits for the skin: use in an infusion to refresh tired skin, or add to hand and face cream to nourish and protect.

Carthamus tinctorius,
SAFFLOWER
Hardy annual with shaggy, thistle-like, red-yellow flowerheads and long ovate leaves. A tea, infused from fresh or dried flowers, induces perspiration, helping to reduce fevers, and is mildy laxative. Infusions can also be applied externally to treat bruises, skin irritations, inflammation and measles. **Caution:** Avoid usage during pregnancy.

Centaurea cyanus,
CORNFLOWER
Tall annual, with bright blue shaggy flowerheads. The flowers were used traditionally to make eyewashes for tired or strained eyes, but are more commonly prized today for their aromatic properties. The petals produce a bitter tonic, and the mildly laxative seeds help to relieve constipation in children.

Chamaemelum nobile,
CHAMOMILE
Evergreen perennial with feathery leaves and white daisy-like flowers. This antiseptic and anti-inflammatory plant is soothing when used as an infusion or essential oil. The famous tea alleviates nausea, indigestion and promotes sleep. As a steam inhalation, it eases asthma, sinusitis or catarrh.

Citrus aurantium,
BITTER ORANGE
This evergreen tree with shiny, ovate leaves produces a fragrant white blossom and bitter orange fruits. Essential oil can be made from all three components: neroli from the flowers, oil of petitgrain from the leaves and twigs, and oil of orange from the rind. Oils are rich in vitamins A, B and C, and have a calming effect. **Caution:** None of the essential oils given above should be taken internally.

Cnicus benedictus,
HOLY THISTLE
Annual with red, hairy stems, spiny leaves and yellow flowers. Leaves and tops are used for their antiseptic, antibiotic qualities, but are very bitter. Infusion or tincture is an effective tonic, and can help to stimulate the appetite. Holy thistle was traditionally used for fevers and settling stomach.

Crataegus laevigata,
HAWTHORN
Common deciduous shrub/small tree, with thorny branches. Produces white, scented flowers and red, globe-shaped fruits, known as haws. Bioflavonoid content makes it a valuable, slow-working "food for the heart". It lowers blood pressure and eases hypertension.

Crocus sativus,
SAFFRON CROCUS
A perennial crocus which produces lilac flowers with three red styles. The styles are dried to make saffron, which is known to have digestive properties, improve circulation and reduce high blood pressure. It is used widely in cooking and is a rich source of vitamin B2.

Echinacea purpurea
CONEFLOWER
Hardy perennial with large pinkish-purple, daisy-like flowers. The dried roots are made into capsules and powders to treat the common cold. Recent research has shown echinadea to have a beneficial effect on the immune system. Taken as a tea, it helps kidney infections, or is used as a compress for boils and abscesses.

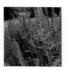

Echium vulgare,
VIPER'S BUGLOSS
A bushy and bristly biennial with prickly leaves and violet-blue flowers. In medieval times it was held that, because it resembled a snake's skin and tongue, it must be an antidote to adder bite or other poisons. Today, it is used for its skin-healing abilities. **Caution:** May cause stomach upset if ingested, and irritate the skin upon first contact. To be used by qualified herbalists only.

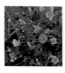

Eschscholzia californica,
CALIFORNIA POPPY
Annual or perennial poppy with bright orange, yellow or pink flowers. A sedative plant that relieves pain and is taken internally as an infusion, for anxiety, nervous tension and insomnia. Good for children, for bedwetting or sleeping problems.

Eupatorium cannabinum,
HEMP AGRIMONY
A hard and woody perennial with red stem and pinkish-white flowers (a local name was "raspberries and cream"). Used as a diuretic and as a tonic and for flu-like illnesses. Its alkaloid content means that caution should be exercised in usage. Applied externally to ulcers and sores.

Euphrasia officinalis,
EYEBRIGHT
An annual, semi-parasitic herb which grows on grasses and has white flowers double-lipped with yellow throats. Infusion used externally as a bath for sore or itchy eyes, skin irritations; internally it helps to relieve hayfever, allergic rhinitis, catarrh and sinusitis.

Filipendula ulmaria,
MEADOWSWEET
This perennial of damp meadows has sweet-smelling creamy flowers and was traditionally used to make aspirin. Both leaves and flowers are now used as an infusion for excess acid, gastric ulcers, rheumatism, arthritis and urinary infections. Safe remedy for children with upset stomachs.

Galega officinalis,
GOAT'S RUE
A bushy perennial with mauve, white or bicoloured flowers resembling those of a sweetpea. Has sedative properties, and infusions are taken to relieve irritability and insomnia. A diuretic, it can improve liver function and has a tonic effect on the system.

Galium odoratum or *Asperula odorata,*
SWEET WOODRUFF
Spreading perennial with spear-shaped leaves and small, white star-shaped flowers. Used as infusion for soothing nerves and insomnia, as a diuretic to improve liver function, and for varicose veins. **Caution:** Avoid usage during pregnancy.

Geranium maculatum,
CRANESBILL
Hardy perennial with round, purplish-pink flowers, native to North America. Whole plant dried for infusions, powders and tinctures; used as astringent to control bleeding and discharges, for diarrhoea and haemorrhoids. Used externally for wounds and as gargle for sore throats and mouth ulcers.

Geum urbanum,
WOOD AVENS
A hardy perennial with small, five-petalled yellow flowers. Whole plant is used: the flowers in infusions, the roots in decoctions. Treats digestive upsets, sore gums and mouth inflammations; can also be used externally to remedy haemorrhoids. The old name, herb bennet, recalls "benedict" (blessed) and the belief that it repelled evil spirits.

Glycyrrhiza glabra,
LICORICE
A plant with ovate leaves and long seed pods, licorice is famed for its use in confectionery. The root has more active medicinal properties, and as an anti-inflammatory agent is used to soothe stomach disorders, sore throats and respiratory infections. **Caution:** Seek advice before using as can raise blood pressure. Avoid usage during pregnancy.

Helianthus annuus,
SUNFLOWER
Tall, impressive and showy annual with large yellow flowerheads and brown disc florets at the centre. The whole plant is used for extracts and tinctures; the seeds are used in the production of sunflower oil. This is an excellent source of vitamin E (an anti-oxidant) and polyunsaturates, which maintain cell membranes and lower blood cholesterol.

Hypericum perforatum,
ST JOHN'S WORT
The yellow flowering tops of this plant are used fresh or dried in infusions, creams and oils. Has antiseptic and anti-inflammatory properties and can be applied to ease burns and muscular pain, including sciatica. Although originally prescribed as an anti-depressant, research now suggests that St John's wort may interact adversely with many other prescribed medicines. **Caution:** Should never be taken internally without first consulting a qualified medical practitioner.

Hyssopus officinalis,
HYSSOP
Semi-evergreen with flowers in blue-pink spikes. Leaves and flowers used in infusions, as an expectorant, for promoting sweating and as an anti-catarrhal and anti-bacterial remedy. Its essential oil is restricted in some countries.

Jasminum officinale,
JASMINE
Evergreen rambler, with sweet-scented white flowers used in calming infusions. The essential oil is used externally on dry skin and in the bath or massage oil. **Caution:** Oil should not be taken internally.

Lavandula angustifolia,
LAVENDER
Cultivated for so long that it now has numerous hybrids, common lavender was the first aromatherapy oil and remains an excellent first aid remedy for skin problems, headaches and nervous digestion. Taken in tea, it relieves headaches and promotes sleep.

Leonurus cardiaca,
MOTHERWORT
A pungent perennial with mauve-pink, double-lipped flowering tops, used in infusions and tinctures. Mildly sedative, with a calming effect on the heart and on palpitations. **Caution:** Avoid usage during pregnancy.

Lilium candidum,
MADONNA LILY
This perennial has pure white, fragrant, trumpet-shaped flowers. The juice from the roots and flowers is used externally in ointments to treat burns, and skin inflammations and disorders.

Lonicera periclymenum,
HONEYSUCKLE
Hardy climber with fragrant, creamy white or yellow flowers, followed by poisonous red berries in Autumn. The leaves were traditionally favoured as an expectorant, the bark as a diuretic and the flowers for asthma. These days its chief use is as a Bach remedy for nostalgia.

Lycopus europaeus,
GIPSYWEED
A perennial mint-like herb which lacks aroma. Astringent and sedative, gipsyweed was once used to treat haemorrhaging, palpitations and menstrual problems; still thought to have sedative properties. Its black dye, said to be used by gypsies to darken their skin, gave this plant its common name.

Lythrum salicaria,
PURPLE LOOSESTRIFE
A perennial with erect stems and crimson-purple flowers. Continues to be recommended by modern herbalists for relief of diarrhoea, dysentery, haemorhaging and excessive menstrual flow.

Marrubium vulgare,
HOREHOUND
Hardy, tall perennial with small white flowers, and a common weed. Usage is controlled by law in some countries. The stems are used as a bitter infusion for non-productive coughs, colds and chest infections.

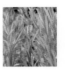

Melaleuca alternifolia,
TEA-TREE
Evergreen with thin, pointed and leathery leaves, and bottle-brush shaped flowers. An antiseptic, anti-bacterial and antifungal, the oil is diluted in carrier oil and used externally to treat burns, stings, insect bites and acne. Undiluted, it is said to be effective against dermatological conditions such as warts and verrcuas.

Melilotus officinalis,
MELILOT
An erect, straggly biennial with yellow, honey-scented flowers. Dried flowering stems are used in infusions or tinctures, as a sedative and anti-inflammatory agent, to treat sleeplessness, tension headaches, flatulence and menopause. **Caution:** If improperly dried, the plant is toxic. Consult a qualified practitioner before use.

Melissa officinalis,
LEMON BALM
The rough-textured green leaves of this busy perennial release a fresh lemony scent when crushed. Infusions of the fresh leaves are sedative and soothing, good for treating headaches, indigestion, nervous tension, anxiety and depression. Externally, it can be used in creams to soothe the skin or as an insect repellent.

Mentha,
MINT
There are many varieties of mint and each has its own properties. Peppermint is taken as a tea for colds, and to aid digestion. The essential oil has decongestant properties and can be used as an inhalant to relieve colds, chest infections, catarrh and asthma.

Monarda didyma,
BERGAMOT
An aromatic hardy perennial with red or mauve flowers. A native of North America, the leaves were made into Oswego tea by early settlers. Bergamot essential oil, extracted from the bergamot orange, *Citrus bergamia*, is still used to flavour Earl Grey tea. The leaves and flowers aid digestion.

Nepeta cataria,
CATMINT
A hardy perennial mint with coarse leaves and whitish-mauve flowers, irresistible to cats. An anti-inflammatory and mild sedative, leaves, flowers and stems make an infusion for feverish colds; used externally for cuts and bruises. Mild enough for children.

Ocimum basilicum,
BASIL
This aromatic annual has soft, ovate, bright-green leaves. Basil has soothing, antiseptic properties and leaves are best used fresh. They can be rubbed on to insect bites, used in steam inhalations, or made into cough syrups with a little honey. Basil produces a safe essential oil which is used in massage, and to treat anxiety.

Oenothera biennis,
EVENING PRIMROSE
Not related to the primrose, this plant is so named because its bright yellow flowers open in the evening. The seeds are pressed to produce an oil which is used for boosting the immune system and hormones. It is taken internally for PMS, menopause and allergies, and externally for skin tone.

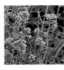

Origanum majorana,
SWEET MARJORAM
Half-hardy aromatic perennial with small lilac pink clusters of flowers. A warming, relaxing, antiseptic herb, it is taken internally as an infusion to treat nervous tension, headaches, insomnia, bronchial complaints, digestive problems and painful periods. The essential oil is diluted and applied to stiff muscles, and joints.

Passiflora incarnata,
PASSION FLOWER
A hardy, tropical perennial climber, with a woody stem and creamy-white, or lavender-blue, intricate flowers. The whole plant is used in herbal medicine. Leaves and flowers are dried for use in infusions, tinctures and tablets. A gentle sedative, it is useful as a mild tranquillizer to treat nervous conditions and insomnia.

Pelargonium graveolens,
GERANIUM

A bushy aromatic perennial with pink flowers, also known as a rose geranium, this African flower is now a universal house plant. Contains a volatile oil used in perfumery, and dried leaves go into various scents and aromatics. Astringent and anti-depressant, it is good in teas for tension and exhaustion.

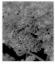

Petroselinum crispum,
PARSLEY

This well-known frost-hardy perennial grows on a short taproot and produces three-pinnate leaves. Parsley is rich in Vitamins A and E, and acts as an antioxidant. Parsley tea is sometimes used to treat coughs and jaundice, but it should not be used in excess as can be toxic.

Primula veris,
COWSLIP

A spring perennial bearing clusters of tubular yellow flowers. Becoming rare in the wild, but flowers and roots are used traditionally as part of a sedative infusion for children and as expectorant. Cowslip aids insomnia, chronic respiratory tract infections and also rheumatism. **Caution:** Avoid usage during pregnancy, or if taking aspirin.

Primula vulgaris,
PRIMROSE

A perennial with clusters of saucer-shaped, pale yellow flowers in early spring, primrose has similar healing properties to cowslip. Flowers (cultivated only, as wild form is rare and protected) are used as an infusion for easing anxiety, insomnia and respiratory tract problems.

Prunella vulgaris,
SELFHEAL

This aromatic herb has tall, violet, two-lipped florets which are dried for use in infusions, tinctures and ointments. Selfheal's common name reflects its traditional usage as a wound herb, to stop bleeding, for bites, bruises, sore throats and inflamed gums. It is still used to soothe burns, skin inflammations and sore gums.

Rosa, ROSE

A deciduous bush of multiple types, roses have been used medicinally since antiquity as water, ointment, syrup, vinegar, conserve and candies. Their main therapeutic use is now in aromatherapy: the essential oil ("attar of roses") is used to relieve nervous depression and anxiety. Mildly sedative, rose essences are also used to treat sensitive skin and sore eyes. Rosehips, a rich source of Vitamin C, are used in cooking to make vinegars, syrups, wine and preserves. They can also be added to teas as a useful immunity booster.

Rosmarinus officinalis, ROSEMARY

This evergreen shrub, with aromatic, needle-like leaves and small pale blue flowers, is prized for its culinary, medicinal, aromatic and cosmetic uses. The leaves and flowers form the basis of infusions for colds, flu and headaches; tinctures for depression and nervous tension; essential oil for massages to relieve rheumatic, muscular pain;

in therapeutic baths to ease fatigue; and in hair products to reduce dandruff. **Caution:** Avoid usage during pregnancy.

Salvia, SAGE

An evergreen, highly aromatic shrub, sage has downy, rough-textured leaves which are both antiseptic and anti-bacterial. Use in a gargle or mouthwash for bad breath, or to treat sore throats, gums and mouth ulcers, and ease laryngitis and tonsillitis. Sage tea is a tonic that aids indigestion and menopausal problems. Applied externally as a compress, sage can help to treat wounds.

Sambucus nigra, ELDER

This small, deciduous tree produces creamy white flowers and clusters of black fruits. Infusions of the flowers are taken for colds, sinusitis, and hayfever; berries make cough syrups. The flowers can be used for home-made skin toners, and the leaves are used in insecticides. **Caution:** Leaves are toxic and should not be taken interally.

Solidago virgaurea,
GOLDEN ROD
This hardy perennial with branched stems and profuse spikes of yellow flowers has antioxidant, diuretic and astringent properties. The leaves and flowers are used to make lotions, ointments and poultices to treat wounds, bites and rashes. Internally, infusions help to ease urinary problems.

Stachys officinalis,
BETONY
A hardy perennial, with magenta-pink flowers. Both leaves and flowers were used historically in infusions, ointments and lotions to ease headaches. Its application today extends to remedies for anxiety and PMS. Externally, betony is good for cuts and bruises. **Caution:** Avoid usage in pregnancy and note that leaves are toxic if used in excess.

Symphytum officinale,
COMFREY
This wild, furry-leaved plant has blue or white flowers, and was historically used as a healing agent for fractures. Today, comfrey leaves are still used externally, as poultices, compresses and ointments to be applied to bruises, varicose veins, inflamed muscles and tendons.

Syzgium aromaticum,
CLOVE
A tropical evergreen which is named after the French word "clou", meaning nail, which the green buds (cloves) resemble. A stimulant, antiseptic and digestive remedy, it relieves nausea and controls vomiting. Oil of cloves is a dental analgesic, and sucking a clove can help to alleviate toothache.

Tanacetum parthenium,
FEVERFEW
With its green foliage and daisy-like flowers, this busy perennial is particularly successful in treating migraine – two or three leaves should be taken orally, with honey or another sweetener as they are very bitter. It is also taken in tablet form to ease rheumatism. **Caution:** Prolonged consumption may cause mouth ulcers.

Taraxacum officinale,
DANDELION
Perennial flowers with well-recognized yellow rosettes followed by fluffy seed heads in Autumn. Although dandelions are often thought of as growing in the wild, they are also cultivated for use in moist, fertile soil and the leaves and flowers have many medicinal properties, both fresh and dried. An effective diuretic, dandelion is taken internally for urinary infections and helps to treat diseases of the gall bladder and liver. It is also beneficial for rheumatic complaints and gout, and – while in itself a rich source of vitamins A and C, and of metals such as magnesium and iron – is said to promote appetite.

Tilia cordata,
LIME
This hardy, deciduous tree has heartshaped leaves and fluffy pale yellow flowers. Newly opened flowers are harvested and dried for linden teas, which are soothing and sweat-inducing. Mix with honey and lemon to treat colds, catarrh, fevers, anxiety and palpitations. Lime is also used to help combat high blood pressure.

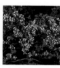

Thymus vulgaris,
THYME
There are many varieties of thyme, but *Thymus vulgaris*, with its white flowerheads, is the only one with acknowledged medicinal uses. As a mouthwash, it helps to combat mouth ulcers, and as a tea it soothes coughs, colds and sore throats. It also produces an essential oil that eases tense muscles, and a sachet of the dried leaves is used as an aid to sleep.

Trifolium pratense,
RED CLOVER
This rather short-lived perennial has pink, circular flowerheads which are used as part of an infusion of blossoms to treat coughs and eczema. Externally, the flowers are applied to skin complaints such as ulcers, burns and sores. Red clover was formerly used for cataracts as its white leaf halo suggested this "signature". Red clover is still used to help control blood sugar.

Tropaeolum majus,
NASTURTIUM
A half-hardy annual with circular leaves and yellow-orange single flowers. Native to Peru, it is widely used in Andean herbal medicine as a disinfectant and expectorant. The leaves, flowers and seeds are all edible, often used fresh to flavour salads and vinegars, and are high in vitamin C content. The seeds are anti-bacterial and can be used in infusions to clear urinary infections and catarrh.

Tussilago farfara,
COLTSFOOT
A small creeping perennial with cheering yellow blossoms which emerge in spring. The leaves or flowers of this herb contain a substance known as mucilage, which is used to produce soothing tonics for mucous membranes. Flavoursome and popular in salads, it is still used in infusions for coughs and can be applied externally, either as a paste of fresh leaves mixed with honey, or as a compress, to treat sores, ulcers and bites **Caution:** Avoid usage during pregnancy.

Urtica dioica,
STINGING NETTLE
A tough, spreading perennial covered in stinging hairs, the common nettle may be known as a bothersome weed, but for centuries it has been viewed as a nutritious and medicinal herb. Its high vitamin C content promotes the absorption of iron, which makes it a suitable remedy for anaemia. It is also diuretic, helping to rid the body of uric acid, promotes circulatory health, and can be used in a compress against rheumatoid aches. Decoctions of roots and leaves are applied to the scalp to alleviate dandruff, and it is even said to help prevent baldness.

Valeriana officinalis,
VALERIAN
Not to be confused with its other herbal relative, the purely ornamental red valerian (*Centranthus ruber*), this perennial with toothed leaflets and white, sometimes pinkish, flowers has strong sedative properties and can be taken as a tea for insomnia, headaches and nervous tension.

Verbena officinalis,
VERVAIN

A hardy, rather straggly perennial with dull green, slightly hairy leaves and small, sparse, lilac flowers, vervain was traditionally thought of as a holy herb (*herba sacra*), as it was supposedly used to staunch Christ's wounds at the Crucifixion. While still believed to have hypnotic and aphrodisiac powers, it is medicinally linked with disorders of the stomach, kidneys, liver, and gall bladder. Externally, vervain can be used in compresses and lotions for skin complaints, and as a gargle for sore gums and mouth ulcers.

Vinca major,
GREATER PERIWINKLE

A trailing evergreen perennial with glossy dark-green leaves and five-petalled violet blue flowers. Both the leaves and flowering stems are processed to extract an alkaloid which helps to dilate the blood vessels and reduce blood pressure. **Caution:** All parts of the plant are poisonous, and self-treatment is not advised.

Viola odorata,
SWEET VIOLET

A low-growing hardy perennial with a tall, basal rosette of heartshaped leaves and drooping flowers that yield an aromatherapy essential oil. Other parts of the plant make a gentle infusion or syrup for coughs, colds and rheumatism.

Viola tricolor,
WILD PANSY

Annual or perennial, with violet, yellow and white triangular flowers. Also known as heartsease, in reference to its older use as a heart tonic. Today, wild pansy is used in infusions as an expectorant for coughs and colds, and externally to treat skin complaints.

Zingiber officinale,
GINGER

Used in China since earliest times, this reed-like perennial has dense cones bearing yellow-green flowers. It is a stimulant, expectorant and antiseptic, often used as a cold remedy to promote sweating, eliminate toxins and dispel catarrh.

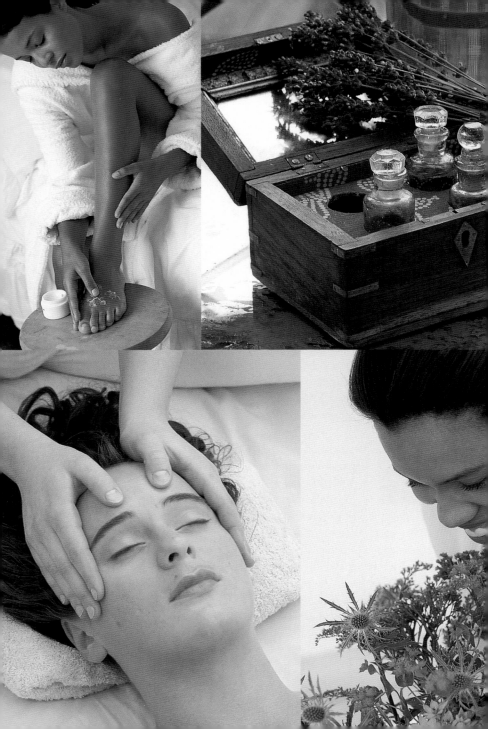

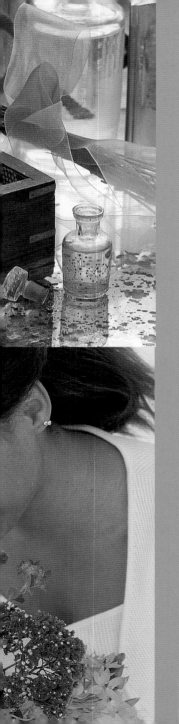

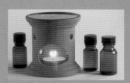

HEALING WITH
AROMA-
THERAPY

Since the dawn of human history, people have used scented products in religious ceremonies, bathing and massage, and for scenting the hair and body. In the 10th century, physicians learned how to distil essential oils from plants, and the practice of aromatherapy was born.

Essential oils can be extracted from a wide variety of plants, including citrus fruits, shrubs, vines, herbs and spices, and are used to relax, sedate, refresh or stimulate, according to need. In addition to affecting moods, however, these essential oils boast considerable healing powers and can soothe aches and ease skin conditions. It is not surprising, then, that so much use is made of aromatherapy in conventional medicine today.

Essential oils

Essential oils are natural, volatile substances that evaporate readily, releasing their aroma into the air, as happens, for example, when someone brushes against an aromatic plant. The oils have many beneficial properties.

A widely used method of employing essential oils in the home is to fragrance the rooms by means of a vaporizer or oil burner. Although vaporizers come in many forms, they all work on the same principle. The reservoir is filled with water, to which are added a few drops of essential oil. The reservoir is then heated, which causes the oil and water to evaporate. The heat must be fairly low to allow slow evaporation of the oil and a longer-lasting scent.

Adding a few drops of essential oil to a bowl of hot water is an effective way of adding scent to a room, especially in a dry atmosphere.

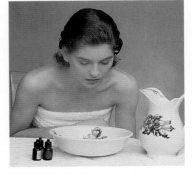

▲ ADD ESSENTIAL OILS TO HOT WATER FOR A BENEFICIAL STEAM INHALATION.

Choose an attractive bowl and place it out of reach of children. Use an oil that you really like, as its fragrance will linger for some time. You can also use the bowl of scented water for an uplifting or calming steam inhalation. Essential oils can be used to make a luxurious addition to the bath, whether they are chosen to aid recovery from an illness, to lift the spirits, or to promote relaxation after a stressful day.

▶ OIL BURNERS CAN MAKE ATTRACTIVE ROOM ORNAMENTS.

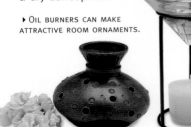

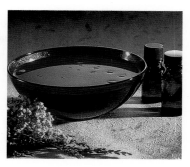

▲ A FEW DROPS OF ESSENTIAL OIL IN HOT WATER WILL PERFUME A ROOM.

The essential oils recommended for the bath affect the body as they are inhaled in the steam, but some also penetrate the skin pores that open in the warmth.

In order to add oils to the bath safely it is important to dilute them in vegetable oil, cream or full-fat (whole) milk. Add the blend to the bathwater, just before the bath has filled to the desired depth, pouring it slowly under the hot water tap so the oil disperses through the water.

▼ SLOWLY ADD DILUTED OIL TO BATHWATER.

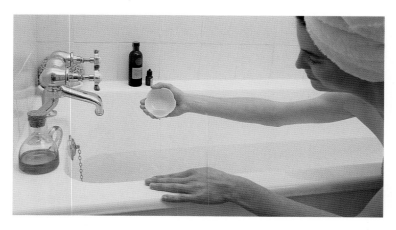

Mixing and storing essential oils

When essential oils are used for aromatherapy massage, different oils are combined to increase their therapeutic effect. Once you have mixed your oils, store and use them immediately, as they are perishable.

Aromatic essential oils may be used in a number of ways to maintain and restore health, and to improve our quality of life with their scents. Essential oils are concentrated substances and as such they need to be diluted for safety and optimum effect.

The ratio of essential oil to carrier oil varies, but, as a rule, ten drops of essential oil in 20ml/4tsp carrier oil is enough for a body massage. This gives a standard 2.5 per cent dilution, recommended for most uses.

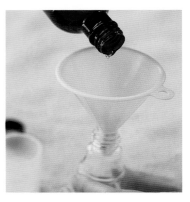

▲ USE A FUNNEL TO AVOID SPILLAGE.

Experiment with different types of vegetable oil to find the ideal blend for your massage style. Add a teaspoonful of another vegetable oil as well as the essential oils for an exotic and personal mixture.

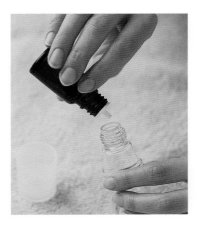

◀ BLEND OILS ONE DROP AT A TIME.

▶ STORE OILS IN DARK BOTTLES.

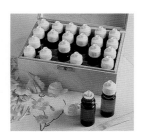

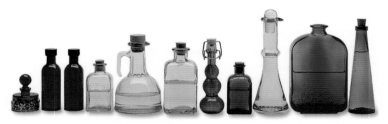

To blend essential oils for massage, first pour the vegetable oil into a blending bowl. Then add the essential oil a drop at a time and stir gently with a cocktail stick (toothpick) to blend. Test the fragrance before beginning, as it may need adjusting.

Essential oils are liable to deteriorate through the action of sunlight, so should be stored in a cool, dark place and away from direct heat. They should always be bought in dark-coloured glass

▲ STORE CARRIER OILS CAREFULLY TO ENSURE THEIR FRESHNESS.

bottles with a stopper that dispenses them a drop at a time. Only blend a small quantity of oils at a time to prevent the mixture deteriorating. Citrus oils tend to go off more quickly than other oils, so it is best to buy them in small amounts as you need them.

▼ USE AROMATHERAPY BLENDS IMMEDIATELY OR STORE IN SEALED BOTTLES AS ESSENTIAL OILS EVAPORATE QUICKLY.

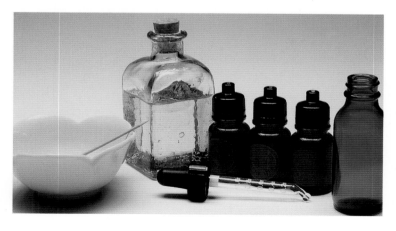

Citrus oils

Many citrus fruits yield essential oils, and they tend to have similar properties. In general they are refreshing, stimulating oils, good for the morning bath, leaving you feeling cleansed and alive.

ORANGES

The bitter, or Seville, orange is the source of three different oils, from the fruit, the blossom (also known as neroli) and the leaf (also called petitgrain). All have a mellow, warming and soothing effect, and are a good tonic and mood lifter, raising the libido.

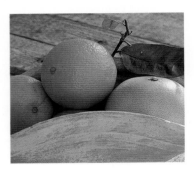

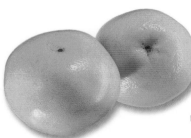

GRAPEFRUIT

This uplifting oil, taken from the fruit's fresh peel, helps to digest fatty foods, and combat cellulite and congested pores. It also soothes headaches and nervous exhaustion.

NEROLI

This oil is particularly effective for nervous tension, headaches, insomnia and other stress-related conditions. It can also be used to create a feeling of peace and is useful during times of anxiety, panic, hysteria or shock and fear. It can also help in the development of self-esteem and self-love.

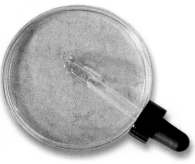

Limes

Oil of lime is good for stimulating a sluggish system and may be used when a tonic is needed, in massage or in the bath.

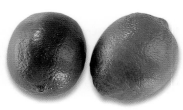

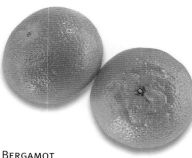

Mandarins

Refreshing and cleansing, this sweetly scented oil is especially good for skin problems such as acne. It also helps digestion, soothing heartburn and nausea.

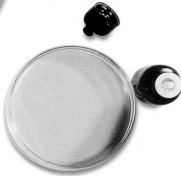

Bergamot

The peel of the ripe fruit yields an oil that is mild and gentle. It is the most effective antidepressant oil of all, best used at the start of the day. The oil can be used on a burner for lifting the atmosphere. Do not use on the skin in bright sunlight, as it can cause irritation.

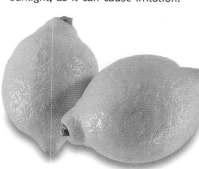

Lemons

Possibly the most cleansing and antiseptic of the citrus oils, lemon oil is useful for boosting the immune and respiratory systems, and for use in skin care. It can also refresh and clarify thoughts, preventing feelings of bitterness or anger about life's injustices.

Shrub and vine oils

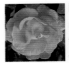 Essential oils can be extracted from many different parts of plants. Rose and jasmine oils are obtained from the flowers, the oil of black pepper comes from the fruit of a tropical vine, and geranium oil is taken from the plant's leaves.

JASMINE
One of the most wonderful aromas, jasmine has a relaxing, euphoric effect, and can lift the mood when there is debility, depression and general listlessness. Use in the bath or in massage oils.

BLACK PEPPER
The essential oil of black pepper is warming and comforting and can often add mysterious depth to a blend. It is particularly effective for treating muscular aches and pains, and relieving colds and fevers.

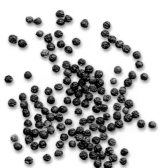

GERANIUM
Rose-scented geranium oil is obtained from the shrub's leaves. It has a refreshing antidepressant quality, which is good for nervous tension and exhaustion, and can combine a blend to make a more harmonious scent.

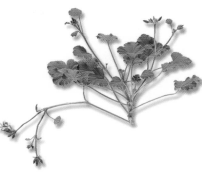

LAVENDER

Extracted from lavender flowers, this oil is the most versatile of all essential oils. It has been used for centuries to bring freshness and fragrance to the home, and as a remedy for stress-related ailments.

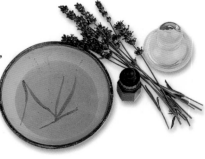

JUNIPER

Good for strengthening the spirits and purifying the atmosphere, this oil is obtained from juniper berries. Its most important use is as a detoxifier, but it is also effective for cystitis, cellulite, water retention, and absence of or painful menstrual periods.

ROSE

Probably the most famous of all oils, rose is good for sedating, calming and as an effective anti-inflammatory. Use in the bath or add to a base massage oil to soothe muscular and nervous tension.

ROSEMARY

This stimulating oil, taken from the plant's leaves, has been used for centuries to help relieve nervous exhaustion, tension headaches and migraines. It improves circulation to the brain, and is an excellent oil for mental fatigue and debility. It is also an effective remedy for fluid retention.

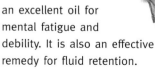

Herb and spice oils

The essential oils of many herbs and spices contain powerful healing properties, which should be enjoyed but also respected. Nature provides an abundance of therapeutic compounds to help restore health and vitality.

CLARY SAGE

This essential oil, taken from the leaves, gives a euphoric uplift to the brain; be careful how much you use, however, as it can leave you feeling very intoxicated! Its relaxing and antidepressant qualities have contributed to its reputation as an aphrodisiac.

PEPPERMINT

The plant's leaves are used to produce this oil which is a classic ingredient in inhalations for relieving catarrh. Peppermint's analgesic and antispasmodic effects make it very useful for rubbing onto the temples to ease tension headaches; ideally dilute a drop in a little base cream or oil before applying.

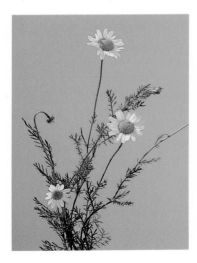

CHAMOMILE

The flowering parts of Roman and German chamomile are used to obtain essential oils with very similar properties. Chamomile oil is relaxing and antispasmodic, and helps to relieve tension headaches, nervous digestive problems and insomnia. It is also a gentle sedative oil for people who are highly strung and over-enthusiastic.

MARJORAM

Obtained from marjoram leaves, this oil has a calming and warming effect, and is good for both cold muscles and for cold and tense people who might also suffer from headaches, migraines or insomnia.

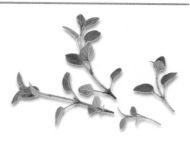

GINGER

Extracted from the ginger root, this oil is known for its warm and comforting nature. It is a balancing oil and counteracts ailments caused by dampness, being particularly effective for muscular aches and pains, catarrh and other symptoms of coughs and colds.

NUTMEG

With its warming, stimulating and euphoric effects, this oil, taken from the fruit of the nutmeg tree, aids poor circulation, muscular aches, sluggish digestion, loss of appetite and the early stages of a cold. It can also be comforting to those who feel emotionally isolated.

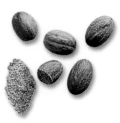

PALMAROSA

Taken from the leaves of this herbaceous plant, palmarosa is a gentle and comforting oil. It is particularly effective for acne, dermatitis, scars, sores and other skin inflammations, as well as weak digestion, headaches and nervous exhaustion.

Tree oils

Oils can be obtained from a variety of trees; with some, for example, cedarwood, the oil is extracted by steam distillation from the wood, whereas with others, such as ylang ylang, the oils come from the flowers.

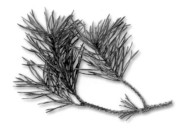

Pine

The pine oil used in aromatherapy generally comes from the Scots pine. It helps to clear the air passages when used as an inhalation, and is also good for relieving fatigue. Tired, aching muscles can be eased with massage using diluted pine oil.

Eucalyptus

Extracted from eucalyptus leaves, this is one of the finest oils for respiratory complaints, eucalyptus is found in most commercial inhalants. Well diluted in a base vegetable oil, eucalyptus can be applied to the forehead to help relieve a hot, tense headache linked with tiredness.

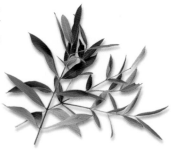

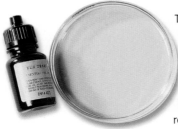

Tea tree

Vigorous and revitalizing, tea tree oil is effective in fighting infectious organisms. It is also a powerful immune stimulant, increasing the body's ability to respond to these organisms.

SANDALWOOD

Probably the oldest perfume in history, sandalwood has been used for 4,000 years. It has a heavy scent, and often appeals to men as much as to women. It has a relaxing, antidepressant effect on the nervous system, and where depression causes sexual problems, sandalwood can be used as a genuine aphrodisiac.

CEDARWOOD

Thought to be one of the earliest known essential oils, cedarwood oil is effective for long-standing complaints rather than acute ones, such as acne, dandruff, arthritis, rheumatism, bronchitis and chest infections. This uplifting oil is useful for treating lack of confidence or fearfulness, and can help to eliminate mental stagnation. Its relaxing and soothing properties can be a good aid to meditation. Cedarwood is also an aphrodisiac.

CYPRESS

With a rich scent similar to the scent of pine needles, cypress oil is useful for treating conditions that cause excess fluids, such as diarrhoea, water retention and watery colds. The oil, extracted from the tree's cones, can be uplifting in cases of sadness or self-pity, and can help to soothe anger.

YLANG YLANG

The flowers of this tropical tree, native to Indonesia, produce an intensely sweet essential oil that has a sedative yet antidepressant action. It is good for many symptoms of excessive tension, such as insomnia, panic attacks, anxiety and depression.

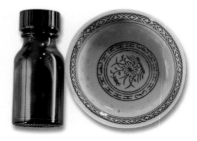

Aromatherapy massage

Massage is a wonderful way to use essential oils, suitably diluted in a good base oil, for your partner or family. Use soft, thick towels to cover areas of the body you are not massaging, and make sure that the room is warm.

Anyone will benefit from regular massage as it eases tense muscles and also helps us feel warm and relaxed. Although quite different and inevitably limited, self-massage is also an excellent way to help yourself relax and can help clear tension headaches and ease a stiff neck and shoulders.

Ideally, massage should be carried out just before a bath or when you can lie down in a warm place. Suitable base oils for massage include sweet almond oil (probably the most versatile and useful), grapeseed, safflower, soya (a bit thicker and stickier), coconut and even sunflower. For very dry skins, a small amount of jojoba, avocado or wheatgerm oils (except in cases of wheat allergy) may be added. Essential

▾ THE NURTURING TOUCH OF MASSAGE IS ENHANCED BY THE AROMA OF ESSENTIAL OILS.

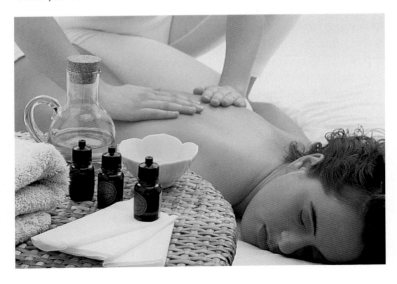

oils may be blended at a dilution of 1 per cent, or one drop per 5ml/1tsp base oil; this may sometimes by increased to 2 per cent, but take care that no skin reactions occur with any oil.

If someone has sensitive skin or suffers from allergies, try massaging with one drop of essential oil per 20ml/4tsp base oil to test for any reaction. Seek medical advice before massaging a pregnant woman.

Prepare for massage by playing some soft music, lowering the lights or lighting candles and ensure your partner is lying comfortably on the floor with a clean towel spread beneath them.

The oil for the massage, blended with essential oil, should be poured into a small, clean bowl from where you can take more oil from time to time without disturbing the rhythm of the massage. It is always a good idea to stand the bowl of oil on a towel in order to protect the underlying surface from spills.

MIXING OILS FOR MASSAGE

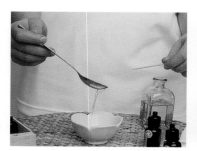

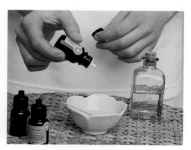

1 Pour about 10ml/2tsp of your chosen vegetable oil into a blending bowl.

2 Add the essential oil, one drop at a time. Mix with a clean dry cocktail stick or toothpick.

Aromatherapy blends

A selection of blends of essential oils for everyday circumstances is given below. These few suggestions are to be used as a guide. If you already have a favourite blend, there is no reason why you should not use it.

Choose up to four essential oils to make an appropriate blend. Mix with a carrier or base oil.

▸ THE VARIETY OF CARRIER OILS INCLUDES ALMOND, SUNFLOWER, SESAME AND JOJOBA.

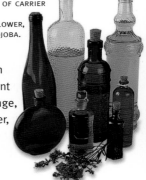

TO AID RELAXATION

For a relaxing massage choose three or four oils from the following list: bergamot, clary sage, lavender, sandalwood and German chamomile. Inlcude one of the citrus oils, to add an uplifting note to the blend.

REMEDY FOR OVER-INDULGENCE

A gentle massage using three or four of any of the following oils may help to restore balance following an over-indulgent period: orange, black pepper, geranium, juniper and ginger.

▾ CAREFULLY MEASURE OUT THE CORRECT QUANTITY OF BASE OIL.

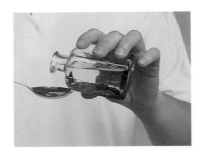

TO DISPEL GLOOM

Try making a blend of three or four of the following essential oils: black pepper, cypress, eucalyptus, ginger, grapefruit, jasmine, juniper, lemon, nutmeg, peppermint, rosemary and tea tree.

FOR STIFF MUSCLES

Everyone suffers from minor muscular aches and pains from time to time. Warming essential oils are the most helpful for stiff muscles. You can choose from any of the following: black pepper, ginger, clary sage, eucalyptus,

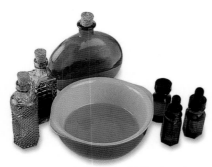

◄ MIX YOUR BLEND OF ESSENTIAL OILS WITH A CARRIER, OR BASE, OIL IN A SMALL BOWL READY FOR USE.

peppermint, grapefruit, jasmine, juniper, lavender, lemon, orange, marjoram and nutmeg.

AN APHRODISIAC BLEND

Tension, anxiety, worry, depression – all these can affect your sexual energy. This can result in a downward spiral of anxiety about sex, and cause reduced enjoyment. Try to take time out of your hectic life to spend time together with your partner and have fun: add to your sensual pleasure with an intimate massage session, using one of these blends to release tensions and allow your natural sexual energy to respond.

Use a blend that appeals to you both – either five drops rose and five drops sandalwood or four drops jasmine and four drops ylang ylang and include in a massage oil. Use gentle, stroking movements all over the back, buttocks, legs and front.

SENSUAL MASSAGE

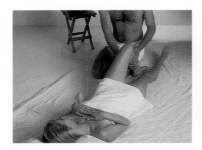

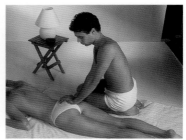

1 Use rose and sandalwood, or jasmine and ylang ylang oil to massage gently all over the body.

2 Apply a firmer pressure when massaging large muscles such as the buttocks.

Facial massage

A face massage dissolves anxiety and stress, eases away headaches, and enhances relaxation. Let your strokes be firm but gentle, following the natural symmetry of the bone structure and facial features.

Receiving a face massage is a wonderful way to finish a body massage, or combined with the chest, neck and head strokes, it can be a deeply satisfying and effective session in its own right.

When giving your partner a face massage, you should try to focus your total attention on to your hands and fingers so that each touch is feather like and made with great sensitivity.

GENTLE STROKES

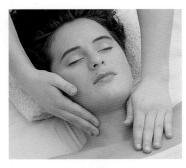

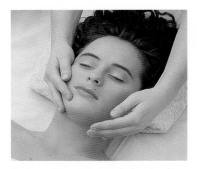

1 Add a very small amount of oil to your hands to ensure a smooth glide over the skin. Then softly stroke your hands, one following the other, up over the chest, neck and sides of the face, moulding them to the natural contours of the face.

2 A gentle caress of the jawline will be comforting to your partner. With slightly cupped hands, stroke one hand after the other in alternating movements along both sides of the face. Move from the point of the chin round towards the ears.

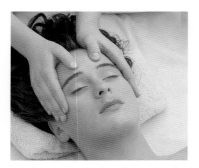

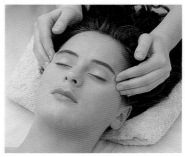

1 Place your thumbs on the forehead, while your hands cradle the face. Draw the thumbs towards the side, finishing with a sweep around the temples.

2 Keeping your hands relaxed and cupped, use your fingertips to stroke the temples very softly several times in a clockwise circular movement.

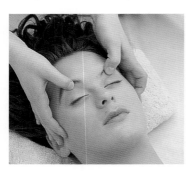

TIP
Choose the blend of oils for the massage according to your partner's needs: if they are tense and over-tired, a relaxing blend of lavender, chamomile and clary sage oils could be helpful; if they need to be revitalized, geranium and bergamot oils will give them an energizing boost.

3 The hollows under the ridge of the brow are sinus passages. Gentle pressure on these points can help to release tension headaches. Press sensitively up under the ridge, on one spot at a time, with your thumb pads.

Continue to hold the pressure under the ridge for a count of five before releasing it slowly. Move from the inner to the outer edge of the eyebrows.

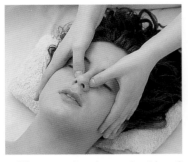

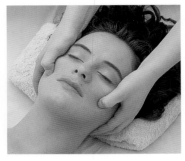

1 Slip your thumbs each side of the bridge of the nose, while wrapping your hands against the sides of the cheeks. Slide both thumbs down each side of the nose to the edge of the nostrils.

2 Without breaking the flow of motion, draw your thumb pads out under the cheekbones, indenting them slightly up under the ridge of the bone.

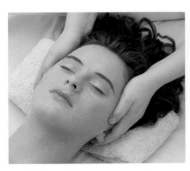

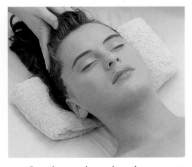

3 Soften the pressure in your thumbs as they reach the sides of the face, and begin to pull both hands soothingly up towards the top of the head.

4 Continue by drawing your hands and fingers out through the head and hair until they pull away from the body. Bring your hands back to the first position of the stroke. Repeat twice.

EASING THE CHEEKS AND JAW

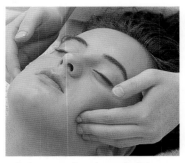

1 Relax your hands and sink your fingertips into the cheek muscles. Rotate them, counter-clockwise, several times on one area before moving to the next fleshy area.

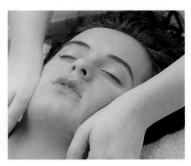

2 Gently press and rotate the heels of your hands in continuous but alternate movements on the cheeks to increase suppleness and to loosen the muscles surrounding the mouth.

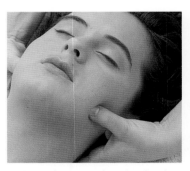

3 To reduce tension in the jaw muscles, slip your fingers behind the neck, and sink your thumbs into the muscle before rotating them on one spot at a time.

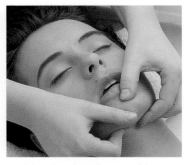

4 Grip the jaw bone with your fingers and use your thumbs to stroke over the chin in small circles, applying more pressure on the down and outward slide.

Self-massage

Give yourself a real treat with these simple self-massage techniques. Choose an appropriate blend of essential oils, and add at 1 per cent dilution to a base oil such as sweet almond. Oil your hands before spreading it on to your skin.

Self-massage is an excellent way to help yourself relax and can help clear tension headaches and ease a stiff neck and shoulders. There is an undoubted sensuality about massage, the feel of oil on the skin and the gradual easing of tension, so enjoy this opportunity to pamper yourself. The benefit is not only from the gentle application of massage oil but also from the time taken to care for yourself and your needs.

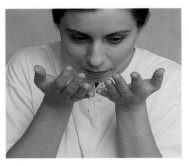

▲ DEPENDING ON THE OIL USED, THE AROMA OF AN ESSENTIAL OIL MASSAGE CAN HELP TO RELAX AND EASE TENSION OR UPLIFT YOUR MIND AND ENERGIZE YOUR BODY.

THE FACE

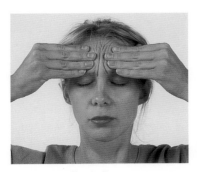

1 Use small circling movements with the fingers, over the forehead, temples and cheeks.

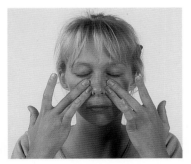

2 Work across the cheeks and along each side of the nose, then out to the jaw line.

THE HANDS

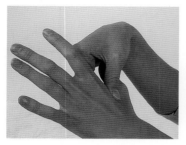

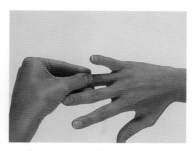

1 You can help to reduce any tension in your hands by firmly squeezing the fleshy area between each finger with the thumb and fingers of the other hand, rolling the flesh a little to give a kneading effect.

2 Squeeze and gently stretch each finger one after the other, working from the base of your finger out towards the tip. Now repeat this exercise on the other hand.

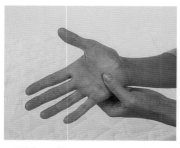

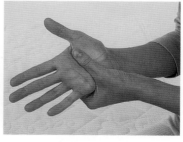

3 With a firm movement, knead the palm with the thumb of your other hand, making strong circular strokes. This squeezes and stretches taut, contracted muscles, and should be a fairly deep action.

4 Continue this kneading action as you work steadily across the palm of your hand, maintaining a firm pressure. Now repeat these movements on the other hand.

THE LEGS

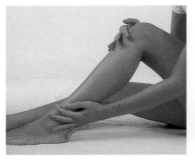 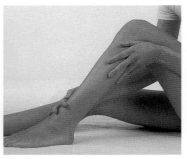

1 Sit with one leg bent, so that you can comfortably reach down as far as the ankle.

2 Sweep up the leg from ankle to knee, using alternate hands. This helps to move venous blood back towards the heart.

THE FEET

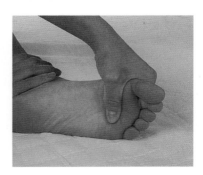

1 Sit so that you can comfortably reach a foot, and with quite a firm grip use small circular strokes all over the sole with your thumb. Pay special attention to the arch of the foot, stretching along the line of the arch with your thumb.

THE ARMS

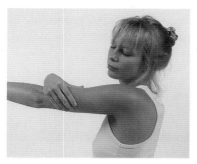

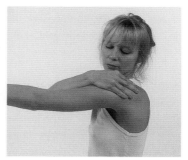

1 Grip your arm at the wrist and squeeze. Repeat this action up the length of the arm.

2 Continue up the arm to the shoulder. Switch arms and repeat the exercise.

THE SHOULDERS

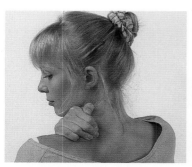

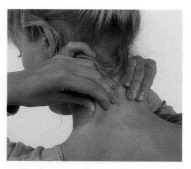

1 Firmly grip your shoulder and use a squeezing motion to loosen the tension, moving along the shoulder several times. Repeat on the other side.

2 Work up as far as the base of the skull, squeezing the neck muscles with your fingertips, and work your way down again.

Massage with a partner

One of the best ways to remove stress and tension from your partner is by massage. The effects of the following simple massage movements can be enhanced greatly by adding essential oils at 1 per cent dilution to the base oil.

When using essential oils in massage with a partner, you are sharing the therapeutic effect, so choose a blend that you both like.

Prepare the massage space beforehand so that it is warm and relaxing. Ensure that your partner is lying comfortably: use cushions or pillows for support if necessary, and cover them with towels, if needed, for warmth. Always warm the oil in your hands before applying it to the skin.

For a relaxing massage, begin with the back, move to the face, then finish with the arms and feet. This should ease headaches and tension and promote a feeling of deep and utter relaxation. Always use gentle strokes.

THE BACK

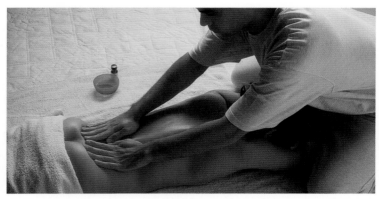

Place your hands on either side of the spine, on the line of muscles that run down the back. Move down the back using a slow gliding motion. Take your hands further out to the side and glide back up towards the shoulders, before repeating this stroke.

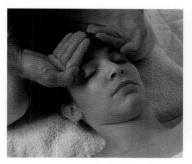

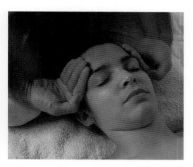

1 Smooth across the forehead with the back of your hands. Start the stroking motion at the centre of the forehead and move towards the temples.

2 These movements can often ease a headache, especially when it is still at an early stage, and are very calming.

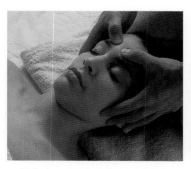

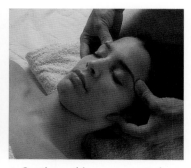

3 Using your thumbs or fingers, work steadily over the forehead in small circles, moving out over the temples to help to ease tight, tense muscles.

4 Continue this movement down the temples to the jaw line for an even greater relaxing effect. Use firm pressure, squeezing the skin with each circle.

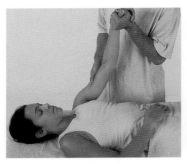

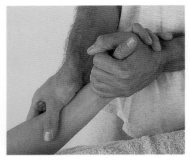

1 Support your partner's arm, raising it into the air and squeeze down the whole length of the arm with your thumb and fingers to encourage the blood and lymph to flow back towards the heart.

2 Let the upper arm rest on the floor, then work on the forearm with stroking movements from the wrist to the elbow – you may need to swap your hands to work around each side of the arm.

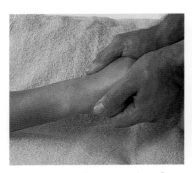

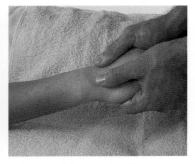

3 To help relieve tension from your partner's hands, hold one hand, palm down, in your hands and apply a steady stretching motion over the back of the hand.

4 Repeat this stretch a few times, with a firm but comfortable pressure on the hand. Repeat all these movements on the other arm and hand.

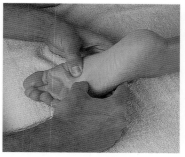

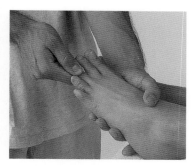

1 Use your thumbs to press firmly in small circles all over the sole. Keep the movements slow and deep, and finish with long lines running from the toes to the heel.

2 Hold one of the toes and give a squeeze and pulling action. Repeat for all the toes.

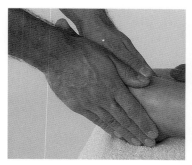

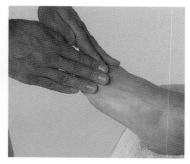

3 Smooth all the way up and down the upper side of the foot with both hands.

4 Extend the stroking from the ankle to the toes, then return to the centre; smooth back up the foot. Repeat on the other foot.

Baby massage

All babies thrive on being cuddled, touched, and massaged. Skin-to-skin contact is essential to the nurturing of infants, helping them to bond with their parents, and to develop emotional and physical health.

SOOTHING AND FEATHERING

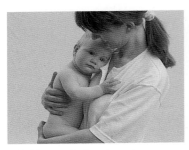

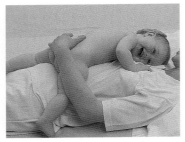

1 Hold your baby close to you, so they can feel the warmth of your body, the beat of your heart, and the rhythm of your breathing, enabling them to be comforted.

2 Babies love to lie against the softness of your body. Soothe them by placing one hand over the base of the spine, while gently stroking the head.

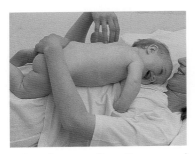

3 Running your fingertips up and down your baby's back will make them giggle as the feather-like touches brush their delicate skin.

OILS FOR BABIES AND YOUNGSTERS

Choose from the following essential oils:

Newborn infants: chamomile, geranium, lavender, mandarin and eucalyptus.

Infants 2–6 months old: as above plus neroli and peppermint.

Infants 6–12 months old: as above plus grapefruit, palmarosa and tea tree.

Flexing and wiggling

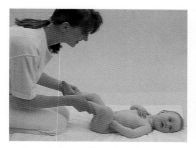

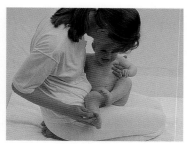

1 Your baby will enjoy this game of passive movements. Bend the knee towards the body and then straighten out the leg. Carry out the same action on the other leg. Repeat several times.

2 Babies never seem to lose interest in their fingers and toes; add to this fascination by wiggling and rotating the little joints one by one.

Effleurage

Kneading and squeezing

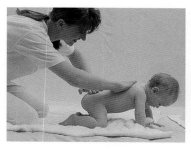

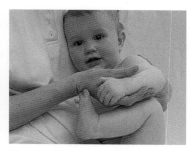

If your baby can keep still for long enough, you can rub nourishing oil into the skin while massaging. Soft effleurage strokes on the back, such as fanning and circles, will delight them.

Chubby little arms and legs are made for gentle squeezing and kneading. Press the limbs softly between your thumb and fingers.

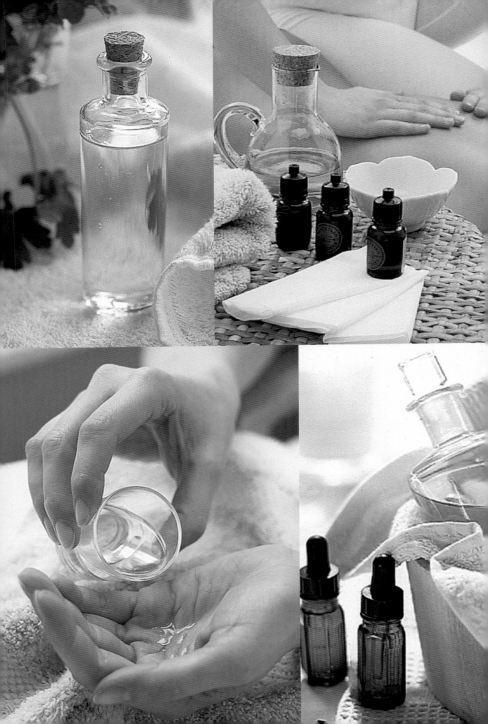

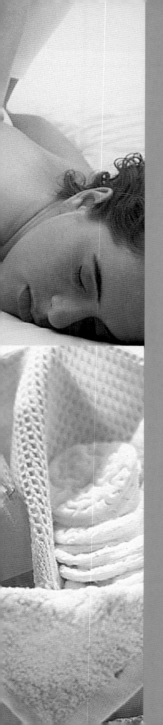

AROMATHERAPY
TREATMENTS

Now that you understand the properties of essential oils, and have learned how to blend them for use in aromatherapy massage, you can apply this knowledge to a wider range of home treatments for everyday complaints.

Aromatherapy works on every level to cleanse the body and calm the mind, and it can be used in response to issues such as stress, headache, poor digestion, low vitality, skin complaints, menstrual pains and muscular aches. In addition to massage therapies, try out inhalations, compresses, hair rinses and a range of pleasurable soaking remedies perfect for soothing the feet or whole body. These simple and effective treatments can easily be incorporated into a daily routine.

Energizers

There are unfortunately times in all our lives when we get depressed, whether due to a specific event or from chronic tiredness. As part of a programme of recuperation and restoring vitality, aromatherapy can be very effective.

UPLIFTING OILS

For a strong, but relatively short-lived effect, try four drops bergamot and two drops neroli in the bath, ideally in the morning. After the bath, gently pat the skin with a soft towel. Do not rub vigorously. A gentler effect, which can pervade the atmosphere all day long, is to use bergamot or neroli oils in an essential oil burner – probably just one drop of each oil at a time, repeating as needed.

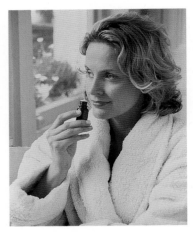

▲ ESSENTIAL OILS CAN PROVIDE AN INSTANT PICK-ME-UP.

INVIGORATING OILS

Chronic tension all too often leads to a feeling of exhaustion, when we just run out of steam. At these times we need a boost, and many oils have a tonic effect, restoring vitality without over-stimulating. As a group, citrus oils are good for this purpose, ranging from the soothing mandarin to the refreshing lemon oil.

Have a warm bath, with four drops mandarin and two drops orange or four drops neroli and two drops lemon. Alternatively, just add a couple of drops of

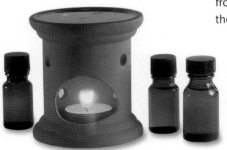

◀ VAPORIZED OILS CAN HAVE A VERY UPLIFTING EFFECT ON THE SPIRITS.

◀ LEMON OIL
REFRESHES AND
CLEARS THE MIND.

▶ ROSEMARY IS
USEFUL FOR MENTAL
FATIGUE OR LETHARGY.

any of these oils to a bowl of steaming water and gently inhale to help to lift tiredness and raise your spirits.

Steam inhalation is a valuable and simple way to receive the benefits of essential oils when time or circumstance prevents massage or a bath.

REVITALIZING OILS

In today's high pressure world, trying to juggle with too many demands leads nearly all of us to reach a state of "brain fag" at some point, when mental fatigue and exhaustion grind us to a halt.

Rather than reach for the coffee, or worse still alcohol, which may seem to relax but actually depresses the central nervous system, try using these revitalizing oils to give you an instant pick-me-up and make you feel more alert.

You can use one to two drops of rosemary or peppermint oil in a burner. Alternatively, add three drops rosemary and two drops peppermint to a bowl of steaming water, or use four drops of either oil on their own. Allow the oils to evaporate into the room.

▼ A STEAM INHALATION OF ESSENTIAL OILS
CAN HELP TO UPLIFT YOUR SPIRITS.

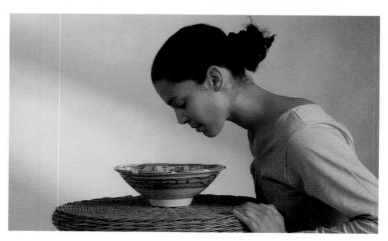

Inhalations

Colds and sinus problems may cause congestion, but we can also feel blocked up and unable to breathe freely through tension. Steam inhalations warm and moisten the membranes, and essential oils help to open the airways.

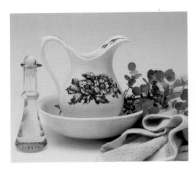

◄ A EUCALYPTUS STEAM INHALATION HELPS TO CLEAR CONGESTION.

CAUTION
If you have either high blood pressure or asthma you should seek medical advice before using steam, and in any case do not overdo an inhalation.

▼ INHALE THE STEAM DEEPLY.

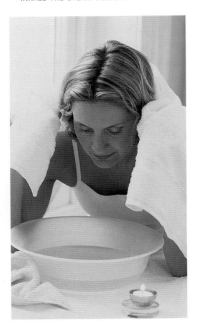

For a stuffed-up feeling, maybe combined with tiredness, try using three drops eucalyptus and two drops peppermint oil in a bowl of steaming water.

For tension causing poor breathing, relax the airways with four drops lavender and three drops frankincense.

Steam inhalations are helpful for respiratory complaints. Use a total of ten drops for a strong medicinal effect, in cases of colds and chestiness, or just five drops for a gentler relaxing effect. Inhale the steam deeply while holding a towel over your head to slow down the rate of oil evaporation.

Sprains and swellings

Hot or cold compresses are excellent ways to use oils for problems such as sprains and muscular aches. To make a compress, add essential oils to iced or hot water and soak a pad in it before placing on the affected area.

Cold compresses are suitable for use on acute injuries such as a strain or sprain, with swelling or bruising. For older injuries, for chronic muscle aches such as backache and menstrual pain, and for arthritic or rheumatic pain, a hot compress may be more useful.

The ideal oil for a cold compress is lavender, which is useful in many first-aid situations. Use four drops to a bowl of iced water. Keep the pad on for at least 20 minutes. Raise the affected limb if a swelling occurs.

For muscular aches, try using two drops of both rosemary and marjoram in a bowl of hot water. Apply for 30 minutes.

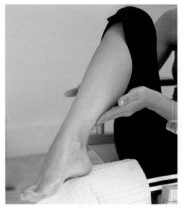

▲ MUSCULAR ACHE CAN OCCUR AS A RESULT OF FAILING TO WARM UP BEFORE EXERCISE.

▼ A COLD COMPRESS IS GOOD FOR SOOTHING STRAINS AND SPRAINS.

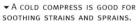

▼ COMPRESSES CAN STIMULATE CIRCULATION.

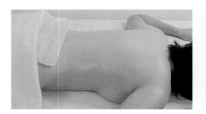

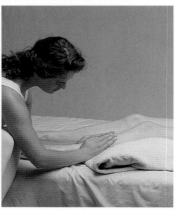

Backache relievers

So often people carry around their tensions in the form of a stiff, aching or knotted back. Symptoms can range from tight shoulders to lower backache. The best way of using oils to relieve backache is in massage of the taut muscles.

When massaging your partner's back to relieve pain, long sweeping strokes along the length of the back and a deep kneading action with the hands will loosen areas of muscle spasm, while the aromatic essential oils will work their magic and relax tension.

Two essential oil blends that will help to work on deeper tensions and knotted muscles are three drops pine and three drops rosemary oil, or four drops lavender used with three drops marjoram oil mixed with the base oil. The oil for the massage should be poured into a small, clean bowl close to hand, from where you can take more oil from time to time as you need it without disturbing the rhythm of the massage.

▸ PENETRATING ROSEMARY OIL
IS PARTICULARLY BENEFICIAL
FOR RELIEVING MUSCULAR ACHES.

RELAXING TENSE BACKS

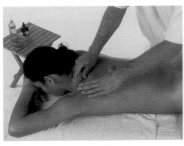

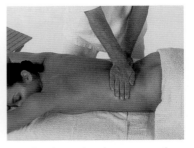

1 Knead the shoulders and neck to ease stiff, tense muscles.

2 Apply steady, sweeping movements down the back with your hands. Finally, stroke firmly down the back with both hands.

Muscular ache relievers

When you are under stress for any length of time, your body stays permanently tense. This can make any or all of your muscles ache and feel tired or heavy. Massage with a blend of essential oils will begin to relieve symptoms.

Gentle but firm massage is a wonderful reviver of tired, tender or tense muscles, especially when the aches are smoothed away with a fragrant oil. As the massage movements start to work on the aching muscles, the oils are being absorbed and get to work on inner tension too.

For the best effect, use a blend of three drops pine, three drops marjoram and two drops juniper oil for a variety of soothing massage strokes. Other warming oils that help to relieve aching muscles include: black pepper, clary sage, eucalyptus, ginger, grapefruit, jasmine, lavender, lemon, peppermint, orange, nutmeg and rosemary. You can also try experimenting with different blends of essential oils to discover which ones suit you best.

▸ A MASSAGE WITH PINE OIL IS IDEAL FOR INVIGORATING TIRED MUSCLES.

MASSAGING ACHING BACK MUSCLES

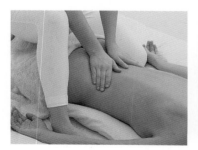

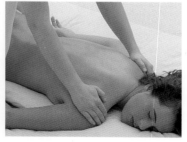

1 Rest your hands on the lower back on either side of the spine. Lean your weight into your hands and stroke firmly up the back. Mould your hands to the body as you go.

2 As your hands reach the top of your partner's back, fan them gently out towards the shoulders using a smooth, flowing motion.

Headache soothers

Tension headaches are a common feature in many people's lives, and may come from long hours at the computer or even longer hours with small children! Whatever the cause, gentle massage can help.

To relieve headaches, gentle massage of the temples and forehead at the earliest moment can help to stop headaches from getting a tight grip. Another option is the application of a warm compress soaked in hot water blended with essential oils.

If your head feels hot, try using an oil with four drops of peppermint. If warmth feels helpful, then you could try applying six drops of lavender oil. Another option for soothing a headache caused by congestion or tension is to use four drops of chamomile oil.

RELIEVING A HEADACHE

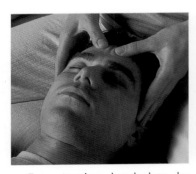

1 Ease tension headaches by massaging aromatherapy oils into the forehead. With your thumbs, use steady but gentle pressure to stroke the forehead.

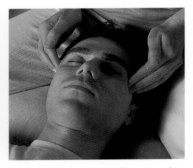

2 Gently massage the temples with your fingers, using slow rotating movements, in order to ease aches and pains caused by too much stress and tension.

◄ Marjoram

◄ Clary sage

One of the most complex of health problems, migraines are nature's way of shutting our systems down when life has been too demanding. The triggers that spark off a migraine attack are highly individual and professional treatment is really needed to try to understand the causes for each person.

At the first sign of a migraine, try using a blend of two drops rosemary, one drop marjoram and one drop clary sage, diluted in a base oil and gently massaged into the forehead and temples. Alternatively, use a drop of each essential oil in a bowl of warm water and apply a warm compress to the forehead.

Alleviating a migraine

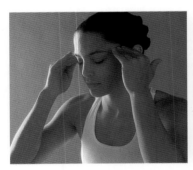

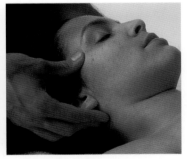

1 Many migraine sufferers have a heightened sense of smell at the onset of the attack and may find any aroma intolerable, so use oils sparingly. For self-help, gently massage the temples with small circling movements.

2 Receiving a gentle head massage from a partner allows you to lie back and relax your body completely and can therefore be even more effective than a self-massage at soothing the pain.

Menstrual pain easers

Painful periods can be due to several factors, but tension will certainly add to muscle spasm and cramping pains. If there is no organic or structural cause of the discomfort, try using essential oils as a hot compress or in the bath.

Some essential oils have a reputation for improving the menstrual cycle in ways other than as a compress or added to a hot bath; seek advice from a professional aromatherapist for longer-term treatments.

For a hot compress, soak a pad in hot water mixed with one drop each of rose, geranium and clary sage essential oils. Apply the compress over the lower abdomen to relieve menstrual pain. Alternatively, a fairly hot bath with three drops of rose, three drops of geranium and two drops of clary sage oil will quickly relax the cramped or aching muscles.

▲ ROSE

▼ A HOT BATH WITH OILS IS RELAXING.

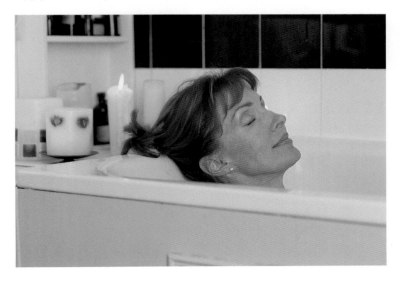

For many women the days leading up to a period can be fraught with mood swings, irritability and other symptoms. Professional treatment may be needed for full assistance; however, you could try this blend of essential oils if before each period you feel very tense and critical of those around you, or you just want to devour a box of chocolates!

Add three drops rose, three drops jasmine and two drops

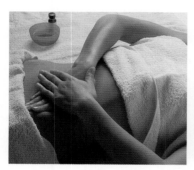

▶ JASMINE

clary sage essential oil to a hot bath and lie back, allowing its aroma to soothe you, and the warm water to soak away any tension in your body. Alternatively, you could try using this mixture in a massage oil and rub it gently into your lower abdomen for a soothing and relaxing effect.

PREMENSTRUAL TENSION SOOTHER

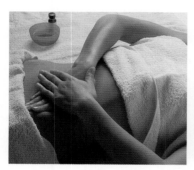

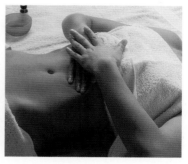

1 Slowly and firmly massage the lower abdomen with your hands. Close your eyes and continue the massage until you feel relaxed.

2 Move your hands in a clockwise direction, working up towards the chest; try to remain relaxed during this time so that the tension drains away.

Settling the stomach

Nervousness often results in an upset stomach. It has been said that our digestive organs also digest stress, and can end up storing emotions, causing discomfort and indigestion. The key is to let our bodies release anxieties.

Aromatherapy can help a great deal to achieve relaxation and calmness, allowing our bodies to release stress which may affect the digestive organs. One of the easiest ways to use oils in this context is to make a hot compress and place it over the abdomen, keeping the area warm for up to ten minutes.

To make the hot compress, add either two drops orange and three drops peppermint oil to a bowl of hot water, or you can use three drops chamomile and two drops orange essential oils. Soak a flannel in the scented water, wring it out, and apply it over the abdomen as directed above. The heat from the compress will soothe away stress and tension, and relax the abdominal muscles. Use the compress as often as necessary for relief, ensuring the flannel remains hot.

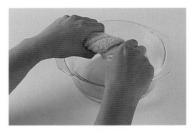

▲ SOAK A FLANNEL IN HOT WATER.

▼ LAY THE COMPRESS OVER THE ABDOMEN.

▼ SOOTHING PEPPERMINT TEA.

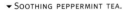

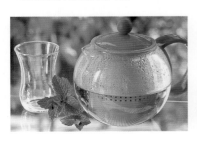

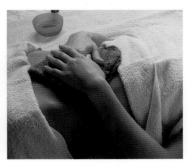

Travel calmers

It is said that travel broadens the mind; unfortunately, for some people it contracts the mind into a series of worries. Is this plane safe? Will I be sick? Try one of the following essential oils to calm the mind and stomach.

Inhaling essential oils while travelling allows you to enjoy the anticipation of new horizons without being stressed by how to reach them. The simplest way for you to use essential oils when travelling is to put a couple of drops onto a tissue or handkerchief, and to inhale them when you have need. Useful aromatherapy

◀ PEPPERMINT

CALMING OILS

▶ MANDARINS

oils for this purpose include peppermint, mandarin and neroli. In addition to helping overcome travel sickness, peppermint is also useful for muscular aches and pains, nausea and colds. Mandarin oil has an uplifting effect and is also a good oil to use for treating restlessness and nervous tension. Likewise, neroli oil is useful during times of anxiety.

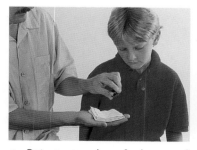

1 Put a couple of drops of aromatherapy oil onto a tissue or folded handkerchief.

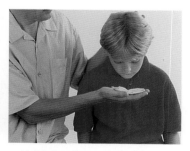

2 Hold the tissue under the nose and lean the head slightly forwards. Inhale. Repeat as necessary throughout the journey.

Hair care

These days there is a bewildering range of products available for every type of hair. However, simpler treatments, which have been tried and trusted over many years, can also make your hair look wonderful.

Good hairdressers recommend a varied programme of hair care because consistently using one product can lead to build-up on the hair and scalp. Herbal hair rinses, shampoos and other treatments use natural ingredients which will leave your hair in really good condition.

The easiest way to make a herbal shampoo is to add 30–45ml/2–3tbsp of a strong herbal infusion to a gentle baby shampoo. Alternatively, you could

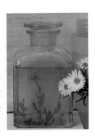

▶ STORE HERBAL HAIR RINSES IN GLASS BOTTLES.

add two to three drops of your favourite oil. For chamomile and orangeflower shampoo, mix 15ml/1tbsp chamomile infusion and five drops neroli essential oil into 60ml/4tbsp mild shampoo just before washing your hair.

HERBAL RINSE

A herbal rinse helps to keep the hair shiny and in good condition. When washing your hair, simply replace the last water rinse with a jugful of herbal rinse, mixed with water 50/50, and leave to dry. Chamomile and rosemary have been combined with vinegar and used in hair rinses for hundreds of years. The herbs enhance the colour of the hair and the vinegar is a wonderful scalp conditioner.

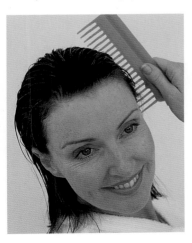

◀ COMB HAIR TREATMENT THROUGH HAIR.

Fair-hair rinse

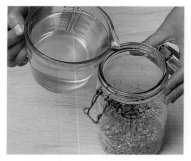

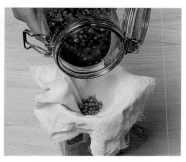

1 Measure 50g/2oz chamomile flowers in a jar. Pour 900ml/ 1½ pints boiled water over them.

2 Seal the jar and leave to stand overnight. Strain through muslin until the mixture is clear.

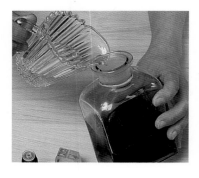

3 Add 50ml/2fl oz cider vinegar and five drops of chamomile essential oil. Store the mixture in a stoppered glass bottle in the fridge and use, within one week, as a final rinse whenever you wash your hair. The chamomile will enhance your hair's natural colour without bleaching.

Dark-hair rinse

This rinse uses the same basic ingredients as the fair-hair rinse but substitutes sprigs of fresh rosemary and rosemary oil for the chamomile flowers and oil. Pregnant women, however, should omit the rosemary essential oil.

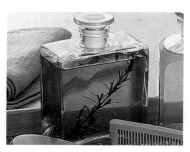

Skin care

When we become stressed, the small muscles close to the skin tend to contract. This can leave our skin undernourished with blood, and our complexion and skin tone suffer. Using essential oils can help counteract this.

Tense skin is frequently much drier than normal skin, and probably the best way to use essential oils is to mix them into your favourite skin cream. Obviously, this is best if the skin cream is originally unperfumed.

To make a reviving skin tonic, add three drops sandalwood and three drops rose oil, or four drops neroli and two drops rose oil to a 25g/1oz pot of skin cream. Mix together and apply to the skin.

To make a fragrant rose lotion which is excellent for all skin types, mix 175ml/6fl oz unscented

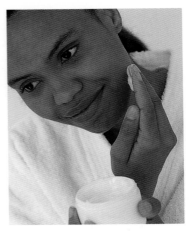

▲ APPLYING OIL-BLENDED SKIN CREAM.

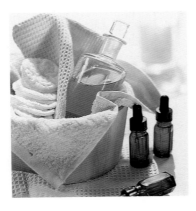

body lotion with ten drops rose essential oil. Pour into a bottle with a tight lid to store. A refreshing, lightly fragranced citrus body lotion can be made in the same way using 175ml/6fl oz unscented body lotion, ten drops grapefruit essential oil and five drops bergamot essential oil; however, do not apply this lotion before going into the sun.

◄ OIL-SCENTED BODY LOTION IS BEST APPLIED AFTER A WARM BATH.

▶ It is best if you only mix up small amounts of cream and oil at a time.

Classic cleansers

Gentle but effective cleansers are easy to make from pure, simple ingredients. Soapwort cleansing liquid is made by placing 15g/½ oz chopped soapwort root (available from herbalists) in a pan with 600ml/1 pint bottled spring water. Bring to the boil and simmer for 15 minutes. Strain the infusion through a paper filter, then stir in 50ml/2fl oz rose water and decant the mixture into a glass bottle. This will keep for one month in the fridge.

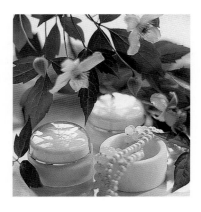

Another classic cleanser is almond oil cleanser, which is a traditional mix of beeswax, almond oil and rose water. Melt 25g/1oz white beeswax in a double boiler and whisk in 150ml/5fl oz almond oil. In a pan, add 1.5ml/¼ tsp borax (available from chemists) to 60ml/4 tbsp rose water and warm gently to dissolve. Slowly add the rose water mixture to the oils, whisking all the time. Add a few drops of rose essential oil. Continue to whisk until the mixture has a smooth, creamy texture. Pour the cleanser into a container and leave to cool. Replace the lid. To use the cleanser, smooth it on to the skin using a circular movement and remove with damp cotton wool.

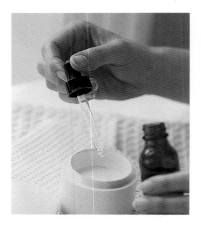

◀ Adding drops of oil to skin cream.

Hand care

Our hands frequently suffer from poor circulation and damage caused from overuse and abuse. Warm hand baths and the application of hand cream relieve poor circulation, soothe the skin and heal any cuts.

HAND BATHS

Circulation to our extremities is affected by tension and stress, among other things. The warmth of the water in a hand bath can help the blood vessels to dilate, which can be helpful in treating tension headaches and migraines, when the blood vessels in the head are frequently engorged with blood. If you regularly suffer from these problems, try a hand bath at the first signs of a headache to drain away the excess stress.

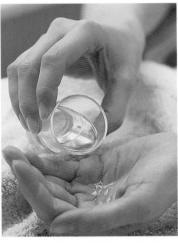

▲ RELAX TIRED HANDS WITH A BLEND OF ROSEMARY AND PINE ESSENTIAL OILS.

▼ A WARM HAND BATH CAN HELP TO RELIEVE POOR CIRCULATION IN THE HANDS.

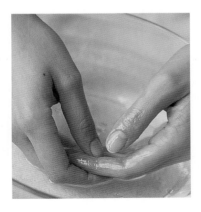

For poor circulation and tense, cold fingers, add two drops lavender and two drops marjoram essential oils to a large bowl two-thirds filled with hot water. Soak your hands in the bowl of water for relief of discomfort.

To relieve over-exertion causing tension and stiffness, try a blend of two drops rosemary and two drops pine in a bowl of hot water.

HAND CREAMS

You can make hand creams by adding suitable essential oils to an unscented cream. Look for a lanolin-rich cream or one that includes cocoa butter as hands benefit from a richer formulation. For a healing cream (see below) blend chamomile, geranium and lemon with unscented hand cream. Store the cream in a plastic bottle.

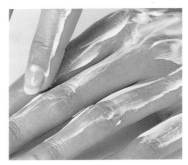

▲ YOU SHOULD ALWAYS TRY TO REMEMBER TO MOISTURIZE YOUR HANDS AT LEAST TWICE A DAY.

PREPARING A HEALING HAND CREAM

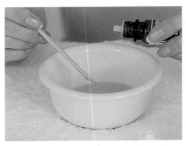

1 Blend ten drops chamomile with five drops geranium and lemon.

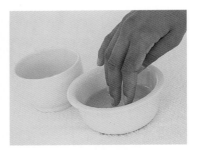

2 Blend the oils with 120ml/4fl oz unscented hand cream.

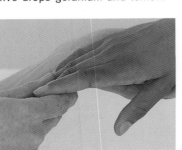

3 Spread the hand cream over the hands and rub it in thoroughly. The cream is healing because the chamomile oil soothes rough skin, the geranium oil helps heal cuts and the lemon oil softens the skin.

Foot care

Feet often suffer from neglect. We take them for granted, and seldom care for them the way we do the rest of the body. Warming foot baths and soothing foot creams are two ways of relieving neglected feet.

FOOT BATHS

Just as hands can be treated with a warm hand bath, feet can also benefit from a foot bath to which has been added three or four drops of essential oil. The warmth of the water helps circulation to improve and soothes aches and pains.

Peppermint essential oil is cooling, counteracts tiredness and is the ideal oil for using in a refreshing foot bath. For hot, aching feet, add two drops peppermint and two drops lemon oil to a large bowl two-thirds filled with hot water. Soak your feet in the water for instant relief.

If you suffer from poor circulation in your toes, add two drops lavender and two drops marjoram oil to a bowl of hot water. Soak your feet until warmed through.

▼ RELAX WITH A WARM FOOT BATH.

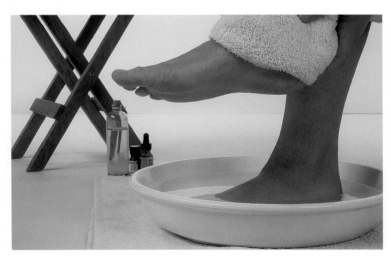

▸ Moisturize your feet with a soothing foot cream blended with essential oils.

Foot creams

You can easily make your own foot cream by adding suitable essential oils to an unscented cream. Tea tree is one of the best essential oils to incorporate in a foot cream. It has healing, antiseptic properties as well as a fungicidal action, which will protect the feet from the various foot complaints that can be picked up at the pool or gym.

To prepare tea tree foot cream, blend 15 drops tea tree essential oil thoroughly into 120ml/4fl oz unscented lanolin-rich cream (or one that includes cocoa butter). Pour the blended cream into a plastic storage bottle using a

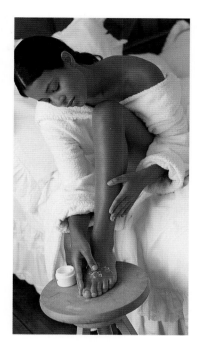

funnel. Although most creams and lotions are best stored in glass or ceramic containers, it is more practical to keep the foot cream in a pump-action plastic bottle.

To use the foot cream, simply press the plunger to release a small amount of cream on to your hands, and rub all over your feet to soothe and heal. Apply as often as required.

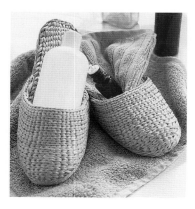

◂ Set aside time to pamper your feet.

Bathing

Imagine soaking in a hot bath, enveloped in a delicious scent of exotic flowers, feeling all the day's tensions drop away . . . well, it can be a reality with aromatherapy. The scented essential oils immediately soothe and relax.

Essential oils make a luxurious addition to the bath, whether they are chosen to aid recovery from a particular illness, to lift the spirits, or to promote relaxation after a stressful day. The essential oils that are recommended for the bath affect the body as they are

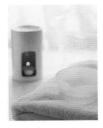

▶ USE ESSENTIAL OIL BURNERS TO ADD THERAPEUTIC SCENTS TO YOUR ROOMS.

inhaled in the steam, but some will also cling to the skin and penetrate through skin pores that have opened in the warm atmosphere. In order to add the oils to the bath safely it is important to dilute them. There are a variety of ways to do this, the most common of which is to use a vegetable oil – any one of the carrier oils used for massage will be suitable. For those who do not need or like an oily bath, a commercial dispersing agent (available from health food shops), some ordinary dairy cream, or full-fat milk can be used instead. These non-slip carriers are especially important in baths for the elderly and young children.

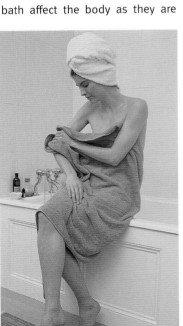

◀ GENTLY PAT YOUR SKIN DRY AFTER A BATH.

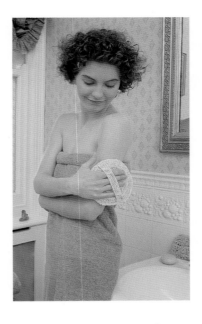

ylang ylang essential oils to add to your bath. For tired, tense and aching muscles, try soaking in a bath to which you have added three drops marjoram and two drops chamomile essential oils.

Add the blend to the water just before the bath has filled to the desired depth, pouring it in slowly under the hot water tap so that the oil is dispersed through the air and the water. After the bath, gently pat the skin dry with a soft towel. Avoid a vigorous rub-down.

Preparation for an aromatherapy bath should include the removal of dead skin cells. Use a massage mitt or a thoroughly dampened loofah, and rub it firmly but gently over the whole body.

SUGGESTED OIL BLENDS

For a refreshing, uplifting bath in the mornings try a blend of three drops bergamot and two drops geranium essential oils.

To relax and unwind after a long day, make a blend of three drops lavender and two drops

▼ CANDLES CREATE A SENSUAL ATMOSPHERE.

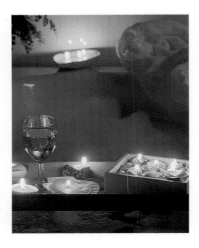

De-stressers

Stress, or rather our inability to cope with an excess amount of it, is one of the biggest health problems today. Regardless of how we react to stress, we can all benefit from the wonderfully balancing effects of aromatic oils.

Our bodies are geared to cope with a stressful situation by producing various hormones that trigger off a series of physiological actions in the body; these are known as the "fight or flight" syndrome, and serve to place the body in a state of alert in a potentially dangerous situation. Extra blood is shunted to the muscles, and the heart rate speeds up while the digestion slows down. These responses are appropriate when we are faced with a physical threat, but can be triggered by quite different kinds of stress and place a strain on our bodies without fulfilling any useful need. In order to help reduce the impact of stress on the whole system, it is necessary to find ways both to avoid getting over-stressed in the first instance and to let go of the changes that occur internally under stress. Aromatherapy can help in each case, the oils helping to keep you calm under pressure and releasing inner tensions following stress, especially in massage. To prevent undue stress, you can try simply inhaling your favourite essential oil at regular intervals throughout the day.

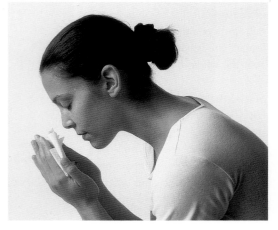

▶ INHALE ESSENTIAL OIL TO RELEASE TENSION.

If possible, use one of the following blends of essential oil in a base oil, and get your partner to massage you, for the perfect antidote to life's stresses. For aiding relaxation, use three drops lavender, three drops geranium and three drops marjoram oils. For calming and soothing, as well as giving a gentle uplift, use four drops rose and three drops jasmine oils. For a more definitely uplifting and energizing effect, try three drops clary sage and four drops bergamot essential oils.

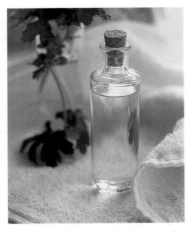

▲ GERANIUM OIL COMBINED WITH LAVENDER AND MARJORAM OILS AIDS RELAXATION.

STRESS-RELIEVING MASSAGE

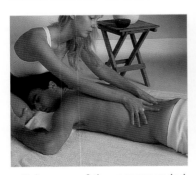

1 Using one of the recommended blends of essential oils, slowly and gently massage the oil into your partner's skin, moving your hands down each side of the spine.

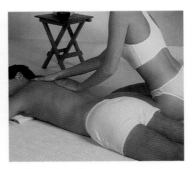

2 For relaxation, use one hand after the other to stroke down the back in a steady rhythm. Continue stroking for several minutes to allow the tension to drain away.

Properties of essential oils

This chart provides a ready reference to those essential oils that are suitable for use in the home, together with some of the more common complaints and disorders they may be used to treat.

	ACHE	ARTHRITIS	ATHLETE'S FOOT	BAD BREATH	BOILS, BLISTERS	BRITTLE NAILS	BROKEN VEINS	BRONCHITIS,	CHEST INFECTIONS	BRUISES	BURNS	CHILBLAINS	COLD SORES	CYSTITIS, URINARY INFECTIONS	DANDRUFF	DERMATITIS	EARACHE	ECZEMA
BENZOIN		•						•				•		•				
BERGAMOT	•			•				•					•	•				•
BLACK PEPPER		•																
CEDARWOOD	•	•						•						•				
CHAMOMILE	•	•			•					•	•	•		•	•		•	
CLARY SAGE	•														•			
CYPRESS								•						•				
EUCALYPTUS		•						•						•				
FENNEL								•										
FRANKINCENSE								•						•				
GERANIUM	•									•	•	•		•	•			•
GINGER		•																
GRAPEFRUIT	•																	
JASMINE																		
JUNIPER	•	•												•		•		•
LAVENDER										•	•						•	
LEMON	•	•			•	•		•		•		•	•					
MANDARIN	•																	
MARJORAM		•						•		•		•						
NEROLI							•	•										
NUTMEG		•																
ORANGE								•										
PALMAROSA	•														•	•		
PEPPERMINT	•			•				•								•		
ROSE						•											•	
ROSEMARY	•							•							•	•	•	
ROSEWOOD	•															•		
SANDALWOOD	•							•							•			•
TEA TREE	•		•					•			•		•	•	•		•	
YLANG YLANG																		

	FLU	HEAVY PERIODS	HICCUPS	INSECT BITES	IRREGULAR PERIODS	LACK OF PERIODS	MENOPAUSE	MOUTH ULCERS	NEURALGIA	NOSE BLEEDS	PALPITATIONS	PERIOD PAIN	PILES (HAEMORRHOIDS)	PMS	RASHES, ALLERGIES	RHEUMATISM	SCARS	SKIN ULCERS	SORE THROATS	SPOTS	SPRAINS, STRAINS	THRUSH	WARTS, VERRUCAS	WOUNDS, CUTS, SORES
	•							•							•	•			•					•
	•			•															•	•		•		•
	•										•					•								
																•								
				•	•		•					•			•	•					•	•		
						•						•			•				•					
	•	•					•					•	•			•								
	•			•																				
			•			•	•	•	•					•		•								
	•	•										•				•	•	•	•			•		•
					•		•											•	•					•
	•				•											•			•		•			
		•																		•				
						•						•				•					•			
	•							•	•		•			•										
																•								
	•							•																
												•				•							•	•
	•											•												
						•						•	•					•						
	•			•								•	•			•								
																			•					•
																			•					•
	•			•					•							•			•	•		•	•	•
												•												

properties of essential oils 175

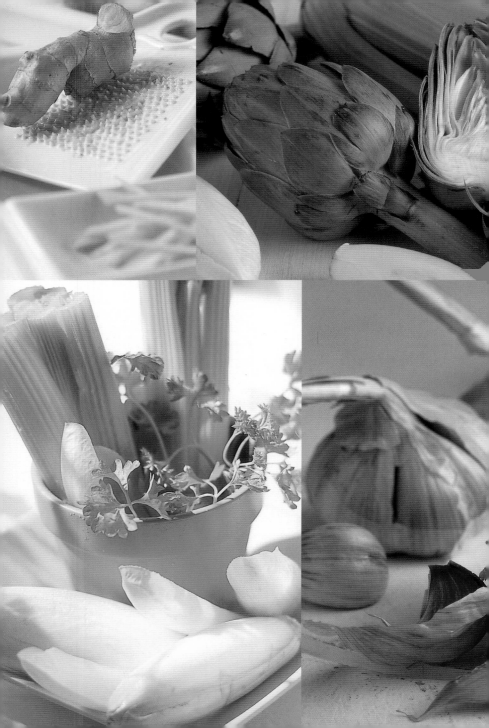

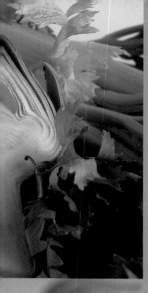
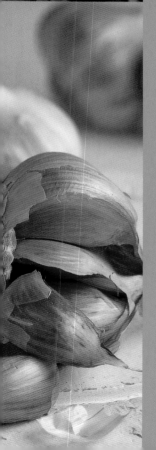

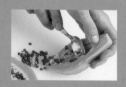

HEALING WITH
FOOD

Eating foods that promote good health makes sense, and is surprisingly simple. This section helps you to make sensible dietary choices, like eating moderate amounts of carbohydrates, sufficient protein, lots of fruits and vegetables, and limiting the amount of salt, sugar and fat you consume on a daily basis.

Aided by the following profiles on fruits, vegetables, pulses, nuts and cereals, you will be able to select the best sources of fibre, protein, vitamins, minerals and antioxidants, and to store and prepare foods to maximize their nutritional value. And what better way to eat for good health than to try out exciting new recipes? The suggestions on the following pages make for simple, easy-to-prepare and delicious fare!

Eating for good health

What we eat has a profound effect on our health and well-being. In a world that is becoming increasingly polluted, and where individuals are subject to high levels of stress, it is easy for our bodies to become out of kilter.

There is ample evidence of a link between poor diet and serious medical conditions like coronary heart disease, cancer and strokes, but it is not just these major health problems that we should be concerned about. A condition does not have to be life threatening to have a huge impact on the way we feel.

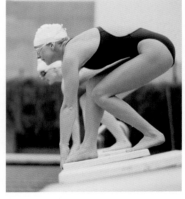

▲ Incorporating exercise into your daily routine will help your body to burn up excess fat, improving body tone.

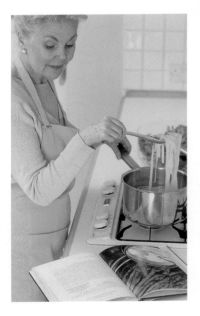

Whatever ails us, whether it is the occasional headache or sore throat, an ongoing condition like diabetes or a digestive problem that causes embarrassment and distress, specific foods can have a positive impact when eaten as part of a sensible, well-balanced diet.

◀ Trying out new, healthy recipes is both rewarding and enjoyable.

▶ A low-fat Mediterranean diet consisting of fish, fresh vegetables and fruit, olive oil and a small amount of red wine promotes good circulation.

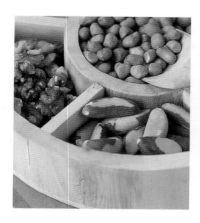

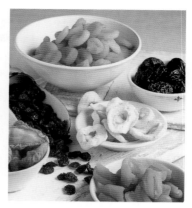

▲ LEFT AND RIGHT: CHOOSE HEALTHY SNACKS THAT NURTURE YOUR BODY, INSTEAD OF REACHING FOR SNACKS WITH EMPTY CALORIES.

Making relatively small changes to our diet, such as eating fruit for a mid-morning snack, can improve matters considerably.

It is important to seek professional advice from a doctor, nutritionist, dietician or state-registered medical specialist before making major changes to your diet, particularly if you are taking any kind of medication.

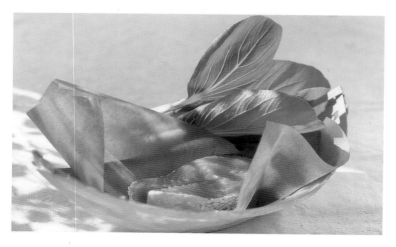

Superfoods

Some foods are such a rich source of concentrated nutrients that they have earned themselves the title "superfoods". Some, such as tofu, are old favourites; others, such as quinoa, have only recently received widespread acclaim.

To understand why these foods are so special, it is useful to look at recent scientific research. One of the most exciting discoveries has been the presence in plants of thousands of different chemical compounds. Each of these compounds – known collectively as phytochemicals – has its own function, and it is believed that some of them may play a crucial role in preventing diseases like cancer, heart disease, arthritis and hypertension. To get the best benefit from phytochemicals, eat at least five different types of fruit and vegetables daily, plus wholegrains, pulses, nuts and seeds.

▼ BUY VEGETABLES IN SMALL QUANTITIES AND EAT THEM AT THEIR FRESHEST.

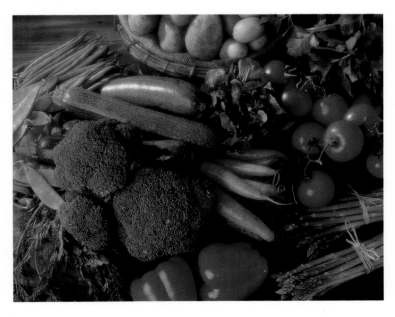

A number of phyto-chemicals also have antioxidant proper-ties. Antioxidants are vital for limiting damage to body cells by unstable molecules known as free radicals. The main antioxidant nutri-ents are vitamins A, C and E, and the minerals zinc and selenium.

When we chew, our bodies produce enzymes. These are protein molecules and are responsible for every aspect of metabolism or the energy we produce. Producing plenty of enzymes improves digestion, detox-ification and immunity, and helps to slow down the ageing process.

◄ Quinoa (left) is a complete protein and has a mild, slightly bitter taste and firm texture. Cook it in the same way as rice. Millet (below) is a highly nutritious gluten-free grain.

Many of the superfoods highlighted in the following pages are useful sources of enzymes and phytochemicals.

Others are included because they contribute valuable minerals, vitamins or omega-3 fatty acids, which are important allies in reducing the risk of heart disease.

▼ Strawberries are rich in B complex vitamins and vitamin C. They contain significant amounts of potassium, and have good skin-cleansing properties.

Good sources of antioxidants
- Sweet potatoes
- Carrots
- Watercress
- Broccoli
- Peas
- Citrus fruit
- Watermelon
- Strawberries
- Nuts and Seeds

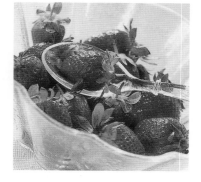

Fruit

What easier way to help yourself to good health than to eat plenty of fruit? There are so many different varieties, with glowing colours and delectable flavours, that eating the recommended portions daily is pure pleasure.

For maximum nutritional value, choose fruits that are ripe and freshly picked, and try to eat as many varieties as you can, as each fruit offers its own special benefits to your health and well-being.

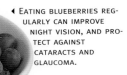

◀ EATING BLUEBERRIES REGULARLY CAN IMPROVE NIGHT VISION, AND PROTECT AGAINST CATARACTS AND GLAUCOMA.

Fruit provides soluble fibre in the form of pectin, which aids digestion and helps to cleanse the liver. All fruits contain generous quantities of antioxidant vitamins C and E, phytochemicals and beta-carotene, which the body converts to vitamin A. These are vital to the health of your heart, helping to

▼ SUMMER PRODUCES AN ABUNDANT CROP OF DELICIOUS SOFT FRUITS.

▼ FRUIT IS THE ULTIMATE CONVENIENCE FOOD, AND AN EXCELLENT SOURCE OF FIBRE.

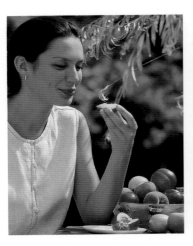

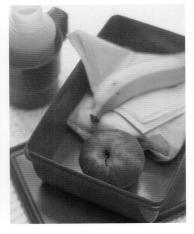

▶ Blackcurrants are usually served cooked and have a tart flavour.

prevent the furring up of the arteries that can lead to atherosclerosis and, in addition, support the body's defence system. The antioxidants in fruit may also ease the discomfort of arthritis sufferers by mopping up free radicals and helping to promote the growth of new cartilage. Mangoes, apricots, apples and bananas are particularly useful in this regard.

Apples contain the flavonoid quercetin, which may reduce the risk of heart attacks and strokes.

Bananas are a good source of fibre, vitamins, and minerals such as potassium, which maintains nerve, cell and muscle function, and can help to relieve high blood pressure. Bananas have a high starch content so provide sustained energy. They are a source of tryptophan, an amino acid that lifts the spirits and aids sleep. Ripe bananas are useful for digestion, strengthening the stomach lining against acid and ulcers.

▼ Fresh fruit salad is a healthy and nutritious dessert.

How much is a portion?

Nutritionists recommend eating five portions of fruit and vegetables a day, but what is a portion?
• One medium apple, banana or orange
• A wine glass of any fresh fruit juice
• One large slice of any type of melon or pineapple
• Two plums or kiwi fruit
• About 115g/4oz/1 cup berries

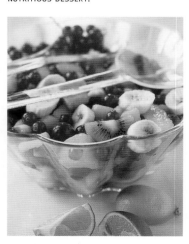

Blackcurrants are high in antioxidants, vitamins C and E, and carotenes. They also contain fibre, as well as the minerals calcium, iron and magnesium. Blackcurrants are also useful for treating stomach upsets.

Citrus fruits, melons and kiwi fruit are rich in vitamin C, offering relief to asthmatics and people suffering from a wide range of respiratory problems. The membranes of citrus fruit contain pectin, which helps to reduce cholesterol, and also bioflavonoids, which have powerful antioxidant properties.

Figs have laxative qualities and are a good source of calcium.

Gooseberries are rich in vitamin C and also contain betacarotene, potassium and fibre.

Mangoes and apricots contain betacarotene, which may help to prevent inflammation of the lungs and airways. Mangoes are used to cleanse the blood, while apricots supply vitamin A.

Papaya or pawpaw contains an enzyme called papain, which assists digestion. This fruit is rich in vitamin C, which promotes healthy skin, hair and nails.

Raspberries are a rich source of vitamin C. Eat them to alleviate menstrual cramps. They cleanse the body and remove harmful toxins.

Strawberries cleanse the skin. They are rich in B complex vitamins and vitamin C.

Tomatoes ripened on the vine have higher levels of vitamin C than those picked when green. They contain vitamin E, betacarotene, magnesium, calcium and phosphorus. They aid digestion, reduce blood pressure and lower the risk of asthma.

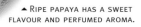

▲ RIPE PAPAYA HAS A SWEET FLAVOUR AND PERFUMED AROMA.

BAKED APPLES

For a nutritious dessert, try these tasty baked apples stuffed with dried fruit and nuts.

INGREDIENTS

4 cooking apples
115g/4oz/²⁄₃ cup mixed dried
  fruit and nuts
20ml/4 tsp soft dark brown
  sugar
butter

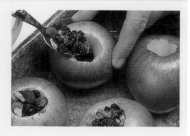

1 Preheat the oven to 180°C/ 350°F/Gas 4. Remove the core from the apples, score them round their middles, then place them in a baking dish.

2 Mix the fruit, nuts and sugar together and fill the centre of each apple. Pour a little water around the apples and top each with a knob (pat) of butter.

3 Bake for 40–60 minutes, until soft and golden. Serve hot, with low-fat yogurt. Serves 4.

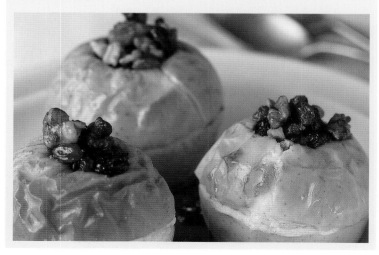

Vegetables

One of the easiest ways of boosting your intake of fibre, vitamins and minerals is to eat plenty of vegetables. Buy organic produce where possible, and make sure it is fresh by purchasing produce from a store with a fast turnover.

Box schemes, run by independent suppliers or co-operatives, are an excellent idea. You state how much you want to spend and how often you would like a delivery, and boxes of beautiful produce arrive on your doorstep regularly. You may be able to specify what they contain, but it can be more fun to have a little of whatever is being harvested. That way you get to try some unfamiliar vegetables.

Like fruit, all vegetables contain phytochemicals, the plant compounds that stimulate the body's enzyme defences against carcinogens (the substances that cause cancer). The best sources are broccoli, cabbages, kohlrabi, radishes, cauliflower, Brussels sprouts, watercress, turnips, kale, pak choi (bok choy), mustard greens, spring

▾ CRUCIFEROUS VEGETABLES ARE PACKED WITH PHYTOCHEMICALS.

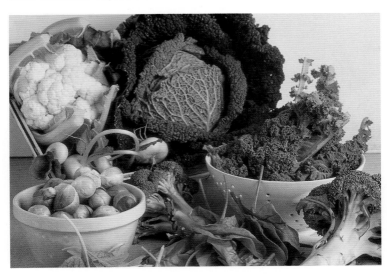

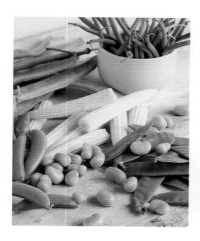

▲ BEANS, PEAS AND CORN CAN BE ENJOYED ALL YEAR ROUND, FRESH OR FROZEN.

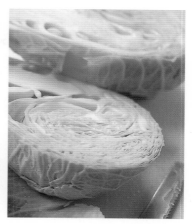

▲ CABBAGE IS BEST EATEN RAW. IT IS A VALUABLE SOURCE OF VITAMINS C AND E.

greens (collards), chard and swede (rutabaga). Vegetables are also a good source of antioxidants.

Artichokes are good liver cleansers. A source of vitamins A and C, fibre, iron, calcium and potassium, they are used in natural medicine to treat high blood pressure.

Asparagus has anti-inflammatory properties and helps to soothe painful joints.

Beetroot (beet), when eaten raw, helps to cleanse the liver and is good for detoxifying the skin.

Cabbage has antiviral and antibacterial qualities and is particularly useful raw or juiced. It is thought to speed up the metabolism of

oestrogen in women and may protect against breast cancer or cancer of the womb.

Carrots and sweet potatoes are rich in betacarotene, which may help to prevent inflammation of the lungs and airways, and may also ease painful conditions of the joints, such as arthritis.

Chillies are very high in vitamin C. They can help to thin mucus and relieve congested airways, and also stimulate the circulation.

Fennel aids digestion, is a diuretic and has a calming and toning effect on the stomach.

Garlic has been found to lower blood cholesterol levels, reduce

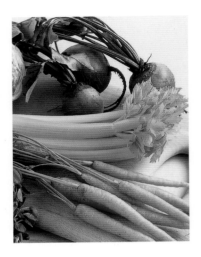

▲ CARROTS AND BEETROOT (BEET) HELP THE LIVER TO DETOXIFY THE BODY.

possibly prevent asthma attacks. Onions also contain quercetin, an anti-inflammatory that can ease painful joints.

Peas and beans are a good source of protein and fibre. They also contain vitamin C, iron, thiamine, folate, phosphorous and potassium.

Peppers contain plenty of vitamin C, as well as betacarotene, some B complex vitamins, calcium, phosphorous and iron.

Salad leaves are largely composed of water, but are worth eating for

blood pressure and help to prevent the formation of blood clots. An antiviral and antibacterial allium, garlic strengthens the immune system. It is a nasal decongestant. It is best eaten raw, but cooking does not radically decrease its decongestant properties.

Green vegetables that are rich in folic acid may help to lower the risk of heart disease by reducing levels of the amino acid, homocysteine. (High levels are linked to increased risk of coronary heart disease.)

Onions have long been considered a folk cure for respiratory problems. They help clear the airways and

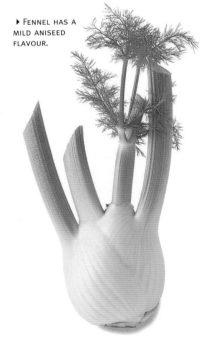

▶ FENNEL HAS A MILD ANISEED FLAVOUR.

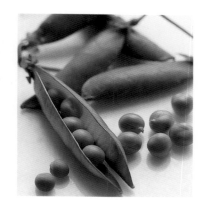

the vitamins and minerals they contribute to the diet. Choose the outer, darker leaves of lettuces, as they are more nutritious than the pale leaves in the centre.

▲ PEAS PICKED AND EATEN FRESH FROM THE POD HAVE A DELICIOUS SWEET TASTE.

▼ ASPARAGUS HAS MILD DIURETIC AND LAXATIVE PROPERTIES.

Spinach is a rich source of cancer-fighting antioxidants, fibre and vitamins C and B6. It also contains calcium, potassium, folate, thiamine, zinc and four times more betacarotene than broccoli.

▼ GARLIC IMPARTS A STRONGER FLAVOUR INTO COOKING WHEN USED CRUSHED.

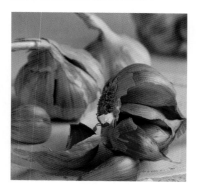

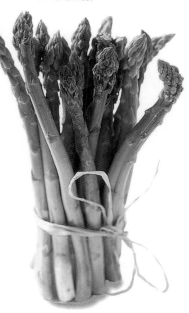

Sprouted grains, seeds and pulses

Sprouted seeds are powerhouses of nutrition. Once the seed, pulse or grain germinates, the nutritional value rockets – by as much as 30 per cent in the case of B vitamins, and 60 per cent for vitamin C.

Sprouts supply plenty of protein, vitamin E, potassium and phosphorus. You can buy sprouts from supermarkets, but they'll be fresher – and cost less – if you grow them. Children love watching them germinate, they taste good in fresh and cooked dishes, and they are very easy to digest.

Many seeds, pulses (legumes) and grains can be sprouted successfully. Here are some of the best.

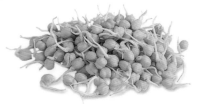

▲ CHICKPEA SPROUTS

Chickpea sprouts are deliciously nutty, but take longer to sprout than small beans. They must be rinsed four times a day.

▼ LENTIL SPROUTS

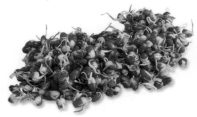

▲ ADUKI BEANSPROUTS

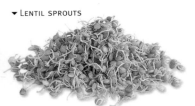

Lentil sprouts are slightly spicy and peppery. Use whole (not split) red,

Aduki beansprouts are said to be good for cleansing the system. These fine, feathery sprouts have a sweet, nutty flavour.

Alfalfa sprouts are wispy little sprouts with a nutty, mild flavour. They are best eaten raw.

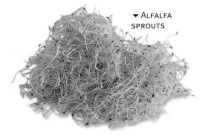

▼ ALFALFA SPROUTS

green and brown lentils. They are best eaten when young.

▼ MUNG BEANSPROUTS

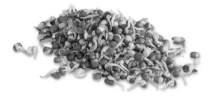

Mung beansprouts are large, with a delicate flavour and crunchy texture. They are great in salads.

▼ WHEAT BERRY SPROUTS

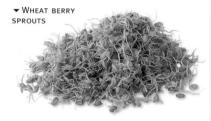

Wheat berry sprouts are sweet and crunchy. They taste great in breads.

STORING SPROUTS

Use sprouts as soon as possible after growing or buying. If you must store them, put them in a plastic bag or sealed tub in the refrigerator. They will keep for 2–3 days. Wash and drain bought sprouts before using them.

SPROUTING

There's nothing simpler than sprouting seeds. It's the fastest way to grow your own organic produce. Most seeds are ready to eat in 3–4 days.

1 Rinse 45ml/3 tbsp seeds, pulses (legumes) or grains, drain and place in a clean jar. Fill with lukewarm water, cover with muslin and fasten securely. Leave in a warm place overnight.

2 Pour off the water, leaving the muslin in place. Refill with water, shake gently, then drain as before. Leave the jar in a warm place, away from direct sunlight.

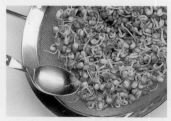

3 Rinse and drain three times a day until they have grown to the desired size. Remove from the jar, rinse, drain and discard any that haven't germinated.

Sea vegetables

For centuries, Asian cooks have known about the health benefits of sea vegetables such as arame, laver and kombu, but the Western world is just waking up to the potential of including these valuable superfoods in the diet.

Sea vegetables are an excellent source of betacarotene and contain some of the B complex vitamins. They are rich in minerals. Calcium, magnesium, potassium, phosphorus and iron are all present, and are credited with boosting the immune system, reducing stress and helping the metabolism to function efficiently. Eating sea vegetables regularly can improve the hair and skin, and the iodine they contribute improves thyroid function and prevents goitre.

Sea vegetables can be used in many different ways. Try toasting them and crumbling them into stir-fries or salads, or add them to soups and casseroles.

Arame is sold as thin, wiry strips. It is mild and slightly sweet.

Dulse is a purple-red sea vegetable which is chewy and tastes spicy. It is rich in potassium, iodine, phosphorous, iron and manganese.

◄ ARAME

Kombu is very versatile, and forms part of the Japanese stock, dashi. It has a strong flavour and is a rich source of iodine.

Laver is a rich source of minerals and vitamins. Cans of laver purée are available from health food stores. Spread it on hot toast.

Nori is a delicately flavoured seaweed that is processed into thin sheets, to be used as wraps. Toast it under a grill (broiler) before use.

Wakame is a versatile sea vegetable, rich in calcium and vitamins B and C. It can also be toasted and crumbled over food.

▼ DULSE

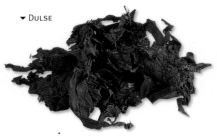

SIMPLE SALMON SUSHI

Sushi is a healthy snack. The rice contributes complex carbohydrate, the fish is a good source of protein and omega-3 fatty acids, and the nori wrapper is a source of iodine.

INGREDIENTS
25ml/1½ tbsp granulated sugar
5ml/1 tsp sea salt
30ml/2 tbsp Japanese rice
  vinegar
250g/9oz/1¼ cups sushi rice
3 sheets yaki nori (toasted
  nori)
175g/6oz very fresh salmon
  fillet, cut into fingers

1 Mix the sugar and salt in a bowl. Add the vinegar and stir until dissolved.

2 Cook the rice according to the instructions on the packet. Drain, add the vinegar mixture and stir well, fanning the rice constantly. Cover with a damp cloth. Cool.

3 Cut the yaki nori in half lengthways and place a half-sheet, shiny side down, on a bamboo mat.

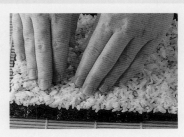

4 Spread with a layer of vinegared rice, leaving a 1cm/½ in clear edge at top and bottom. Arrange fingers of salmon across the centre.

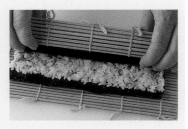

5 Roll up the yaki nori into a cigar. Wrap in clear film and chill.

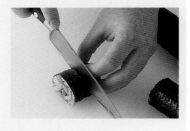

6 Cut into 24 slices.

Cereal grains

The seeds of cereal grasses, grains are packed with concentrated goodness and are an important source of complex carbohydrates, protein, vitamins and minerals. Grains are inexpensive and versatile.

Wheat, rice, oats and barley have always been an important part of the diet, but it is some of the less well-known grains that are currently causing excitement. Two of these are quinoa and millet. Both have been cultivated for centuries, but it is only comparatively recently that the full extent of their nutritional value has been realized.

Millet is highly nutritious. Low in fat, it is easily digested. The grains are a good source of iron, zinc, calcium, manganese and B vitamins.

Oats have been found to lower blood pressure. They provide insoluble fibre, which can reduce blood cholesterol levels when part of a low-fat diet. Oats are a source of vitamin E, an anti-inflammatory.

Quinoa is the only grain that is a complete protein, possessing all eight essential amino acids. Low in saturated fats and high in fibre, it is an excellent source of calcium, potassium, zinc, iron, magnesium and B vitamins. It is cooked like rice, but the grains swell to four times their original size. As the grain cooks, the germ that surrounds it forms a spiral that resembles a bean sprout. This stays firm and crunchy, providing a tasty contrast to the soft, creamy grain. Use quinoa in pilaffs, bakes, stuffings and as a breakfast cereal. It is also available in flakes and as flour.

◀ CLOCKWISE FROM TOP: ROLLED OATS, OATMEAL, WHOLE OATS AND OATBRAN.

◄ BROWN AND WHITE RICE

Rice is a good source of fibre, vitamins and minerals. Eat brown rice where possible, as it retains the husk, bran and germ in which most of the nutrients reside.

Wheat is a nutritious grain, but not everyone can tolerate it. It is best eaten unprocessed, as wholewheat. It is a very good source of dietary fibre, most of which is in the bran. It also contains B vitamins, vitamin E, iron, selenium and zinc. Wholegrains are a source of phytoestrogens, which may also help to protect against breast cancer.

RECIPE SUGGESTION

TABBOULEH
A quick and easy way to boost your dietary fibre intake.

INGREDIENTS
175g/6oz/1 cup bulgur wheat
30ml/2 tbsp each chopped fresh
  mint and parsley
6 spring onions (scallions), sliced
½ cucumber, diced
60ml/4 tbsp extra virgin olive oil
juice of 1 large lemon
salt and ground black pepper

1 Place the bulgur wheat in a bowl. Pour on boiling water to cover. Leave to stand for 30 minutes, so that the grains swell.

2 Drain well, removing as much water as possible. Tip the wheat into a bowl.

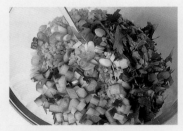

3 Add all the remaining ingredients and toss well. Chill for 30 minutes to allow the flavours to mingle. Serve as a salad, or as a filling for warm wheat tortillas, with guacamole. Serves 4–6.

Pulses

Low in fat and high in complex carbohydrates, vitamins and minerals, pulses are economical, easy to cook and good to eat. They are a valuable source of protein and good for diabetics, as they help to control sugar levels.

LENTILS AND DRIED PEAS

There are several varieties. All these pulses (legumes) are low in fat and rich in protein. They are a good source of fibre and are reputed to help lower levels of harmful LDL cholesterol.

▾ YELLOW AND GREEN SPLIT PEAS

DRIED BEANS

These are packed with protein, soluble and insoluble fibre, iron, potassium, manganese, magnesium, folate and most B vitamins. Soya beans are the superfood here, containing all the amino acids essential for the renewal of cells and tissues. Including dried beans in your diet regularly can lower cholesterol levels, reducing the risk of heart disease and strokes. Beans contain phytoestrogens, which can protect against cancer of the breast, prostate and colon. There are plenty of other varieties too, including aduki beans, black beans, black-eyed beans (peas), borlotti beans, broad (fava) beans, butter (lima) beans, flageolet or cannellini beans, chickpeas, haricot (navy) beans, pinto beans, red kidney beans and ful medames. Canned beans are not as nutritious as dried beans, but contain appreciable amounts of nutrients.

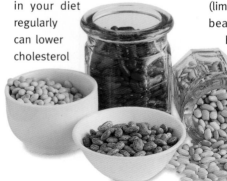

◂ CLOCKWISE FROM LEFT: HARICOT (NAVY) BEANS, KIDNEY BEANS, FLAGEOLET (CANNELLINI) BEANS AND PINTO BEANS.

Split pea mash

This purée makes an excellent alternative to mashed potatoes, and is particularly good with winter pies and nut roasts. Serve warm with pitta bread.

Ingredients

225g/8oz/1 cup yellow split peas, soaked overnight

1 bay leaf

8 sage leaves, roughly chopped

15ml/1 tbsp olive oil

4 shallots, finely chopped

5ml/1 tsp cumin seeds

1 large garlic clove, chopped

50g/2oz/¼ cup butter, softened

salt and ground black pepper

1 Drain the split peas, put them in a pan with cold water to cover and bring to the boil. Skim, add the herbs and simmer for 10 minutes.

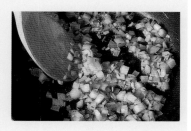

2 Heat the oil and fry the shallots with the cumin seeds and garlic for 3 minutes. Add to the pan and simmer for 30 minutes more. Drain, reserving the cooking water.

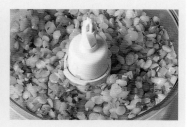

3 Remove the bay leaf, then process the split peas with the butter and enough of the cooking water to form a coarse purée. Season, serve warm with diced tomatoes and olive oil. Serves 4–6.

Protein foods

An essential nutrient, protein is converted by the body into amino acids, which are vital for the growth and repair of body cells. The body manufactures some amino acids, but eight cannot be manufactured.

Eating a good variety of proteins is important because the eight amino acids have to come from our food. The other 12 amino acids can all be synthesised from the food that we eat. Good sources of protein are red meat, poultry, fish, milk, eggs, quinoa, lentils and beans, especially soya beans and their derivatives. Tofu, an excellent source of protein, is a rich source of B vitamins, essential fatty acids,

▾ EAT A VARIETY OF PROTEIN TO ENSURE YOU GET THE MAXIMUM NUTRIENTS.

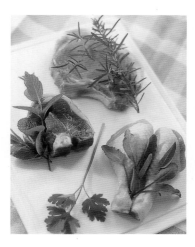

zinc and iron. It contains phyto-estrogens that help to regulate hormone levels, and can lower cholesterol levels if eaten regularly.

Although protein is so important, we do not need to eat vast amounts of it; eating too much protein, especially animal protein, can lead to weight gain and osteoporosis. Far better to balance a moderate amount of animal protein with protein from plant sources, such as tofu, quinoa, rice and pasta. There is also protein in bread and breakfast cereals.

Limit red meat to four 115–175g/ 4–6oz servings a week, and try not to eat more than three eggs. Milk, cheese and yogurt provide protein, calcium and vitamins B12, A and D. Choose low-fat products and consume in moderation.

Eat fish twice a week. Choose oily fish for preference. Herrings, sardines, mackerel, salmon and tuna provide omega-3 fatty acids, which can help to reduce the risk of heart disease.

MOROCCAN SPICED MACKEREL

A spicy marinade is the perfect foil for rich, oily fish.

INGREDIENTS

150ml/¼ pint/⅔ cup sunflower oil
15ml/1 tbsp paprika
5–10ml/1–2 tsp chilli powder
10ml/2 tsp ground cumin
10ml/2 tsp ground coriander
2 garlic cloves, crushed
juice of 2 lemons
30ml/2 tbsp chopped fresh mint
30ml/2 tbsp chopped fresh coriander (cilantro)
4 mackerel, cleaned
salt and ground black pepper
lemon wedges and mint sprigs, to serve

1 Whisk the oil, spices, garlic and lemon juice. Add the herbs.

2 Slash each mackerel in several places, then place in the dish. Turn to coat in the marinade.

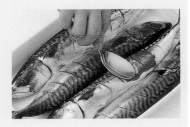

3 Cover with plastic wrap and chill for 3–5 hours. Grill (broil) for 5–7 minutes on each side. Turn once and baste often. Serve with lemon and mint. Serves 4.

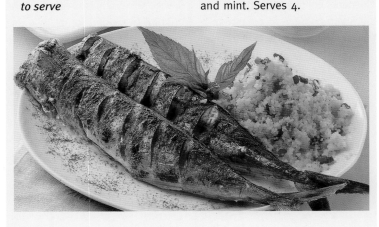

Nuts and seeds

Seeds and nuts make a valuable addition to the diet. Most nuts make delicious snacks, and are tasty sprinkled on salads and desserts. A few almonds, dry-roasted in a frying pan, make a wonderful topping for grilled chicken.

Nuts are an excellent source of B complex vitamins and vitamin E, an antioxidant that has been associated with a lower risk of heart disease, stroke and certain cancers. They are a useful source of protein, but are high in calories, so don't have too many of them.

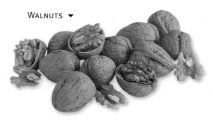

WALNUTS ▼

IN A NUTSHELL

Brazil nuts are high in saturated fat, but cholesterol-free. They are a rich source of selenium, which is a mood enhancer.

Chestnuts contain very little fat and are a good source of potassium.

Peanuts are high in fat, but a good source of potassium. Eat sparingly.

Pecan nuts have a very high fat content, so eat only occasionally.

Walnuts supply omega-3 fatty acids, which help to keep the heart healthy. Fatty acids thin the blood, which helps to prevent blood clots (DVT) and reduce blood cholesterol levels. They can also reduce inflammation in painful joints. Walnuts are also rich in potassium, magnesium, iron, zinc, copper and selenium.

▼ UNSALTED NUTS OF ANY KIND MAKE A HEALTHY SNACK FOR ANY TIME OF DAY.

CAUTION
• Always inform guests if you've included nuts in a dish, as some people are highly allergic to them.
• Never eat rancid nuts, as they have been linked to a high incidence of free radicals.

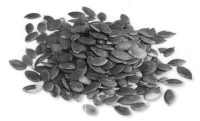

▲ PUMPKIN SEEDS

SEED CATALOGUE

Packed with vitamins and minerals, as well as beneficial oils and protein, seeds make delicious snacks, or can be sprinkled over food to boost the nutritional benefits.

Linseed has abundant levels of omega-3 and omega-6 fatty acids, good for strengthening immunity and easing digestive problems.

Pumpkin seeds are rich in iron and an excellent source of zinc.

Sesame seeds are tiny white or black seeds and are rich in iron.

Sunflower seeds are delicious when dry-roasted. They are a good source of vitamin E and B vitamins and boost flagging energy levels.

▼ LINSEEDS (LEFT) AND HEMP SEEDS

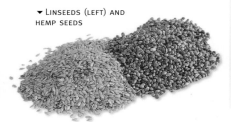

RECIPE SUGGESTION

SALAD AND ROASTED SEEDS
A nutritious light lunch or supper dish.

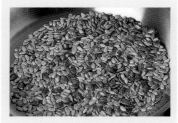

1 Dry-fry 50g/2oz/6 tbsp mixed pumpkin seeds and sunflower seeds in a frying pan, over a high heat, for 3 minutes until golden, tossing frequently to stop them from burning. Set aside to cool slightly.

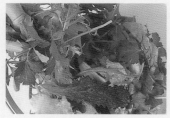

2 Mix about 175g/6oz salad and herb leaves in a bowl. Add the roasted seeds and toss with 30ml/2 tbsp vinaigrette to combine. Serves 4.

Herbs and spices

Herbs and spices are invaluable in the kitchen, not only because they help to make our food taste good without the need for excessive amounts of salt, but also because they are healing foods. Many herbs aid digestion.

Basil helps to relieve stomach cramps, nausea and constipation.

Chillies are an excellent source of vitamin C and a good source of other antioxidants. The spice stimulates the body and is a powerful decongestant.

Cinnamon aids digestion.

Fennel calms the digestive system.

Ginger is an expectorant that helps to fight coughs and colds. It also soothes stomach cramps. Fresh root ginger is an anti-inflammatory, and may help to ease painful joints.

Parsley delivers betacarotene, vitamin B12, ample amounts of vitamin C and a host of minerals, including iron. It aids digestion, can be used as a breath freshener, purifies

◀ ROSEMARY AND SAGE

the blood and supports the liver and the kidneys.

Peppermint is good for digestive problems. A tisane of peppermint and basil can alleviate flatulence.

Rosemary tea is effective against cold symptoms, fatigue and headaches.

Sage is an antiseptic, antibacterial herb. Sage tea eases indigestion and menopausal problems.

Turmeric is an earthy spice that is valued for its antibacterial and anti-fungal properties. Including it in the diet may reduce the risk of certain cancers. It has anti-inflammatory properties, and may ease painful joints.

▼ CHILLIES

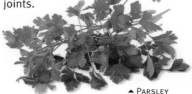

▲ PARSLEY

Foods to avoid

Cut down on foods that are high in saturated fat, including high-fat dairy products, fatty meat and hydrogenated or trans fats found in margarine and processed foods. Drink alcohol in moderation and eat less salt.

If you have respiratory problems, avoid wine, beer, cider, salt, dairy products, wheat, food additives, yeast and red meat. For a weak or compromised immune system, avoid or eat in moderation, dairy products, caffeine, alcohol and processed foods. To ease digestive problems, avoid bran, spicy foods, alcohol and processed foods.

Arthritis sufferers may benefit from cutting down on or eliminating saturated fat and acidic foods, such as citrus fruits. Caffeine, red meat, sugar, alcohol, aubergines (eggplant), tomatoes and potatoes can exacerbate symptoms, so try eliminating these by degrees.

If you are anxious or stressed, avoid or cut down on stimulants, including nicotine, which can deplete the body of valuable nutrients. Alcohol leads to dehydration, and robs the body of vitamins A, C, the B vitamins, magnesium, zinc and essential fatty acids. Tea and coffee inhibit the absorption of iron, magnesium and calcium.

▼ ALCOHOL CAN INHIBIT THE ABSORPTION OF ESSENTIAL VITAMINS AND MINERALS.

▼ CUT DOWN ON THE AMOUNT OF SATURATED FATS THAT YOU EAT.

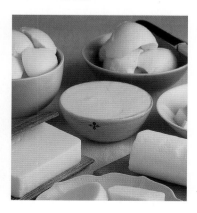

Maximizing nutritional value

To get the most nutritional value from your food, especially fruit and vegetables, it should be as fresh as possible, and any preparation or cooking should ensure that as many nutrients as possible are retained.

• If you grow your own fruit and vegetables, or buy from a farm where the produce is picked or pulled as needed, freshness is guaranteed. If not, make sure your supplier has a rapid turnover.

• Transport produce home quickly. Remove any plastic wrapping. Store produce in a cool larder or in the refrigerator crisper.

• Avoid buying fresh produce from a supermarket or store that has installed fluorescent lighting over displays, as this can cause a chemical reaction, depleting nutrients in fruit and vegetables.

• Buy organic produce where possible, and do not peel it unless absolutely necessary, since nutrients are concentrated just below the skin. Instead wash produce thoroughly. Although prepared vegetables are convenient, it is not a good idea to peel or slice

▼ Buy loose produce when you can: it is easier to check than pre-packed food.

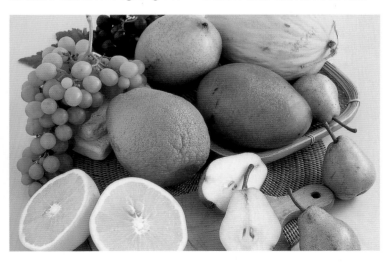

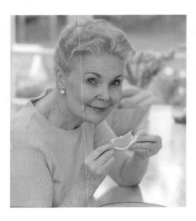

▲ An orange a day supplies an adult with the daily requirement of vitamin C.

produce until you are ready to use it, as the nutritional value diminishes rapidly after preparation.

• Try to eat most of your vegetables and fruit raw. Otherwise, use a steamer in preference to boiling vegetables since soluble vitamins, such as thiamine and vitamin C and B vitamins leach into the water. If you must boil vegetables, use just a little water, and save the water to use in a soup or sauce.

• Buy nuts and seeds in small quantities. Store them in airtight containers in a cool, dark place. Herbs, spices, pulses (legumes), flours and grains should be kept in the same way. Store oils in a cool, dark place to prevent oxidation.

STORAGE TIPS

Apples Store in a cool place, away from direct sunlight.
Bananas Store bananas at cool room temperature, away from other fruit.
Berries Store in a tub lined with a paper towel, in the refrigerator. Use the same day if possible.
Celery Store in the salad drawer of the refrigerator for 1–2 weeks.
Fennel Keep for 2–3 days in the salad drawer of the refrigerator.
Grapes Store unwashed in the refrigerator for up to 5 days.
Squash Can be kept for several weeks in a cool, dry place. When cut, wrap and store in refrigerator.
Tomatoes Store at room temperature; chilling spoils the taste and texture.

▼ To ripen bananas, store them in a brown paper bag with an already ripe fruit. Keep in a cool, dark place.

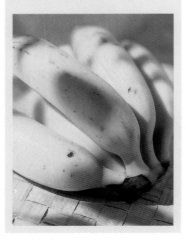

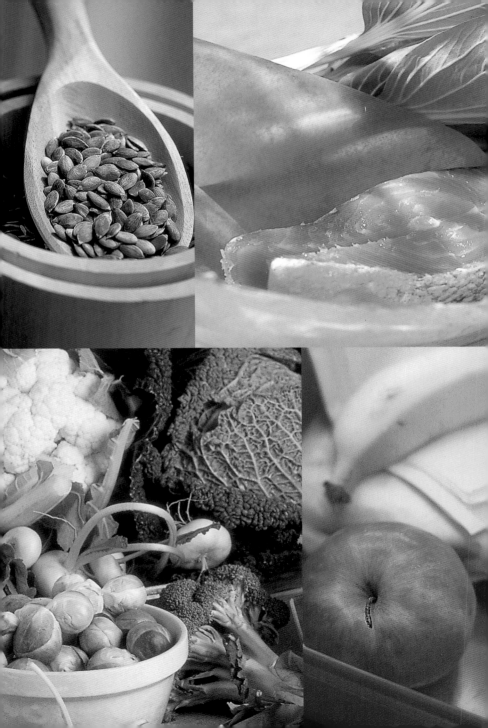

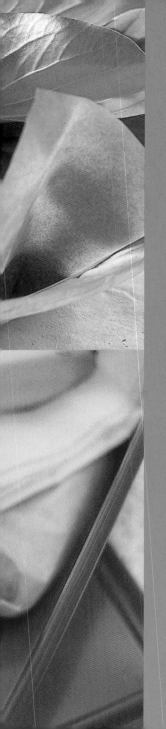

FOODS
THAT HEAL

By thinking more about the food you eat, you are likely to find that your general well-being improves: your skin and hair are in top condition, your body shape finds its natural proportions, you have lots of energy and are seldom ill. Even so, there are times when we all succumb to minor illnesses like coughs and colds or headaches, or just wake up feeling a bit tired or down in the dumps.

The good news is that eating specific foods can be of enormous help in easing all sorts of everyday ailments, either by helping the immune system to work more efficiently, supplying essential nutrients that have been lacking in the diet, or by helping to restore balance to a body system that is under stress.

Easing the symptoms

If you are not in peak physical condition, the signs often show in the body. Dull, lifeless locks don't necessarily mean merely a bad hair day; they may signal that something more serious is wrong.

Thin or brittle nails, successive mouth ulcers, digestive upsets – all these are indications that all is not as it should be. The problem may be something minor, a health hiccup if you like, but it is also possible that there is a more serious underlying cause. Always see your doctor if symptoms persist or are particularly severe. This book offers some suggestions that may help to prevent certain conditions from developing, and ease those that have, but it is not our intention to suggest that diet can ever be a substitute for professional diagnosis and treatment.

Having said that, there are plenty of practical steps you can take to ease unpleasant symptoms. Imagine sipping a glass of papaya juice next time you have a sore throat. As it goes down, the cool

▼ ALTERNATIVE HEALTH PRACTITIONERS CAN HELP YOU COME TO TERMS WITH AN ILLNESS OR CONDITION BY SUGGESTING DIETARY AND LIFESTYLE CHANGES THAT WILL HELP.

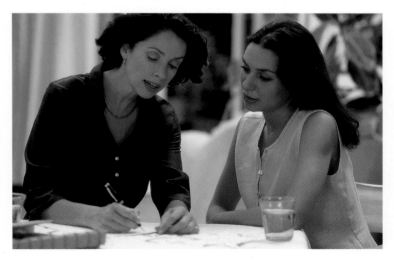

liquid will soothe and comfort, and an enzyme in the fruit will help to alleviate your discomfort. If you have had a bout of diarrhoea, eating live yogurt can help to balance the microflora in the gut. A ripened banana can boost potassium levels and help to bring down high blood pressure.

Nature provides a wonderful natural pharmacy of fruits, vegetables, herbs and spices, which can be of great benefit alongside conventional medical treatment.

▼ EXERCISING HELPS TO KEEP YOU FIT, REDUCES STRESS AND TENSION AND MAKES YOU FEEL BETTER PSYCHOLOGICALLY.

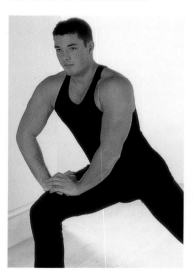

RECIPE SUGGESTION

PAPAYA JUICE SOOTHER
This reviving juice helps the throat, liver and kidneys.
INGREDIENTS
1 papaya
½ cantaloupe melon
90g/3½ oz white grapes

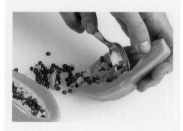

1 Halve and skin the papaya, remove the seeds and cut into rough slices. Cut open the melon and remove the seeds. Slice the flesh away from the skin, then cut into rough chunks.

2 Blend the fruit in a processor.

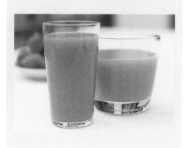

Headaches and migraine

Having a headache is no fun, and when headaches occur regularly, or are particularly severe, they can be worrying as well as unpleasant. If you notice a recurring pattern to your headaches, you need to take action.

If your doctor has ruled out any underlying medical condition, making changes to your diet can make you less prone to headaches, particularly if they are triggered by low blood sugar levels. Erratic eating habits can be a factor, so eat small amounts of healthy food at regular intervals, and don't skip meals.

If you wake up with a thumping headache after a night out, you may be dehydrated so drink plenty of water. Coffee and cola contain caffeine, which affects the blood supply to the brain, and can cause headaches, so drink in moderation.

Tension headaches – the kind that make you feel as though your head is trapped in a vice – may be caused by stress. Make sure you are getting your quota of B vitamins by eating wholegrains, dairy products, lean meat, seafood, green vegetables, nuts and seeds. Vitamin C is depleted in times of stress, so eat an orange or a couple of kiwi fruit every day.

MIGRAINE

Some migraine attacks appear to be triggered by a reaction to a specific food, with chocolate, cheese, coffee and citrus fruits the main culprits. Alcohol, especially red wine, may also be implicated, and there are suggestions that stock cubes, processed meats containing nitrates and even pulses (legumes) can be problematical for some sufferers. Food allergies can be a trigger; if you think this may be the case, seek advice.

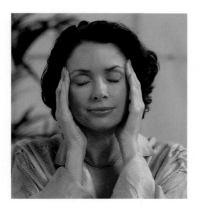

◀ DON'T IGNORE A HEADACHE, PARTICULARLY IF YOU ARE A REGULAR SUFFERER.

Colds and sore throats

Colds are especially common in winter, and characterized by streaming eyes, a sore throat, blocked nose, headaches, aching muscles and a high temperature. Getting plenty of rest and taking care of your health will speed your recovery.

A healthy lifestyle, plenty of exercise and a balanced diet won't stop you getting coughs and colds, but it will help to build up your resistance. You are also likely to recover more rapidly than someone who is below par. If you do succumb, the best advice is to drink plenty of fluids, alternating water with fresh citrus juices. There is some evidence that foods that are rich in zinc can help you fight off a cold. Oysters are the best source, but may not slide down a sore throat all that readily. Try soft scrambled eggs, another source of zinc.

A hot toddy with lemon is an old favoured recipe based on sound nutritional sense. Lemons, like limes, are rich in vitamin C, and have potent antiseptic qualities, making them ideal for combating sore throats and sniffles. Alternatively, try papaya juice, which is great for soothing a sore throat. Reduce dairy produce, which tends to increase mucus production.

If your throat is fine, and you just have a heavy cold, a curry may be just what you need. Include ginger, which is an expectorant, and chilli, a powerful decongestant.

▾ Regarded as one of life's luxuries, oysters are rich in zinc.

▾ Eggs provide B vitamins, vitamins A and D, and iron.

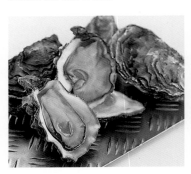

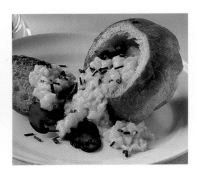

A healthy digestive system

To break down food we need friendly bacteria and digestive enzymes. These are produced by the stomach and small intestine and can get out of balance due to poor diet, stress, antibiotics, food intolerances or toxin overload.

If we suffer these conditions then food remains semi-digested and conditions such as constipation, nausea, flatulence and indigestion can arise. If you are prone to digestive problems, avoid spicy foods, alcohol and processed foods, which can all irritate the gut.

CONSTIPATION

This is a common problem. If there is no underlying medical condition, it may be the result of poor diet, inadequate fluid intake and a

▼ GINGER CAN HELP TO SOOTHE STOMACH CRAMPS. TRY A GINGER AND PEPPERMINT TEA.

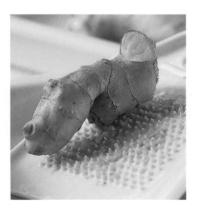

sedentary lifestyle. If you make sure you get enough fibre, drink plenty of water and take some exercise, symptoms can often be alleviated naturally, which is better than resorting to laxatives.

Fresh fruit and vegetables, which are good sources of soluble fibre, stimulate the digestive system, but avoid beans, cabbage and Brussels sprouts, which can cause flatulence and indigestion. Other foods that can boost your fibre levels are brown rice, dried fruit, wholegrain bread and pasta. Bananas are also useful. They are a natural, gentle laxative, and can help to prevent and treat indigestion, and also ulcers.

Eating live natural yogurt can improve the condition of the gut and treat gastro-intestinal disorders. Live yogurt contains active, beneficial bacteria, which balance the intestinal microflora and promote good digestion, boost the immune system and increase resistance to infection.

Irritable bowel syndrome (IBS)

 It is important to see a doctor if you think you may be suffering from IBS, as similar symptoms may indicate other medical conditions. Symptoms include stomach cramps, bloating, constipation and diarrhoea.

If you have been diagnosed with IBS, there are several steps you can take, such as eating live yogurt, which may make you more comfortable. Have plenty of fruit and vegetables, which contain soluble fibre, but avoid cabbage, lentils and beans. Avoid insoluble fibre, such as wheat bran, particularly in break-fast cereals. Also make sure you drink six glasses of water every day.

Linseed can be helpful. Dissolve 15ml/1 tbsp linseeds in 250ml/8fl oz/1 cup warm water and leave overnight. Next morning, strain into a mug and drink the liquid.

In some people, IBS may be linked to food intolerance. If you suspect this, seek professional advice. An elimination diet may help to pinpoint the problem – a nutritionist should advise you.

> ## TIP
> To treat a digestive upset, try grated apple or a glass of apple juice.

▼ HERBAL TEAS AND TISANES, ESPECIALLY CHAMOMILE OR PEPPERMINT, CAN HELP IBS.

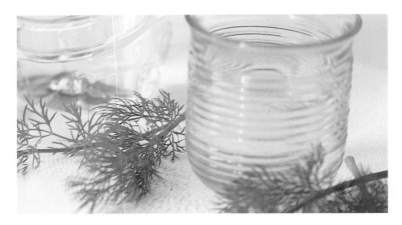

Healthy hair and scalp

Glossy, shiny hair is synonymous with good health, a fact that manufacturers of shampoo capitalize upon. The first step to beautiful hair and a healthy scalp is to eat a well-balanced diet, with plenty of fresh fruit and vegetables.

Aim for a good balance of protein foods, including dairy produce, nuts and pulses (legumes). Your shopping list should include organic artichokes, sweet potatoes, carrots, spinach, broccoli, asparagus and beetroot (beet). Choose apricots, citrus fruits, kiwi fruit, berries and apples. Have plenty of oily fish, and shellfish. Drink six glasses of water a day, and limit sugar.

Dry hair and an itching, flaky scalp may be the result of zinc deficiency. The most efficient way to address this is to swallow an oyster (a single oyster yields 18mg zinc, more than most people consume in a day). Other forms of shellfish are good sources of zinc, too, as are red meat and pumpkin seeds. Essential fatty acids in vegetable oils, nuts and oily fish can also improve the condition of the scalp, while the minerals in sea vegetables, such as kombu and arame, help to make hair lustrous.

Vitamins A and B are important if hair is to be shiny and healthy. Eating liver once a week is a great way of boosting your intake of vitamin A (retinol), provided that you are not pregnant. Fish liver oils are the richest source of retinol, but it can be obtained from eggs and full-cream milk. Also eat carrots, spinach, sweet (bell) peppers, sweet potatoes, peaches and dried apricots on a regular basis. These contain betacarotene, which the body converts to vitamin A.

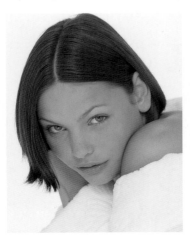

◀ GLOSSY HAIR IS ONE OUTWARD SIGN OF A HEALTHY PERSON.

Improving your skin

The skin is the largest organ of the body, and is especially vulnerable to the effects of modern living. The most useful thing you can do to improve the quality of your skin is to drink water; ideally six to eight large glasses every day.

Also of benefit is regular exercise and plenty of fresh air, so a bracing walk in the country is ideal. If you have a specific skin condition, such as eczema or acne, it is important to consult your doctor, but if you merely think your skin is looking a bit lifeless and could do with a lift, you may find the following advice helpful.

Eat fresh vegetables, especially carrots, spinach, broccoli and sweet potatoes, which deliver the antioxidant betacarotene. Citrus fruit, kiwi fruit, berries (especially strawberries), avocados, vegetable oils, wholegrains, nuts, seeds and some types of seafood provide the antioxidant vitamins C and E, selenium and zinc, which help to transport nutrients to the skin and maintain collagen and elastin levels. Zinc-rich foods, such as liver, pate and eggs, can improve conditions such as psoriasis and eczema.

Apples are rich in pectin, which helps to cleanse the liver, thus aiding detoxification of the skin.

Artichokes are good liver cleansers, too, along with asparagus and raw beetroot (beet). Fish, meat and eggs provide B vitamins, which promote a glowing complexion and combat dryness. Similar benefits are to be gained from eating oily fish such as mackerel, salmon, tuna, sardines and herrings. The fatty acids these fish contain (also found in nuts, seeds and vegetable oils) soften and hydrate the skin.

▼ A GLASS OF WATER WITH YOUR MEAL AIDS DIGESTION AND BENEFITS THE SKIN.

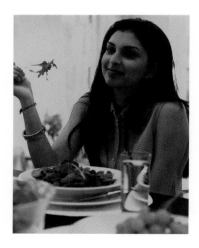

Mouth ulcers

Having a mouth ulcer may not be a major life problem, but it can make you feel pretty miserable as you worry it with your tongue, or try to avoid chewing close to the affected area and biting it with your teeth.

What causes these agonizing little spots is not always clear. They can be the result of an iron deficiency, or failure to take in enough B vitamins, but they might be linked to pre-exam nerves or a similar stressful event. Ill-fitting dentures may be to blame, or a broken tooth. They can also be triggered by a food intolerance.

If you suffer from recurrent clusters of mouth ulcers, it is a good idea to see your doctor, as they may be symptoms of disease.

Take a look at your diet, too. It may be helpful to increase your intake of B vitamins by eating more wholegrains, pulses (legumes), meat and milk. Liver is particularly useful, and will also boost your iron intake, especially if eaten with a source of vitamin C. Liver also contains folate, which is essential for the formation of new body cells, and helps to keep the lining of the mouth healthy. Other sources are pulses, wholegrain cereals and green vegetables.

▼ WHOLEGRAIN CEREALS ARE KNOWN TO HELP PREVENT MOUTH ULCERS.

▼ YOU MAY BE MORE SUSCEPTIBLE TO MOUTH ULCERS IF YOU ARE FEELING LOW.

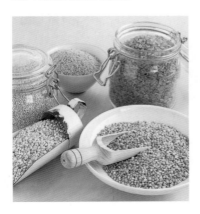

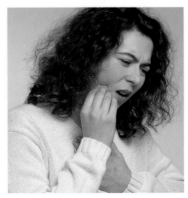

Healthier nails

Our nails reveal quite a lot about our state of health. Ideally, they should be strong, well shaped and flexible. The nail bed should be pale pink, indicating that the blood is adequately oxygenated.

The best way to ensure nails are strong and healthy is to eat a balanced diet, with plenty of fresh fruit and vegetables.

◀ SEAWEED AND SHELL-FISH CONTAIN ZINC.

so a meal of braised liver with onions and cherry tomatoes once a week may work wonders. Chickpeas and tofu are a good choice for vegetarians. It used to be thought that drinking milk – or eating cheese – was good for nails, because of the calcium these foods deliver, but this is inaccurate. Nails are made of a protein called keratin and contain little calcium.

Drink lots of water, and make sure that you get enough iron, which helps to prevent the nails from thinning. Foods that are good sources of iron include liver and other red meat, fish, poultry, green leafy vegetables, dried apricots, prunes and wholegrain cereals. To optimize iron absorption, eat suitable foods with ingredients that deliver vitamin C, such as tomatoes or potatoes, or drink orange juice with your meal. Avoid drinking tea, as the tannin impairs iron absorption.

If your nails are dry and brittle, you may not be getting enough zinc. Seafood (especially oysters), eggs and liver are good sources,

Wide ridges on the nails can indicate a deficiency of selenium, which is closely associated with the function of vitamin E in the body. Good sources are meat, especially liver, fish and shellfish, chicken and wholegrain cereals. Don't worry if you find little white spots on your nails – these are not sinister, and probably indicate minor damage, such as knocking against a table.

Anxiety and stress

It is almost impossible to avoid stress. A hectic workplace, unrealistic demands on our time, trying to juggle a job and care for a family, facing a life change such as retirement – all these elements make it increasingly difficult to cope.

If you are severely stressed, it is all too easy to bottle it up. Counselling can be beneficial or you may need medication. There are also some simple ways you can help yourself. A nutrient-rich diet combined with regular exercise and a healthy lifestyle can help to reduce anxiety levels. Your diet should include wholegrains, dairy products, liver, green vegetables, seafood, lean meat, nuts, seeds, yeast extract, pulses (legumes), eggs and fortified breakfast cereals. These are all good sources of B vitamins, which help the body cope with stressful situations, and correct poor sleep patterns. Vitamin C is depleted in times of stress, so eat citrus fruit, kiwi fruit, broccoli, potatoes and green leafy vegetables. Magnesium levels may be low, too: wholegrain cereals, nuts, pulses, sesame seeds, sea vegetables, dried figs and leafy green vegetables can help to restore the balance. Eating oily fish can also be beneficial, especially if you include the bones. This delivers a double benefit: omega-3 fatty acids and calcium for efficient functioning of the nerves.

Being stressed can affect health in many different ways. The most immediate, and obvious, is its effect on digestion. Taking time over meals, making sure you are relaxed when eating, eating a balanced diet with plenty of fresh fruit and vegetables, and drinking lots of water can only help.

▲ SARDINES ARE A HEALTHY OILY FISH.

Minor depression

It is no coincidence that we crave sweet foods when we are feeling down. Studies show that sweet, carbohydrate foods, like biscuits, chocolate and cakes, help in the production of seratonin, a neurotransmitter that is said to lift the spirits.

Bingeing on sugary foods affects blood sugar levels, and a quick high will soon be followed by a deep low. The answer is to eat complex carbohydrates, like wholemeal (whole-wheat) bread, muffins or scones, cereal bars, brown rice or wholemeal pasta, which are broken down slowly in the body. They will give you a seratonin lift, but its effects will be even and last longer.

The amino acid tryptophan, which the body converts to seratonin, is found in lean meat, poultry, eggs, soya beans and some other pulses (legumes), dried dates, broccoli, low-fat dairy products, bananas and watercress, so next time you are feeling just a bit blue, chop up a banana with a couple of dried dates and eat it with a spoonful of low-fat yogurt. Sprinkle over a few Brazil nuts and you add selenium, a mood enhancer.

Not getting enough iron can lead to mild depression, so make sure you are getting enough of this valuable mineral, remembering that vitamin C is needed if the body is to absorb it properly.

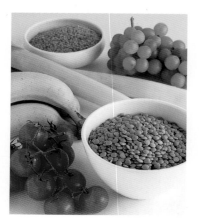

◄ FRUIT, PULSES (LEGUMES) AND VEGETABLES HELP TO KEEP BLOOD SUGAR LEVELS STABLE.

QUICK LIFT
Chillies stimulate the brain to release endorphins, which naturally boost the spirits. Ginger has a similar effect, so a meal of stir-fried chicken, liver or tofu with fresh root ginger and chillies is a savoury solution to feast upon if you are feeling down.

Diabetes

The incidence of diabetes in the Western world is increasing. Many cases of the milder form of this disease are not diagnosed, or are diagnosed too late to prevent some lasting damage, so it is important to be aware of the symptoms.

Diabetes is the result of the body's inability to control the amount of glucose in the blood. An essential form of energy, glucose is produced when we digest starchy and sugary foods. Blood glucose levels rise until a certain level is reached, whereupon the pancreas releases insulin to bring the levels back to normal. If the pancreas fails to produce insulin, Type 1 – insulin-dependant diabetes – is the result. If the body fails to utilize insulin correctly, or the pancreas becomes inefficient, Type 2 – sometimes referred to as adult-onset diabetes – occurs. Symptoms of untreated diabetes include thirst, frequent urination, headaches, blurred vision, weight-loss or nausea.

All diabetics need to control their diet with professional help. To keep blood sugar levels under control, it is vital to eat a balanced, healthy diet, and to lose any excess weight under medical supervision. The diet should be high in high-fibre, starchy carbohydrates, which raise blood glucose levels gradually and maintain them for longer. Wholemeal (whole-wheat) bread, potatoes, rice and pasta are recommended. It is important to eat five portions of vegetables and fruit daily, but very sweet fruit should only be eaten occasionally, because of the fructose they contain. Diabetics who are not overweight may be able to eat very small amounts of sugar in food, but

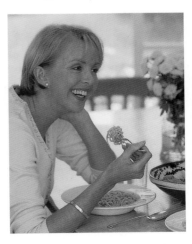

◀ EATING SMALL REGULAR MEALS WILL HELP KEEP YOUR BLOOD SUGAR LEVELS STEADY.

should avoid sweets and sweetened drinks. A low-fat diet is essential, as diabetics have an increased risk of coronary heart disease. Salt should be limited.

It is important to eat regular meals. Grazing – eating little and often – may be a good approach for Type 2 diabetics, helping to keep blood sugar levels steady.

QUICK BEAN FEAST RECIPE SUGGESTIONS

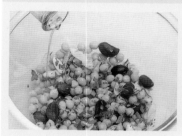

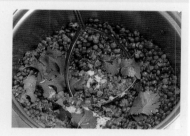

• Mix cooked chickpeas with spring onions (scallions), olives and chopped parsley, then drizzle over a little olive oil and some lemon juice.

• Mash cooked beans with olive oil, garlic and coriander (cilantro) and pile on to toasted wholemeal (whole-wheat) bread. Top with a poached egg.

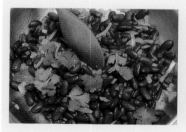

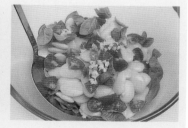

• Heat a little olive oil and stir-fry cooked red kidney beans with chopped onion, chilli, garlic and fresh coriander leaves.

• Dress cooked beans with extra virgin olive oil, lemon juice, crushed garlic, diced tomato and fresh basil.

Restless legs

This may sound like a puppet's problem. The syndrome usually occurs when you sit or lie down. The legs jerk involuntarily and there may be discomfort, "pins and needles" or a burning pain.

The problem is often at its worst at night, making it difficult for sufferers to get to sleep. The cause is unknown, but there is some evidence that RLS (restless leg syndrome) can be inherited. It can also begin at any age. Women who suffer from it may find their symptoms worsen when they are pregnant or in later years during the menopause.

It may help to choose a diet that is rich in iron. Liver, dried apricots, prunes and wholegrain cereals are good sources (avoid liver if you are pregnant). Folate, which is essential for building new body cells, can also ease the symptoms, so eat liver, pulses (legumes), green vegetables and wholegrain cereals. It is also worth increasing your intake of vitamin B12 by eating lean meat and dairy produce.

RLS may worsen as you age. It can be linked to circulatory problems, so the diet should include foods that are rich in vitamin E, such as avocados and beansprouts.

RECIPE SUGGESTION

SPICED APRICOT PURÉE
Try this with natural yogurt.

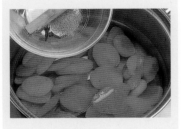

1 Place 350g/12oz/1½ cups dried apricots in a pan with water to cover. Add 1 cinnamon stick, 2 cloves and 2.5ml/½ tsp freshly grated nutmeg. Simmer until soft.

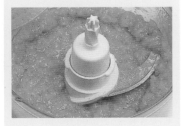

2 Remove the cinnamon stick and cloves. Leave to cool, then purée until smooth.

Fatigue

Are you often exhausted, too weary even to contemplate getting undressed for bed? Do you fall asleep on your desk after lunch? Have you been known to wake up feeling weary or as if you need a good night's sleep?

All the above are typical of chronic fatigue, which can be linked to a medical condition such as diabetes, and must be investigated by a doctor. General tiredness, however, is something all of us suffer from time to time. It may be unavoidable, the result of sleepless nights getting up to a small baby, or studying hard for an exam, or it may be linked to depression or a similar emotional state.

There may be a physical explanation, such as iron deficiency.

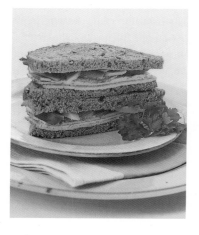

▲ COMPLEX CARBOHYDRATES PROVIDE AND SUSTAIN CONSTANT ENERGY LEVELS. CHOOSE BREADS CONTAINING WHOLEGRAINS.

ENERGIZE

If your energy levels have taken a dive because your blood sugar is low, don't reach for a bar of chocolate or a rich biscuit. The quick energy boost these give will be followed by a slump, and you may end up far more tired than you were at the start. Eat a wholemeal (whole-wheat) salad sandwich instead; the carbohydrate in the bread will give you a more efficient energy fix that will be more prolonged and even.

This can happen when a woman has particularly heavy periods. To redress the balance, eat iron-rich foods such as dried apricots, liver, red meat, pulses (legumes), eggs, green leafy vegetables, fortified breakfast cereals, seeds and wholegrains. At the same time, eat citrus fruit, kiwi fruit or blackcurrants. These are good sources of vitamin C, which is necessary for the uptake of iron into the bloodstream.

Joint problems

Aching joints are a common problem, especially as we get older. The condition may be related to a recognized medical condition, such as rheumatoid arthritis or osteoarthritis, but may simply be down to general wear and tear.

Whatever the cause, aching joints are no fun. Simply straightening up or getting in and out of a car can be very uncomfortable. There is a lot of discussion as to whether diet has any role to play in the prevention or treatment of either condition, but several recent studies suggest that antioxidants and oily fish may help.

▼ DOING TOO MUCH GARDENING, OR TAKING UNACCUSTOMED EXERCISE CAN MAKE YOUR JOINTS STIFF AND UNCOMFORTABLE.

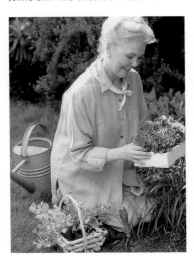

ARTHRITIS

The most common forms of this condition are rheumatoid arthritis and osteoarthritis. The former is a complex condition whose cause is largely unknown. It is an inflammatory condition affecting the joints and is thought to be related to a malfunctioning immune system. It can strike at any age. Osteoarthritis is a degenerative condition of the joints, which most commonly occurs with age, and tends to affect those who are overweight. Certain foods may bring relief to arthritis sufferers, but others can make the symptoms worse. If this happens, an allergy may be implicated. Consult an expert, who may recommend you try an exclusion diet, followed by a tailor-made diet plan.

You can boost your antioxidant intake by eating plenty of green leafy vegetables, also carrots, broccoli, sweet potatoes and avocados, which contain appreciable amounts of vitamins C and E, betacarotene and selenium. Apricots, apples,

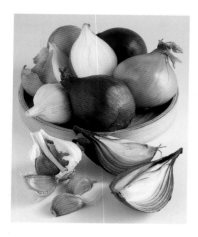

▲ Onions are one of the oldest natural cures. They stimulate the body's antioxidant mechanisms and help arthritis, rheumatism and gout.

sufferers and may help those with osteoarthritis. It is certainly worth eating oily fish more often (about three times a week is recommended) as there are other health benefits too. The vitamin B12 in oily fish is important for a healthy nervous system, and the iodine promotes healthy thyroid function. Fish oils are rich in omega-3 fatty acids, which can help to reduce inflammation. Vegetarians should eat soya beans, tofu, linseeds, wheatgerm, walnuts and rapeseed oil: all good alternative sources of omega-3 fatty acids.

It has been suggested that New Zealand green-lipped mussels may help to reduce inflammation, although there is limited therapeutic evidence of this.

bananas and mangoes are the best fruits to eat. Try eating asparagus and celery, both of which have anti-inflammatory properties, and may help to reduce swelling and ease painful joints. Another anti-inflammatory agent is quercetin, which is found in kelp, onions and apples. Spices that have anti-inflammatory qualities include turmeric and fresh root ginger.

Eat more oily fish
Salmon, tuna, mackerel, sardines and herrings have been shown to offer relief to rheumatoid arthritis

▼ Cook fish the healthy way – try grilling (broiling), poaching or baking it.

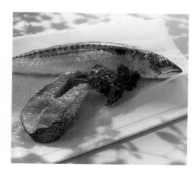

Women's health

Fluctuating hormone levels have a marked effect on women's well-being. Balance can be easier to achieve if you adopt a healthy lifestyle, enjoy plenty of regular exercise and watch what you eat.

PRE-MENSTRUAL SYNDROME (PMS)
Any woman who regularly experiences pre-menstrual syndrome (PMS) will need no explanation of the symptoms. Mood swings, irritability, food cravings, bloating, constipation and diarrhoea can all occur, and when these symptoms are every month, 2–14 days before a period starts, life can be difficult.

Certain foods may offer some benefits. Wheatgerm, wholegrains, bananas, oily fish and poultry are

▼ TAKING PLENTY OF EXERCISE AND EATING A BALANCED DIET WILL HELP RELIEVE PMS.

good sources of vitamin B6, which is especially helpful in combating water retention and breast tenderness. Vitamin B6 can aid the absorption of magnesium, a lack of which causes mood swings and cravings. Magnesium is found in fruits and vegetables. Jacket potatoes (with the skin) are an excellent source, as are avocados and Chinese leaves (Chinese cabbage). Dried apricots, liver, red meat, eggs, green leafy vegetables, seeds and wholegrains are rich in iron, a lack of which can lead to anaemia and

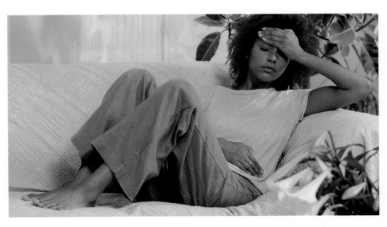

fatigue. To help the body absorb iron, take in plenty of vitamin C, such as kiwi fruit and blackcurrants.

Breast pain can cause discomfort. It may be eased by eating foods rich in essential fatty acids such as oily fish, sunflower oil, rapeseed oil, nuts and seeds, or by eating foods rich in vitamin E such as vegetable oils, nuts, avocados, eggs and wheatgerm.

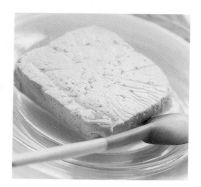

▲ TOFU IS AVAILABLE IN DIFFERENT FORMS, AND CAN BE USED IN SOUPS, SALADS AND STIR-FRIES.

MENOPAUSE

Some women sail through the menopause, but others experience side effects, such as depression, insomnia and anxiety, hot flushes, vaginal dryness and night sweats. These symptoms can be eased by HRT (hormone replacement therapy), but a healthy diet may help.

There is current interest in the role of phytoestrogens – chemicals in plants that act in a similar way to the female hormone, oestrogen. Japanese women, whose diets are high in phytoestrogens, have few menopausal problems and a lower risk of breast cancer. It is hoped that trials will confirm whether eating more phytoestrogen-rich food – soya beans, tofu, soy milk and linseeds – can help Western women.

It is believed that soya products may help to maintain bone density and also reduce the risk of breast cancer. Sweet potatoes contain natural progesterone, and may help to correct hormone imbalance and ease menopausal symptoms. To slow down bone density loss during menopause, eat calcium-rich foods like low-fat dairy products, nuts, seeds, green leafy vegetables, canned fish, pulses, seaweed and bread. Foods rich in vitamin D, zinc and magnesium are also valuable.

Treat yourself to an avocado now and then. This vegetable is rich in potassium, which helps to prevent fluid retention, and is high in vitamin E, which may help to alleviate hot flushes.

A healthy heart

What you eat has a direct bearing on the health and efficiency of your heart and circulation. You may not be able to do anything about hereditary heart disease or stroke, but you can eat sensibly, take exercise and avoid obesity.

Reducing the amount of saturated fat you consume is a vital first step. Limit dairy products, fatty meat and hydrogenated or trans fats found in margarine and processed foods. Foods high in saturated fats are chocolates, cakes, sauces, biscuits (cookies) and puddings. Saturated fat may be listed as hydrogenated vegetable fat or oil.

Eat plenty of fresh fruit and vegetables. The fibre, phytochemicals, antioxidants and vitamins they contribute help to prevent the blocking of the arteries. Green, leafy vegetables and pulses (legumes) are high in folate, which reduces levels of homocysteine. This amino acid has been linked to increased risk of coronary heart disease and strokes. Eat one or two garlic cloves a day. Garlic has been found to lower blood cholesterol levels, reduce blood pressure and help to prevent blood clots forming.

Omega-3 oils have the same effect. You'll find these in oily fish, walnuts, wheatgerm and soya beans. Just one serving of oily fish a week is believed to cut the risk of heart attack by half.

Eat oats, lentils, nuts and pulses. The insoluble fibre they contain can reduce blood cholesterol levels when eaten as part of a low-fat diet.

Red wine, tea and onions all contain the flavonoid quercetin, which may reduce the risk of heart disease and strokes. Drink wine in moderation only.

▼ EATING FOODS HIGH IN VITAMIN E CAN HELP TO IMPROVE THE CIRCULATORY SYSTEM.

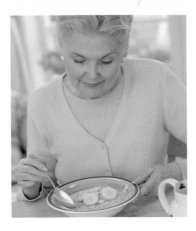

Boosting the immune system

A healthy immune system is the key to maintaining general good health and keeping infections at bay. Poor diet and stress have a negative effect on the immune system, leaving the body vulnerable to colds, flu and disease.

A diet based on unprocessed foods, along with a healthy lifestyle, is essential for maintaining the immune system. Raw fruits and vegetables, especially sprouting seeds, are particularly helpful.

Key protective foods include good sources of the antioxidant vitamins C and E, and betacarotene, which help to boost the immune system. Sweet potatoes and avocados are ideal, as are berry fruit (especially blackcurrants) and citrus fruit. Limes and lemons are also good for colds, coughs and sore throats, and have potent antiseptic properties.

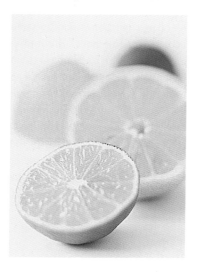

▲ CITRUS FRUITS ARE A RICH SOURCE OF VITAMIN C.

PUMPKIN SEEDS

Boost your zinc intake with pumpkin seeds by
• Sprinkling them over baked goods before cooking.
• Adding them to flapjacks.
• Tossing them into a stir-fry.
• Adding them to a sweet crumble topping.
• Using them to make pesto.
• Scattering them over a salad.

Also good are wholegrains, meat, tuna, salmon, nuts, seeds and bananas, which provide vitamin B. This supports the body's production of antibodies. Zinc is an essential mineral to boost and support a healthy immune system. It can be found in shellfish such as oysters and crab, eggs, beef, turkey, pumpkin seeds, peanuts, cheese and yogurt.

Food allergy and intolerance

Food does not always heal. Food sensitivities – allergies and intolerances – seem to be on the increase, and can cause anything from minor discomfort to more serious risk in susceptible individuals.

An allergic reaction is not the same as a food intolerance. The former occurs when the body reacts to an essentially harmless substance as though it were an invading organism like a bacterium. An immune response is triggered and antibodies are activated to deal with the threat. What happens next depends on the individual, the site of the problem and the allergen itself.

Sneezing and watering eyes are common, as are hives, asthma and eczema. Sometimes the reaction is violent, and can be life threatening, as is the case with peanut allergy.

Food intolerance is more subtle, occurring when the body finds a substance difficult to cope with. Why this should happen is not always clear, but when the offending food is located and omitted

▼ TRY TO ELIMINATE ONE FOOD AT A TIME FROM YOUR DIET AND NOTE ANY CHANGES.

▼ AN ORANGE JUICE ALLERGY DOESN'T MEAN YOU CAN'T EAT OTHER CITRUS FRUITS.

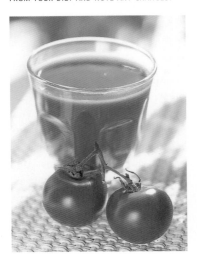

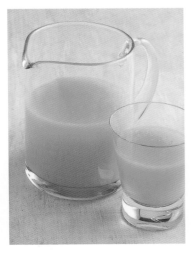

from the diet, the results can be quite dramatic.

There are many different types of food intolerance. Among the common culprits are soya products, caffeine, chocolate, orange juice, tomatoes and food additives. The lactose in cow's milk and the gluten in wheat, rye and barley are often implicated. The symptoms are wide ranging, but can include anxiety, depression, fatigue, headaches, skin disorders, asthma, joint or muscle pain, rheumatoid arthritis and mouth or stomach ulcers. Irritable bowel syndrome can be linked to a food intolerance.

It is one thing to suspect a food allergy or intolerance; quite another to track it down. Seek advice from a doctor, dietician or naturopath.

ALTERNATIVES

If you are lactose intolerant, try switching to soya milk, but make sure you get sufficient calcium from other sources. Live yogurt can often be tolerated, as the bacteria in the yogurt helps to break down the lactose.

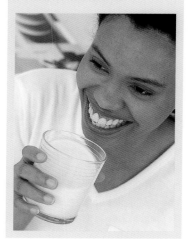

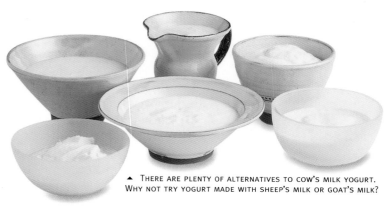

▲ THERE ARE PLENTY OF ALTERNATIVES TO COW'S MILK YOGURT. WHY NOT TRY YOGURT MADE WITH SHEEP'S MILK OR GOAT'S MILK?

food allergy and intolerance **231**

Glossary

Amino acids These are the basic components of proteins. There are 20 in all, 12 of which can be synthesized by the body and eight which must come from our food.

Quinoa, pronounced "keen-wa", is the only known complete food, in that it contains all eight of the essential amino acids that the body cannot make. Usually our bodies obtain them from a variety of foods.

Antioxidants Found in vitamins A, C and E, in co-enzyme Q10 and betacarotene, as well as in minerals like selenium and zinc, these help to mop up free radicals in the body, thus limiting tissue damage.

Betacarotene is what gives fruit and vegetables such as mangoes, apricots, carrots, (bell) peppers and sweet potatoes their bright orange colour. An important antioxidant, betacarotene can be converted into

▲ OYSTERS

vitamin A by the body.

Carcinogens are cancer-causing substances.

Complex carbohydrates These are contained in fresh fruit, wholemeal (whole-wheat) bread, fruit bread, wholemeal muffins or scones, wholegrain cereal, brown rice and wholemeal or buckwheat pasta. The body breaks complex carbohydrates down slowly, providing sustained energy over a long period of time. Complex carbohydrates can also promote sleep if they are eaten towards the end of the day.

Enzymes These are protein molecules that act as catalysts in the body, making it possible for biological processes to take place. Metabolic enzymes are implicated in the building of healthy bones, tissues and muscle. Digestive enzymes, most of which come from the food we eat, ensure that food is digested and made available to the body, or eliminated. Enzymes are vital for every biological function

▼ WALNUTS

and poor enzyme activity can seriously damage our health.

Essential fatty acids Fatty acids are responsible for several bodily processes, including the maintenance of cell walls. The body can manufacture most fatty acids, but two main types – essential fatty acids – must come from food. These are omega-3, found in oily fish, walnuts and rapeseed oil; and omega-6, from corn oil and sunflower oil. These fats are "good" fats, and should be eaten regularly. In effect they help the body to process damaging fats.

Free radicals These are damaging molecules produced by the body as part of a natural process. The chemical structure of a free radical differs from a healthy molecule in that it has an unpaired electron. The electron roams the body searching for a healthy electron to pair up with. This process damages the host molecule, changing its

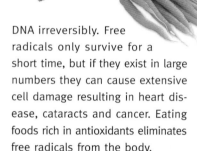
▼ Carrots

DNA irreversibly. Free radicals only survive for a short time, but if they exist in large numbers they can cause extensive cell damage resulting in heart disease, cataracts and cancer. Eating foods rich in antioxidants eliminates free radicals from the body.

Goitre is a painful swelling of the thyroid gland.

Phytochemicals are plant compounds, widely found in fruit and vegetables, which appear to offer protection against diseases like cancer, arthritis, heart disease and hypertension, and may slow down the ageing process. Phytochemicals also have antioxidant properties.

Phytoestrogens These are chemicals found in plants. They mimic the action of the female sex hormone, oestrogen, and can be helpful in reducing menopausal symptoms. Soya beans are a good source.

▼ Sweet potatoes

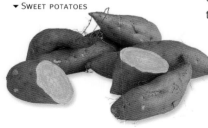

Essential vitamins and minerals

VITAMIN	BEST SOURCES	ROLE IN HEALTH
A (retinol in animal foods, beta-carotene in plant foods)	Milk, butter, cheese, egg yolks and margarine, carrots, apricots, squash, red (bell) peppers, broccoli, green leafy vegetables, mango and sweet potatoes.	Essential for vision, bone growth and skin and tissue repair. Beta-carotene acts as an antioxidant and protects the immune system.
B1 (thiamin)	Wholegrain cereals, brewer's yeast, potatoes, nuts, pulses (legumes) and milk.	Essential for energy production, the nervous system, muscles and heart. Promotes growth and boosts mental ability.
B2 (riboflavin)	Cheese, eggs, milk, yogurt, fortified breakfast cereals, yeast extract, almonds and pumpkin seeds.	Essential for energy production and for the functioning of vitamin B6 and niacin as well as tissue repair.
Niacin (part of B complex)	Pulses, potatoes, fortified breakfast cereals, wheatgerm, peanuts, milk, cheese, eggs, peas, mushrooms, green leafy vegetables, figs and prunes.	Essential for healthy digestive system, skin and circulation. It is also needed for the release of energy.
B6 (piridoxine)	Eggs, wholemeal (whole-wheat) bread, breakfast cereals, nuts, bananas and cruciferous vegetables, such as broccoli and cabbage.	Essential for assimilating protein and fat, to make red blood cells, and a healthy immune system.
B12 (cyanocobalamin)	Milk, eggs, fortified breakfast cereals, cheese and yeast extract.	Essential for formation of red blood cells, maintaining a healthy nervous system and increasing energy levels.
Folate (folic acid)	Green leafy vegetables, fortified breakfast cereals, bread, nuts, pulses, bananas and yeast extract.	Essential for cell division. Extra is needed pre-conception and during pregnancy to protect foetus against neural tube defects.
C (ascorbic acid)	Citrus fruits, melons, strawberries, tomatoes, broccoli, potatoes, peppers and green vegetables.	Essential for the absorption of iron, healthy skin, teeth and bones. An antioxidant that strengthens bones.
D (calciferol)	Sunlight, margarine, vegetable oils, eggs, cereals and butter.	Essential for bone and teeth formation, helps the body to absorb calcium and phosphorus.
E (tocopherol)	Seeds, nuts, vegetable oils, eggs, wholemeal bread, green leafy vegetables, oats and cereals.	Essential for healthy skin, circulation and maintaining cells – an antioxidant.

MINERAL	BEST SOURCES	ROLE IN HEALTH
Calcium	Milk, cheese, yogurt, green leafy vegetables, sesame seeds, broccoli, dried figs, pulses, almonds, spinach and watercress.	Essential for building and maintaining bones and teeth, muscle function and the nervous system.
Iron	Egg yolks, fortified breakfast cereals, green leafy vegetables, dried apricots, prunes, pulses, wholegrains and tofu.	Essential for healthy blood and muscles.
Zinc	Peanuts, wholegrains sunflower and pumpkin seeds, pulses, milk, hard cheese and yogurt.	Essential for a healthy immune system, tissue formation, normal growth and wound healing and reproduction.
Sodium	Most salt we eat comes from processed foods such as crisps, cheese and canned foods. It is also found naturally in most foods.	Essential for nerve and muscle function and the regulation of body fluid.
Potassium	Bananas, milk, pulses, nuts, seeds, wholegrains, potatoes, fruits and vegetables.	Essential for water balance, normal blood pressure and nerve transmission.
Magnesium	Nuts, seeds, wholegrains, pulses, tofu, dried figs and apricots and vegetables.	Essential for healthy muscles, bones and teeth, normal growth and nerves.
Phosphorous	Milk, cheese, yogurt, eggs, nuts, seeds, pulses and wholegrains.	Essential for healthy bones and teeth, energy production and the assimilation of nutrients.
Selenium	Avocados, lentils, milk, cheese, butter, brazil nuts and seaweed.	Essential for protecting against free radical damage and may protect against cancer.
Iodine	Seaweed and iodized salt.	Aids the production of hormones released by the thyroid gland.
Chloride	Table salt and foods that contain salt.	Regulates and maintains the balance of fluids in the body.
Manganese	Nuts, wholegrains, pulses, tofu and tea.	Essential component of various enzymes that are involved in energy production.

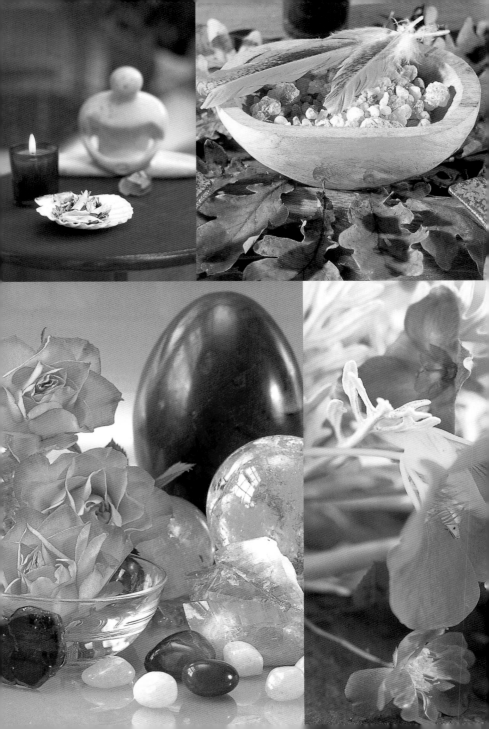

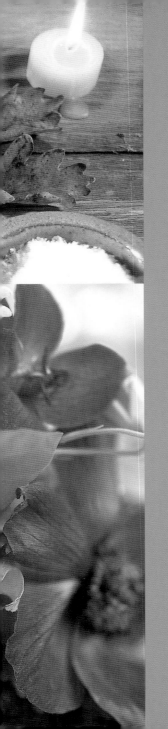

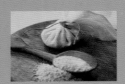

HEALING WITH
AYURVEDA

According to legend, the 52 great Rishis (seers) of ancient India discovered the Veda, or knowledge of how the universe works, in their meditations. These secrets were then organized into a system known as Ayurveda, which means "science of life".

Increasingly popular as a holistic system of healthcare in the West, Ayurveda gives clear instructions on how we can achieve physical and spiritual well-being. Through an understanding of our constitutional type, or dosha, it shows how we can prevent and treat disease by paying attention to diet and lifestyle, and how to strengthen and heal the body using a range of techniques, incorporating yoga, colour healing, crystals, massage and much more.

What is ayurveda?

Ayurveda is the art of living a balanced life. This is the path to good health, happiness and longevity, and Ayurveda teaches a broad-based doctrine of holistic living with practical instructions on how we may best achieve this.

Rooted in the philosophical and spiritual traditions of India, at the heart of Ayurveda is the understanding that everything in the universe is interconnected: we are not isolated individuals but are part of the greater whole, linked to the web of life by invisible energy pathways, or prana, the "breath of life". Similarly, within each of us, every-thing is connected and operating on many different levels. Ayurveda recognizes that our emotions, intellect and physical body, together with our actions and surrounding environment, are all interlinked and influence each other. Good health is achieved when all these aspects are balanced and in proportion with one another. This leads to inner

▼ CRYSTALS HELP TO CHANNEL ENERGY AS PART OF THE AYRUVEDIC HEALING PROCESS.

▼ IN AYURVEDA MEDITATION HELPS TO BALANCE THE THE BODY, MIND AND SPIRIT.

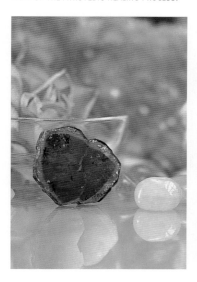

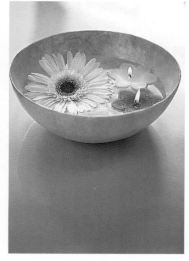

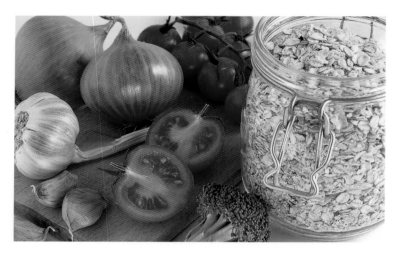

harmony and equilibrium – a feeling of being "at one" with the world and oneself.

There are eight branches to the "tree" of Ayurveda, each one covering various aspects of health and healing, including surgery, gynaecology, paediatrics and medicine. Ayurvedic medicine is the branch responsible for treating our health on a day-to-day basis. Its aim is to prevent and treat ill-health so that we are left free to develop our spiritual potential. This does not mean that you have to have any particular religious belief to benefit from Ayurvedic medicine as the philosophy both acknowledges the uniqueness of the individual, and

▲ CHOOSING A HEALTHY DIET THAT SUITS OUR DOSHA IS THE BASIS OF WELL-BEING.

is also very practical in its applications. It is founded on the belief that all diseases stem from the digestive system and are caused by poor digestion and/or by following an improper diet.

Ayurveda's primary method of treatment is through nutrition, supported by the use of herbs, massage and aromatic oils, but there are also many other outlets, including yoga and meditation, crystals and colour healing. It is about finding what works for you and then applying it to improve your life in whatever ways seem most fitting.

Elemental energies

Everything in the universe is shaped by the cosmic energies of space (or ether), air, fire, water and earth. These forces combine into three fundamental life energies, or doshas, of the human body; vata, pitta and kapha.

The elements are graded beginning with ether, the highest, lightest and most rare, followed by air, then fire and water. The density of earth makes it the heaviest element. Each dosha is a combination of two elements, which predisposes them towards certain principles.

Ayurveda recognizes that each individual is a creation of cosmic energies and a unique phenomenon. No other person has an identical dosha pattern to our own. The combination of vata, pitta and kapha in each of us is determined at conception and is influenced by the season, time of day, and the genetics, diet, lifestyle and emotional state of our parents. Some people are born with a constitution in which all three doshas are equally balanced, which suggests exceptionally good health and a long life span.

However, in most of us, one or two doshas predominate. This unique and specific combination of the doshas is referred to as the "prakruti", our basic nature or constitution. As we experience life's ups

▼ ETHER SUGGESTS A LIGHT AND TRANSIENT STATE. THIS IS THE HIGHEST ELEMENT.

▼ AIR IS HEAVIER THAN ETHER, BUT LIGHTER THAN THE OTHER THREE ELEMENTS.

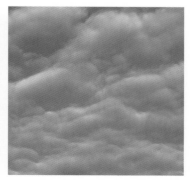

Characteristics of each dosha

dosha	element	cosmic link	character	principle	influence
vata	ether/air	wind	dry/cold	change	activity
pitta	fire/water	sun	hot	conversion	metabolism
kapha	water/earth	moon	moist	inertia	cohesion

and downs, the balance of the doshas in our mind-body system changes. The "vikruti" is our current state of health, influenced by such things as our diet, stress levels, emotional state, physical fitness, and even the weather. If your health is excellent, your vikruti and your prakruti may match. Much more likely, however, is that there will be a discrepancy between the two. The aim of Ayurvedic medicine is to re-establish the balance required by your prakruti.

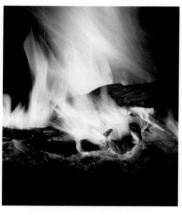

▲ FIRE HAS THE QUALITIES OF HEAT AND DRYNESS. IT IS MIDWAY IN THE ELEMENTS.

▼ WATER SUGGESTS COOL, SMOOTH AND SOFT QUALITIES. IT DESCENDS INTO EARTH.

▼ EARTH IS THE HEAVIEST OF THE FIVE ELEMENTS AND SUGGESTS A SLOW ENERGY.

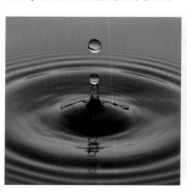

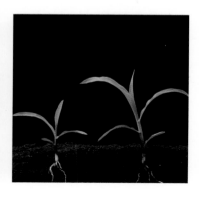

Lifestyle influences

The theory of the doshas is central to Ayurvedic medicine. All bodily, mental and spiritual functions are controlled by the vital forces of vata, pitta and kapha. Health is achieved when these forces are working in harmony.

The subtle energies of vata, pitta and kapha cannot be perceived by any of the senses, yet they are thought to move, increase or diminish, and seem invisibly linked. Changes in the balance of one dosha can have a knock-on effect on the others. In fact the word dosha means "that which tends to go out of balance easily".

Imbalance occurs when we go against our own nature (prakruti) over a long period of time. A modern Western lifestyle and living in an urban environment seems to make us particularly susceptible. Eating an unhealthy or unsuitable diet puts the body under stress. We suffer pollution in our food, air and water, and even the medicines we take have potentially harmful side-effects. We overload our senses by spending too much time on noisy, polluted city streets, working

▼ TAKE TIME TO RELAX AND ENJOY THE COMPANY OF FRIENDS.

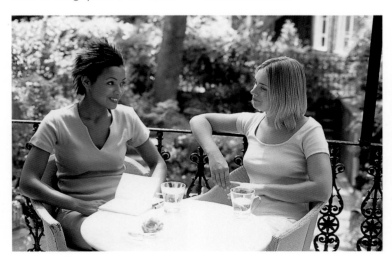

long hours or watching television. There is pressure to live life on the run, eat "fast" food, and overwork in the pursuit of material gain and the realization of goals.

Negative thoughts and emotions affect how we feel, but generally we do not allow ourselves enough time to relax and unwind and to return to mental equilibrium. We tend to forget about the body and its needs and only consider our health when it breaks down and stops us "getting on" with things. When all these factors are taken together, it is hardly surprising that stress-related illnesses are on the increase in the Western world.

However, retreating from life and becoming a hermit is not the answer. Sensory stimulation, desire and challenge are part of life. The approach of Ayurveda is one of balance and it advocates living in tune with nature's laws, paying attention to the rhythms of day and night, the changing seasons and our age. When we get the balance right we live in harmony with our bodies. It is when we go to extremes and pay insufficient attention to the natural patterns of life that we are liable to throw the doshas off balance.

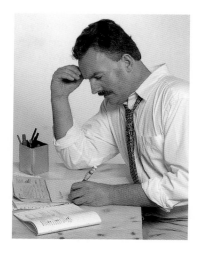

▲ BALANCE YOUR WORKING HOURS WITH RELAXATION, PUTTING THE SAME AMOUNT OF EFFORT INTO EACH.

▼ AYURVEDA TEACHES US TO ATTUNE OUR ATTENTION TO THE NEEDS OF OUR BODIES.

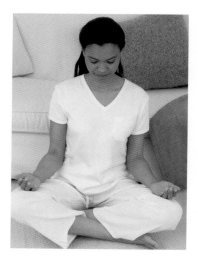

Ayurveda and dis-ease

When the doshas are thrown out of balance their energies become over- or under-stimulated, leading to excess or blocked energy in the body. If these imbalances are left untreated, they will eventually manifest as illness.

The purpose of Ayurveda is to recognize the early warning signs of doshic imbalance so as to "catch" the condition and treat the "dis-ease" before it develops into a serious health problem. If the early warning signs, such as mood swings, low energy levels, persistent aches and pains, or poor digestion over a period of time, are ignored then illness will eventually result.

"AMA"

The main effect of imbalance in the doshas is a build-up of "ama" in the body: these are damaging toxins and waste products. A white coating on the tongue is seen as evidence of ama in the body. The aim of Ayurvedic medicine is to deep-cleanse the system (mind and body) of ama and to restore the balance between the doshas.

▼ DRINKING SEVERAL GLASSES OF WATER EVERY DAY HELPS TO FLUSH OUT TOXINS.

▼ MASSAGE HELPS TENSION TO DISPERSE AND IS PLEASANT TO GIVE AND RECEIVE.

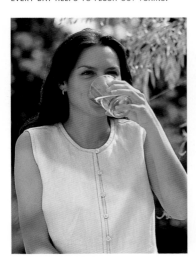

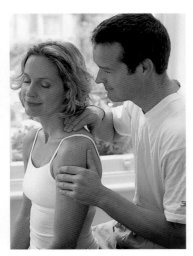

There are many Ayurvedic treatments based on ways to effectively detoxify the system. One simple method is to sip boiled water continuously throughout the day; hot water stimulates the metabolism and encourages the elimination of toxins. Additionally, fasting, eating light meals suitable for your doshic type, meditation and yoga, regular massage and exercise all have a purifying effect on the body and mind. Ayurvedic practitioners advocate moderation in all things to create balance and harmony in the mind and body.

▼ EAT A LIGHT BREAKFAST THAT IS HEALTHY AS WELL AS APPETIZING.

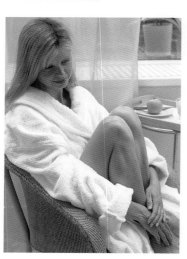

THE SEVEN STAGES TO ILL-HEALTH

Ayurveda sees illness as a gradual process that happens over time and recognizes seven distinct stages. These are states that we are all susceptible to, and some of them are stages that we can actively do something to resolve.

1 Doshic imbalance. This is caused by negative influences, such as poor diet, inadequate rest, environmental pollution or emotional stresses and strains.

2 Aggravation. While the above negative influences continue, the doshas become more seriously unbalanced.

3 Dispersion. The imbalance begins to spread to other parts of the body.

4 Relocation. The affected dosha relocates elsewhere in the body, causing an accumulation of toxic waste products.

5 Mild symptoms. These show in the area where the doshic imbalance is located. It may be at this stage that our attention is brought to our sense of ill-health.

6 Acute illness. In time the symptoms may flare up into an acute condition.

7 Chronic condition. This is the final stage when the symptoms have taken root in the body.

Identifying the doshas

 Vata, pitta and kapha are associated with psychological and physical characteristics that influence how we look, think, feel and function. Ayurveda uses these distinctions to determine our constitution (prakruti) and state of health (vikruti).

The characteristics of the doshas are influenced by the elemental energies that make them up. Ayurveda recognizes specific states: there are hot and cold people, thin and fat people, dry and moist people. These body types will have different tendencies emotionally, mentally and physically, and therefore will be affected by different types of food and need different approaches to treatment.

Ayurveda stresses the importance of following the correct diet and lifestyle for your dosha. A basic approach to Ayurveda is to first identify your dosha, at the levels of both prakruti and vikruti and then learn how to eat and live in accordance with this information. If the vikruti is different from the prakruti,

you should begin by dealing with the vikruti first, following the guidelines for how to heal your current emotional, physical or mental health conditions with the use of diet and other basic Ayurvedic methods. The aim of treatment is to bring you back to your prakruti, where you can then follow the diet and lifestyle guidelines for your dosha type to maintain balance for lasting health and well-being.

Use the self-assessment chart on the following pages to determine your dosha type. Fill it out twice, using a tick for the prakruti, and a cross for the vikruti. For an objective view, you could also ask someone who knows you well to fill it out for you.

◀ VATA PEOPLE ARE LIGHT IN WEIGHT AND TALL OR VERY SHORT.

To determine your vikruti, concentrate upon your current condition and recent health history. To discover your prakruti, base your choices on what seems most consistently true over your whole lifetime. When you have finished, add up the marks under each dosha to discover your balance in prakruti and vikruti. Most people will have the highest score in one dosha. However, if your score is almost equal between two doshas, then you are probably a dual dosha type, or if equal between three, a tri-dosha type.

▶ PITTA PEOPLE ARE OF MEDIUM BUILD.

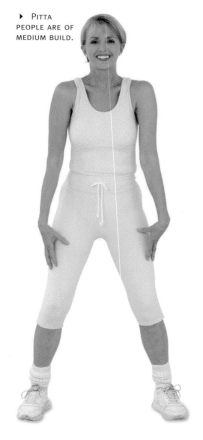

▶ KAPHA PEOPLE HAVE A STURDY BUILD WITH A TENDENCY TO GAIN WEIGHT EASILY.

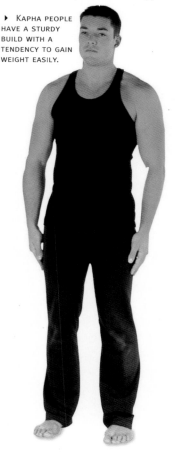

Which dosha are you?

	VATA	PITTA	KAPHA	V	P	K
Height	Tall or short and thin	Medium	Tall or short and sturdy	☐	☐	☐
Musculature	Thin, prominent tendons	Medium/firm	Plentiful/solid	☐	☐	☐
Bodily frame	Light, narrow	Medium	Large/broad	☐	☐	☐
Weight	Light, hard to gain	Medium	Heavy, gains easily	☐	☐	☐
Sweat	Minimal	Profuse, especially when hot	Moderate	☐	☐	☐
Skin	Dry, cold	Soft, warm	Moist, cool, possibly oily	☐	☐	☐
Complexion	Darkish	Fair/pink/ red/freckles	Pale/white	☐	☐	☐
Hair amount	Average	Early thinning and greying	Plentiful	☐	☐	☐
Type of hair	Dry/thin/ dark/coarse	Fine/soft/ red/fair	Thick, lustrous brown	☐	☐	☐
Size of eyes	Small, narrow or sunken	Average	Large, prominent	☐	☐	☐
Type of eyes	Dark brown or grey, dull	Blue/grey/ hazel, intense	Blue, brown, attractive	☐	☐	☐
Teeth and gums	Protruding, receding gums	Yellowish, gums bleed	White teeth, strong gums	☐	☐	☐
Size of teeth	Small or large, irregular	Average	Large	☐	☐	☐
Physical activity	Quick pace, active	Moderate, average	Slow, steady	☐	☐	☐
Endurance	Low	Good	Very good	☐	☐	☐
Strength	Poor	Good	Very good	☐	☐	☐

	VATA	PITTA	KAPHA	V	P	K
Temperature	Dislikes cold, likes warmth	Likes coolness	Aversion to cool and damp	☐	☐	☐
Digestion	Irregular, forms gas	Quick eating causes burning	Prolonged, forms mucus	☐	☐	☐
Stools	Tendency to constipation	Tendency to loose stools	Plentiful, slow elimination	☐	☐	☐
Lifestyle	Variable, erratic	Busy, tends to achieve a lot	Steady	☐	☐	☐
Sleep	Light, interrupted, fitful	Sound, short	Deep, likes plenty	☐	☐	☐
Emotional tendency	Fearful, anxious, insecure	Fiery, angry, judgemental	Greedy, possessive	☐	☐	☐
Mental activity	Restless, lots of ideas	Sharp, precise, logical	Calm, steady, stable	☐	☐	☐
Memory	Good recent memory	Sharp, generally good	Good long term	☐	☐	☐
Reaction to stress	Excites very easily	Quick temper	Not easily irritated	☐	☐	☐
Work	Creative	Intellectual	Caring	☐	☐	☐
Moods	Change quickly	Change slowly	Generally steady	☐	☐	☐
Speech	Fast	Clear, sharp, precise	Deep, slow	☐	☐	☐
Finances	Poor	Spends on luxuries	Rich, good at saving	☐	☐	☐
Resting pulse:						
Women	Above 80	70–80	Below 70	☐	☐	☐
Men	Above 70	60–70	Below 60	☐	☐	☐
			TOTALS	☐	☐	☐

Vata types

Vata is the energy of movement, and regulates all activity in the body, both mental and physiological, from breathing and blinking to the beating of our hearts. All the impulses in the network of the nervous system are governed by vata.

Vata individuals usually have light, flexible bodies and tend not to gain weight easily. Their tendency is towards dry hair and cool skin and, with little fat to protect them, to feel the cold. Most vata types feel

▼ VATA IS A CREATIVE DOSHA — MANY ARTISTS, DANCERS AND WRITERS ARE VATA TYPES.

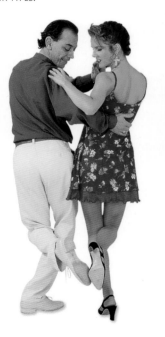

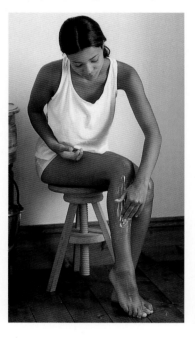

▲ VATA PEOPLE ARE PRONE TO EXCESSIVELY DRY SKIN, CRACKED HEELS AND DRY LIPS.

most comfortable during the spring and summer seasons.

Their constitution is delicate and their levels of energy erratic; they may find it hard to maintain order and structure in their daily lives, quickly becoming bored with routine or mundane tasks. A bundle of nervous energy, the vata type is always on the go, preferring to jog or work out rather than to sit down and take it easy. These individuals may find it hard to relax, which in turn can lead to insomnia and stress-related disorders.

Vata people are clear, quick thinkers, with a highly developed imaginative and intuitive faculty; some may possess clairvoyant abilities. Despite being fearful, anxious types, these people enjoy new challenges and love excitement: they seem to make major life changes, such as change of residence, partner, or employment for instance, much more frequently than other more "grounded" dosha types. This can easily upset their balance and lead to vata disorders.

BALANCED VATA CHARACTERISTICS
- flexible
- artistic, creative
- imaginative, inventive
- changeable
- fresh, light
- emotions: joy and happiness

EXCESS VATA SYMPTOMS
- digestive disorders: constipation, flatulence
- lower back pain, sciatica, arthritis
- nervous disorders
- premenstrual tension
- mental confusion, hyperactivity, restlessness
- emotions: fearful, nervous, anxious, capricious, impatient, irritable

▶ VATA PEOPLE ARE PRONE TO DRY HAIR.

GUIDELINES FOR BALANCING VATA
- keep warm
- slow down and stay calm
- eat regular meals
- eat cooked, rather than raw food
- spend time alone
- keep a regular routine
- put energy into creative pursuits

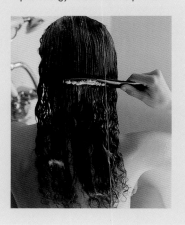

Pitta types

Pitta is the energy of metabolism. It governs all the biochemical changes that take place in the body, regulating temperature and digestion, absorption and assimilation – not only of food, but also environmental, external stimuli.

Pittas have a strong constitution; they enjoy their food and have a healthy appetite. Their body type is usually of average build and nicely proportioned, seldom gaining or losing much weight. Generally they have straight, fine, fair hair and skin that is sensitive to the sun. Their eyes are bright and typically blue, greyish-green or coppery brown. Pittas tend to be

▼ TO BALANCE THEIR WORKAHOLIC NATURE PITTA PEOPLE SHOULD MAKE SURE THEY SPEND TIME IN NATURAL SURROUNDINGS.

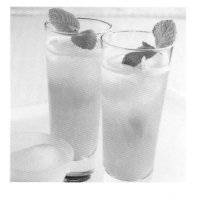

▲ PITTA TYPES MAY NEED TO DRINK MORE IN ORDER TO STAY COOL.

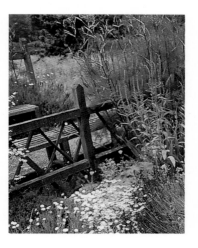

warm and sweat easily, and are aggravated by hot, humid weather.

Pitta types have a keen intellect and a logical, enquiring mind. They love planning and order, and make good leaders and public speakers; they are often attracted to professions such as medicine, engineering and the law, as they enjoy the challenge of going deeply into problems to find a solution. Ambitious, determined and aggressive by nature, their deep-seated fear of failure drives them to succeed. Pitta types are often found reading or working late into the night and many become workaholics, burning their energy through too much mental activity.

Their perfectionist tendencies can make them impatient and intolerant – both towards others and themselves – whereupon they become critical, impatient and judgemental. They are also quick to flare up in anger and are inclined towards jealousy.

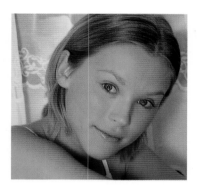

▲ PITTA PEOPLE HAVE A GOOD SENSE OF HUMOUR AND A WARM PERSONALITY.

BALANCED PITTA CHARACTERISTICS
- keen intellect
- meticulous and precise
- capacity for leadership and organization
- enjoys new challenges
- emotions: happiness, humour, warmth

EXCESS PITTA SYMPTOMS
- fevers
- diarrhoea
- inflammatory diseases
- acid indigestion
- skin rashes, eczema
- eye disorders
- premature greying, hair loss
- emotions: anger, hate, irritability, jealousy, envy, fear, bewilderment

▶ PITTA PEOPLE BENEFIT FROM COOLING SHOWERS.

GUIDELINES FOR BALANCING PITTA
- stay cool: cool showers, cool environments, cool drinks
- avoid hot, spicy food
- take time off to relax and slow down
- relax in natural surroundings
- drink more water

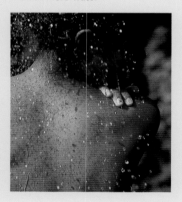

Kapha types

This is the energy of stability, forming the body's structure and supplying the fluids that lubricate the joints, moisturize the skin and heal wounds. It creates and repairs the body's cells, maintains immunity and nourishes our emotions.

The kapha body type is well built, with strong muscles and large, heavy bones. Kapha individuals have thick or fine or wavy hair, smooth skin and large, attractive eyes. They enjoy deep, prolonged sleep and have a steady appetite and thirst, but their slow metabolism and digestion means they have a tendency to gain weight easily, especially if they don't take

enough exercise. Although they are naturally athletic and have plenty of stamina, they are not easily motivated into action – a typical kapha type is happy to sit, eat and do nothing. Winter and early spring are the most difficult seasons for a kapha, when the weather is heavy, wet and cold and it is even more difficult to get motivated to keep exercising regularly.

The kapha individual dislikes change and is happiest following a

▼ KAPHA PEOPLE ARE LOVING AND DEPENDABLE BY NATURE.

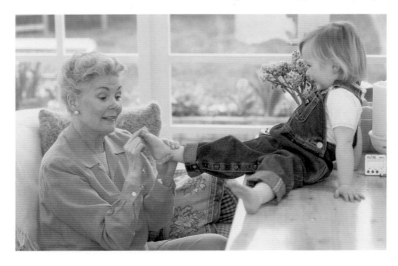

regular routine. They are steady, methodical, practical and pragmatic people – the workers who can be relied upon to get a job done. They have good organizational skills and usually make excellent managers. Additionally, their warm, loving, sensitive nature makes them well suited to the caring professions. Their calm, grounded presence instils confidence in others, acting as a steadying influence on those who are "all over the place".

It is easy for kapha people to get stuck in a rut and fall into lethargy and depression. Once depressed, it becomes even more difficult for them to motivate themselves, and they frequently turn to food for emotional support.

BALANCED KAPHA CHARACTERISTICS

- strength and stamina
- slow and steady
- health and vigour
- good long-term memory
- practical and reliable
- emotions: sweet, loving, sensitive, patient, nurturing

EXCESS KAPHA SYMPTOMS

- congestion
- excess mucus: bronchial/nasal discharge
- sluggish digestion
- slow mental responses
- obesity and fluid retention
- diabetes
- depression
- too much sleep
- emotions: stubbornness, greed, jealousy, possessiveness, lethargy

▸ KAPHA PEOPLE BENEFIT FROM STRONG COLOURS AND REGULAR ACTIVITY.

GUIDELINES FOR BALANCING KAPHA

- wear bright, strong and invigorating colours
- take regular exercise
- avoid heavy, sweet food and dairy products
- vary your routine
- keep active

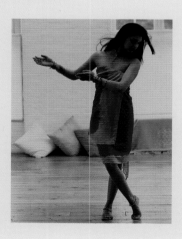

Vata dietary guidelines

Nourishing stews, warming soups and hot, spicy food are good for vata people, whereas cold, raw food is best avoided. To balance their restless nature, they should eat at regular times in a calm, relaxing atmosphere.

HERBS AND SPICES
best source: most of them — particularly warming or sweet herbs; asafoetida helps with the digestion of food.
avoid: caraway.

GRAINS
best source: cooked oats, quinoa, rice, and wheat.
avoid: barley, buckwheat, rye, corn, cereals (cold, dry or puffed), couscous, muesli (granola) and millet.

▼ ALL TYPES OF NUTS AND SEEDS ARE GOOD FOR VATA IF EATEN IN MODERATION.

BEANS, PEAS AND LENTILS
best source: chickpeas, mung beans, red lentils.
avoid: all, except those listed.

MEAT, FISH AND EGGS
best source: beef, chicken, duck, freshwater or sea-fish, shellfish and turkey; boiled or scrambled eggs.
avoid: lamb, pork, rabbit and venison.
• Meat and fish are grounding and strengthening for vata.

▼ ALL FRESH, RIPE FRUITS ARE GOOD FOR THE VATA DIET.

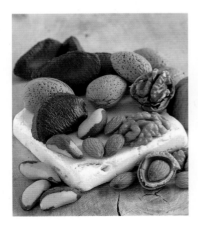

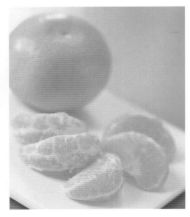

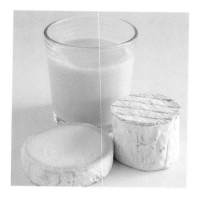

▲ DAIRY PRODUCTS ARE GOOD, ESPECIALLY COW'S AND GOAT'S MILK AND SOFT CHEESE.

VEGETABLES

best source: asparagus, beetroot (beet), carrots, courgettes (zucchini), cucumber, green beans, garlic, leeks, okra, olives, onions (cooked), parsnips, peas, pumpkins, spinach, swede (rutabaga), sweet potatoes and watercress.

avoid: beansprouts, broccoli, Brussels sprouts, cabbage, cauliflower; hot (bell) peppers, mushrooms and white potatoes.

• Cooked vegetables are better than those that are raw or dried.

FRUIT

best source: most ripe, sweet fruit.
avoid: cranberries, dried fruit, pears, persimmon, pomegranate, unripe fruit and watermelon.

COOKING OILS

best source: unrefined sesame oil.

SWEETENERS

best source: in moderation: honey, maple syrup and unrefined cane sugar products.
avoid: white sugar.

DRINKS

best source: some fruit juices, beer or wine in moderation, hot dairy drinks, herbal teas, especially chamomile, lavender, licorice, fresh ginger, peppermint and rosehip.
avoid: black tea, coffee, carbonated drinks, ice-cold drinks – tomato, cranberry, pear and apple juice.

▼ HOT CHOCOLATE IS A GOOD CHOICE OF HOT DRINK IF IT IS MADE WITH MILK.

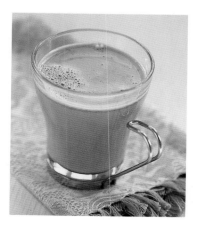

Pitta dietary guidelines

Pitta people should choose cooling and soothing foods, and avoid hot, sour, spicy dishes and fatty, fried or oily food. It is important to eat when hungry, as pitta types easily suffer low blood-sugar levels and become irritable.

HERBS AND SPICES
best source: aloe vera juice (not to be used in pregnancy), basil leaves, cinnamon, coriander (cilantro), cumin, dill, fennel, fresh ginger, hijiki, mint leaves and spearmint.
avoid: all hot spices, cayenne and chilli peppers, garlic, salt, vinegar, mustard seeds and ketchup.

GRAINS
best source: barley, oats, wheat, and rice (especially white basmati).
avoid: brown rice, buckwheat, corn, millet and rye.

▼ CINNAMON IS A MILD, VERSATILE SPICE THAT IS A GOOD CHOICE FOR PITTA PEOPLE.

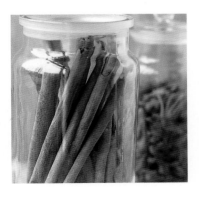

BEANS, PEAS AND LENTILS
best source: all beans, chickpeas, tofu and other unfermented soya products.
avoid: green lentils (except in soup) and red lentils; miso, soy sauce.

NUTS AND SEEDS
best source: almonds, coconut, pumpkin and sunflower seeds.
avoid: all others, particularly cashew nuts and sesame seeds.

MEAT, FISH AND EGGS
best source: in strict moderation: chicken, freshwater fish, rabbit, turkey and venison.
avoid: red meat, all seafood and egg yolk.

VEGETABLES
best source: most, especially asparagus, broccoli, green leaf vegetables, green lettuce, chicory.
avoid: carrots, aubergines (eggplant), spinach, radishes, onions, raw beetroot (beet), green olives, peppers, kohlrabi and tomatoes.

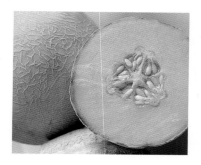

▲ SWEET RIPE MELON IS BENEFICIAL FOR PITTA PEOPLE.

• Include plenty of salads and raw, rather than cooked vegetables in your diet.

FRUIT

best source: fully ripe, sweet, fresh fruit, including apples, apricots, avocados, berries, cherries, dates, figs, mangoes, melons, papaya, pears and plums.

avoid: citrus fruits, fruits with a sour or sharp, tangy taste such as cranberries, rhubarb, strawberries and green grapes.

DAIRY PRODUCTS

best source: most in moderation.

avoid: salted butter, buttermilk, sour cream and yogurt.

COOKING OILS

best source: in moderation: olive, sunflower, soya, coconut and walnut oils.

avoid: almond, corn and sesame oils.

SWEETENERS

best source: most in moderation.

avoid: honey and molasses.

DRINKS

best source: most sweet fruit juices, cow's milk, soya milk, rice milk mixed vegetable juice, beer and black tea.

avoid: hard spirits, wine, caffeinated drinks, sour or sharp fruit juices (such as berry juices), tomato juice and any ice-cold drinks.

▼ PITTA PEOPLE SHOULD EAT HARD CHEESES SUCH AS CHEDDAR IN MODERATION.

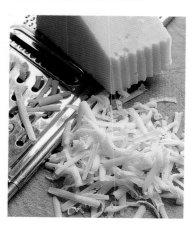

Kapha dietary guidelines

Kapha food should be light, dry, hot and stimulating. Opt for cooked foods in preference to salads but go easy on rich sauces. Dairy products, sweet, sour and salty tastes and an excessive intake of wheat all aggravate kapha.

HERBS AND SPICES
best source: all pungent spices − ginger, black pepper, coriander (cilantro), turmeric and cardamon.
avoid: salt.

GRAINS
best source: barley, buckwheat, corn, couscous, millet, oat bran, polenta, rye.
avoid: oat flakes, pasta, wheat and rice (brown and white).

▼ MOST BEANS ARE GOOD FOR THE KAPHA DIET.

NUTS AND SEEDS
best source: pumpkin and sunflower seeds.
avoid: all nuts.

BEANS, PEAS AND LENTILS
avoid: kidney beans, soy beans (and their products), tofu (cold) and miso.

MEAT, FISH AND EGGS
best source: in strict moderation:

▼ FRESHWATER FISH IS BETTER THAN SEA-WATER FISH FOR KAPHAS.

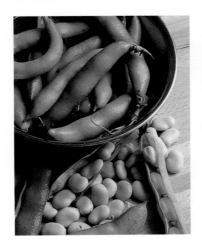

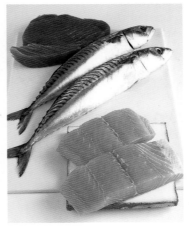

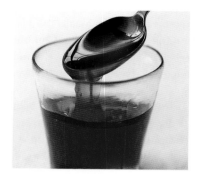

scrambled eggs, poultry, prawns (shrimp), rabbit and venison.
avoid: beef, lamb, pork, seafood (except prawns/shrimp).

VEGETABLES
best source: most.
avoid: sweet vegetables, such as courgettes (zucchini), cucumber, parsnips, sweet potatoes, pumpkin, squash and tomatoes.
• Cooked vegetables are best.

FRUIT
best source: apples, apricots, berries, cherries, cranberries, peaches, pears, pomegranates, prunes and raisins.
avoid: bananas, kiwi fruits, avocados, coconuts, dates, melons, olives, papaya, plums and pineapple.

• Sharp, astringent fruits are better than sweet or sour ones.

COOKING OILS
best source: corn, almond or sunflower oil.
• Use fats and oils sparingly.

DRINKS
best source: fresh fruit and vegetable juices, black tea, herbal teas, hot soy milk drinks, dry red or white wine very occasionally.
avoid: fizzy, caffeinated drinks, coffee, orange juice, tomato juice and iced drinks.

▼ SQUASH IS A SWEET-TASTING VEGETABLE AND SHOULD BE AVOIDED BY KAPHA PEOPLE. SWEET FOODS HINDER A KAPHA'S ENERGY.

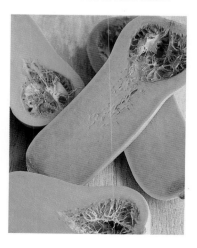

Optimum living

Ayurveda stresses the importance of living a balanced life. It is all very well following the dietary guidelines for our dosha type, but if we neglect to take care of ourselves in the rest of our lives, then our efforts will be less effective.

Regular exercise plays an important role in staying healthy for all dosha types. It keeps the body strong and stimulates the digestive system to work more effectively.

Kaphas will get the most benefit from vigorous exercise, such as running, fast swimming, aerobics and fitness training, which will help to cleanse the body and dispel sluggish, lazy feelings. Kaphas should exercise more when the weather is cold and damp. Pittas require a moderate amount of

▼ THE TYPE OF EXERCISE YOU SHOULD DO IS DETERMINED BY YOUR CONSTITUTION.

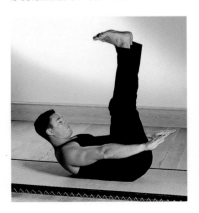

exercise, done for the fun of it rather than to be top dog; jogging, team sports and tai chi are all good. Vata people benefit from gentle, relaxing forms of exercise. They are the most easily exhausted of the dosha types, so they should not overdo things. Walking, yoga and slow swimming are ideal, although vata people can undertake most sports and activities, so long as they don't push themselves beyond their limits.

ROUTINE

Keeping a regular routine for vital activities such as sleeping, eating, exercising, bathing and working helps us to maintain balance in our lives. Ayurveda recommends harmonizing our internal body clock with the natural rhythm of the day. Long-distance travel, working night shifts, and eating at irregular times can all throw our body clock, and the doshas, off balance, making us feel out of sorts and out of harmony with those around us.

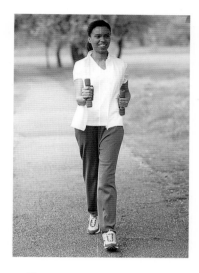

▲ WE ARE AT OUR MOST ACTIVE BETWEEN 10AM AND 2PM.

THE DAILY CYCLE

Ayurveda divides the day into two cycles, which roughly correspond with day and night. Each cycle has three phases, governed by one of the doshas.

DAY

06.00–10.00 kapha time of day. The body is gathering energy to begin the day. This is the best time for purification rituals (shower, cleansing, eliminating), yoga and meditation. Eat a light breakfast.

10.00–14.00 pitta time of day. The appetite is strongest at lunch-time so have your main meal of the day between these hours.

14.00–18.00 vata time of day. This is the most creative and communicative time of the day. Take a regular break to avoid activity turning into stress. The late afternoon is a good time to meditate.

NIGHT

18.00–22.00 kapha time of night. The body tires. Eat a light meal and take a walk to aid digestion.

22.00–02.00 pitta time of night. Avoid strenuous activity. Go to bed at a reasonable hour.

02.00–06.00 vata time of night. The body shuts down.

▼ ALL DOSHAS SHOULD ADOPT A ROUTINE THAT ADHERES TO THE NATURAL RHYTHM OF THE DAY AND NIGHT.

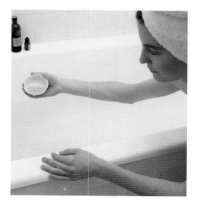

The cycles of life

The seasons of the year show us that life is cyclical; an ever-lasting round of gestation, birth, growth, decline and death. The doshas are inevitably related to these natural laws and follow this regenerative cycle.

The doshas are sensitive to changes in weather conditions, which loosely tie in with the seasons. Vata is highest in autumn and early winter, and at times of dry, cold and windy weather. The pitta season is late spring and summer and during times of heat and humidity. Kapha is highest in the winter months and during early spring when the weather is cold and damp.

Ayurveda recommends that we take these seasonal changes into account when we are planning our eating and lifestyle habits, as the weather can aggravate or cause doshic imbalance. For instance, during the cold, damp months of winter, kapha accumulates. This leads to more "damp" in the body in the form of excess mucus, and is the traditional season for coughs and colds. This is made much more likely if your diet is high in foods that aggravate the kapha condition – lots of dairy products and heavy, rich food – and more likely still if

▼ SPRING IS THE TIME TO CONSIDER A CLEANSING FAST TO CLEAR EXCESS KAPHA.

▼ SUMMER IS THE SEASON OF HEAT. COUNTER IT WITH SOOTHING ACTIVITIES.

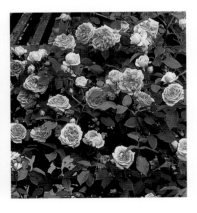

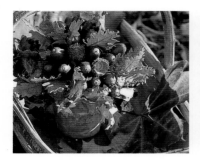

▲ AUTUMN IS THE SEASON OF CHANGEABLE WEATHER AND INCREASED LEVELS OF VATA.

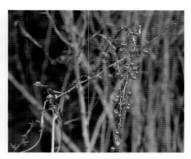

▲ KAPHA PEOPLE FIND IT HARD TO MOTIVATE THEMSELVES IN WINTER.

you are a kapha or have a kapha imbalance (vikruti).

If you are a dual or tri-dosha type, work with whichever dosha predominates at any given time. For example, if you are a vata-pitta type, choose foods from the pitta eating plan during the summer months and from the vata plan during the autumn and winter.

THE STAGES OF LIFE

Ayurveda also sees the human life span in terms of the doshas.

0–30 years – kapha: this is the time of growth and development.

30–60 years – pitta: we apply the skills and knowledge of our kapha years to this time of life.

60+ years – vata: physical decline and spiritual growth.

WEATHER/SEASON	VATA	PITTA	KAPHA	BEST ACTION
warming up (spring)	neutral	accumulating	aggravated	cleansing fast to clear excess kapha
hot (summer)	accumulating	aggravated	decreasing	wear cooling colours, eat raw foods, rest and relax
cooling (autumn)	aggravated	decreasing	neutral	stay warm and comfortable; follow a regular routine
cold (winter)	decreasing	neutral	accumulating	treat kapha dosha with spices and warm drinks

Yoga

An important element of Ayurvedic therapy is yoga as an exercise and a therapy. It is not only a physical discipline that helps to keep the body strong and supple, but it also calms the mind and helps us to find inner peace.

Yoga works with a variety of techniques, including physical postures, breathing exercises, relaxation and meditation. In its purest form it is a preparation for spiritual enlightenment, but it is also an effective therapy in the treatment of stress and chronic disease conditions.

Vata types are particularly suited to the gentle, rhythmic nature of yoga exercise, but all three doshas can benefit from yoga.

STANDING WARM-UPS

Before practising yoga, it is best to warm-up and stretch out the body. Stand relaxed but tall with the spine erect and the feet hip-width apart. Bring your hands together in front of your chest into prayer position. Raise your arms to the sides and come up on to your toes. Breathe in and stretch the arms up. Then breathe out to lower the arms and heels. Get a vigorous swinging movement going, opening the chest, stretching the spine and "waking up" the circulation.

SALUTE TO THE SUN

The following routine is best practised on rising first thing in the morning. The sequence should be repeated between two and six times. It is a good exercise to get yourself moving and release sluggish, tired feelings.

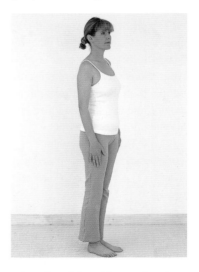

1 Stand upright with your hands at your side, knees and shoulders relaxed and your neck fully extended upwards. Inhale.

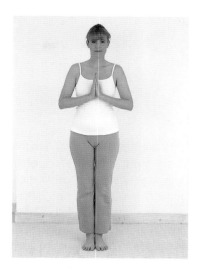

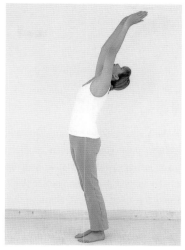

2 Look straight ahead. Breathe out while bringing the palms of your hands together at chest height into the prayer position.

3 Breathe in deeply. Keeping your hands together, raise your hands over your head. Arch your back as far as is comfortable. Exhale slowly.

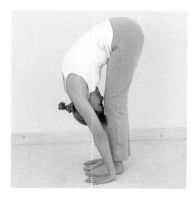

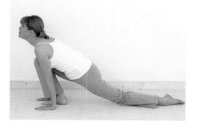

4 Bend forward to touch the floor if you can, at each side of your feet.

5 Breathing in, bend your right knee and slide and extend your left leg out behind you. Your knee rests on the floor. Put the hands on the floor. Extend your neck upwards.

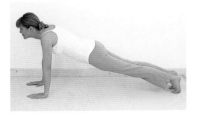

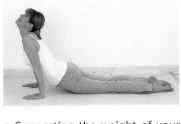

6 With your hands flat on the floor, extend your right leg out to meet your left leg. Take your weight up on to your hands and your toes. Keep the neck straight. Breathe out. Lower the body flat to the ground.

7 Supporting the weight of your upper body on your arms, raise your chest, stomach and pelvic bones from the ground. Extend your neck upwards. Exhale slowly. Breathing in, lower your stomach and pelvis back down to the floor.

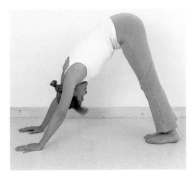

8 In one movement, raise your bottom and pull yourself up into an arch. Extend your arms and legs fully. Lower your heels towards the floor (but don't strain). Bend your left knee so that it touches the ground part way between your right foot and hands. Bring the right foot to the side of the left knee.

TYPES OF YOGA

There are many different types of yoga. The most widely practised in the West is "Hatha" yoga. Hatha yoga is just one branch of yoga and within this branch there are various sub-categories.

• Astanga Vinyasa: a fast series of challenging postures performed using synchronized breathing. This is probably the most aerobic form of yoga.

• Iyengar: alignment and precision of movement are used to enhance posture, breathing and flexibility.

• Kundalini: breathing techniques and prana (life force) are worked on to balance the body's energy and achieve relaxation.

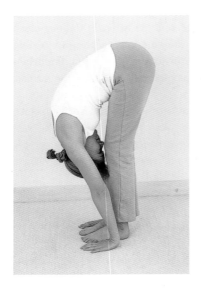

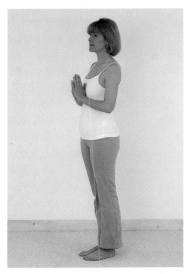

9 Move your hands back to your feet and return to position 4

10 Breathe in deeply as you raise your torso and repeat step 2.

11 Breathe out slowly as you lower your arms and return to the starting position. Look straight ahead, allow your breathing to return to normal, then repeat the whole sequence with the other leg.

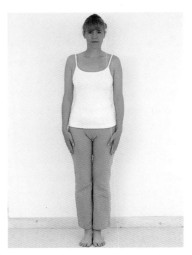

CAUTION
This sequence is not suitable during pregnancy, the menstrual cycle, if you are suffering from any physical injury, or back pain.

Relaxing meditation

Meditation is food for the soul. Its effect is to deep-clean the mind and transform the emotions, leaving us feeling refreshed and calm. It is one of the most important methods in Ayurveda for permanently stabilizing the doshas.

Ayurvedic practitioners believe that toxins (ama) in the body also have their emotional and mental counterparts. Emotional states, such as greed, envy, jealousy and anger, negative thoughts and compulsive behaviour patterns create psychic "dirt" or emotional ama. They are as detrimental to our health as the chemical stress hormones produced by the body.

DAILY MEDITATION
Make meditation a part of your daily routine. Practise it for 10–15 minutes a day. Sunrise and sunset are the best times to meditate, but find a time that is convenient for you and stick to it. Some people like to use a (gentle) alarm to indicate when the session is finished.

1 Find a quiet place where you won't be disturbed. Either sit on a straight-backed chair or cross-legged on the floor. It is important that you are relaxed and comfortable and that your spine is straight.

2 Place your hands, palms upmost, on your thighs. Alternatively, rest your hands on your knees or on a small cushion on your lap.

3 Close your eyes and become aware of your breathing. With every out-breath, think "letting go".

4 Focus your attention inwards, allowing any noises or distractions outside to fade away.

▼ THE CLASSIC YOGA POSE, THE LOTUS POSITION, HAS BECOME SYMBOLIC OF RELAXATION AND MEDITATION. HOWEVER, IT TAKES SUPPLE JOINTS AND PRACTISE TO ACHIEVE IT.

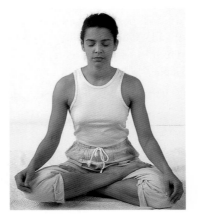

5 Don't try to control your mind – either by trying to hold on to a particular thought, or by rejecting any other. Meditation is all about accepting what you find and just allowing it to be there. Let your mind wander freely.

6 Remember to stay focused on your breath (this will naturally help to quieten the mind) and keep your body relaxed.

7 When you are ready, open your eyes and let yourself return to normal waking consciousness. Slowly get up and have a good stretch, ready to face the world again with renewed vigour.

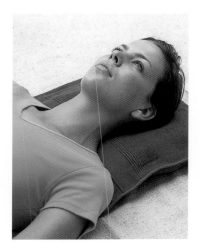

▲ YOU CAN MEDITATE LYING DOWN, BUT DON'T CHOOSE A BED FOR YOUR SURFACE OR YOU MAY FIND YOURSELF FALLING ASLEEP.

▼ AT THE END OF YOUR MEDITATION, HUG YOUR KNEES INTO YOUR CHEST, THEN STRETCH OUT YOUR LIMBS.

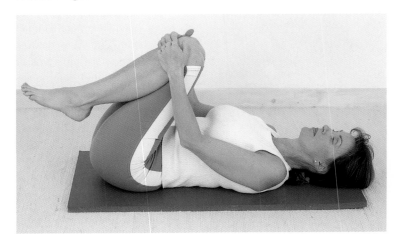

The radiance of colour

Colour is a delight to our visual sense and its subtle vibrations affect us on all levels of our being. Ayurvedic treatments make use of the healing powers of colour to restore or stabilize the balance between the three doshas.

COLOURS AND THE DOSHAS

We can use colour to influence our well-being in the clothes we wear, the food we eat, and in our environment. The vibrations of certain colours help or aggravate each of the doshas.

VATA

Energetic vata individuals benefit from most of the pastel colours and earthy colours that are gentle and warm to look at, such as ochres, browns and yellows. Brown and ochre help to draw energy down through the body's system, stabilizing and grounding the vata personality; yellow is linked to the mind and will help to keep the vata mentally alert. Minimize the use of dark and cool colours, such as blues, browns and black.

PITTA

Excess pitta (such as irritability and impatience) is balanced by wearing cooling and calming colours, such as green, blue, violet, or any quiet pastel shade. Blue is a healing colour and helps the pitta type to remain open without being over-stimulated; green soothes the emotions and encourages harmonious feelings; and violet increases awareness of spiritual issues. Reds and oranges can inflame the pitta dosha, and yellow, gold and black should be minimized.

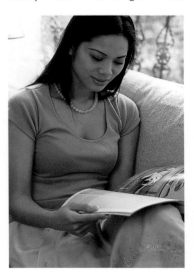

◀ PASTEL COLOURS ARE LIBERATING FOR VATA PEOPLE.

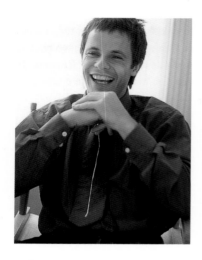

SOOTHING BLUE CALMS A PITTA PERSON.

KAPHA

The lethargy of kapha is balanced by bright, lively, bold colours, especially reds, oranges and warm pinks. Both reds and pinks are energizing and positive but red should be used sparingly as it may be over-stimulating. Orange is a warming, nourishing colour that feeds the sexual organs and helps to remove congestion in the system. Yellow and gold are also good colours for kapha, but greens, dark blues or white are best avoided.

COLOUR INFUSIONS

In Ayurveda colour is an important healing tool. Different colours carry specific energies. To make a colour infusion wrap a piece of coloured fabric or film around a glass of water and leave it to stand in the sun for 4 hours. The water will become infused with the vibrations of that colour, and drinking it is said to bring beneficial results.

KAPHA PEOPLE SHOULD CHOOSE VIBRANT COLOURS TO HELP MOTIVATE THEMSELVES INTO ACTION.

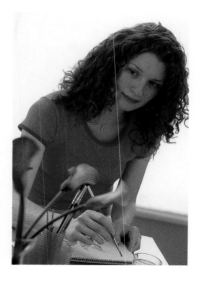

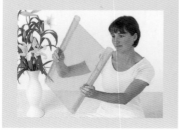

Crystals and gems

All substances in nature are believed to contain the creative intelligence of the cosmos. Gems and crystals have healing energies that enliven the vital energy centres (chakras) in the body, and can be utilized to harmonize the doshas.

Stones are able to act as energy transmitters, having the power to store, magnify and transform energy. This means it is important to always clean any stone before it is used for healing purposes; leave it to soak in salt water overnight and then rinse thoroughly. Once the stone is free from any psychic "dirt", you can then make an infusion by placing it in a glass bowl of spring water and leaving it in sunlight for about 4 hours. Drain off the water and drink it.

VATA

Rose quartz balances excess vata and brings relief to conditions such as nervousness, dry skin and hair, constipation and bloating. Topaz is a warm stone that dispels fear and is ideal for calming vata anxiety; wear it when you want to feel confident and in control. Amethyst has balancing properties and is useful for troublesome emotional states or when clarity of mind is needed.

▼ CRYSTALS ARE IMPORTANT HEALING TOOLS IN AYURVEDA.

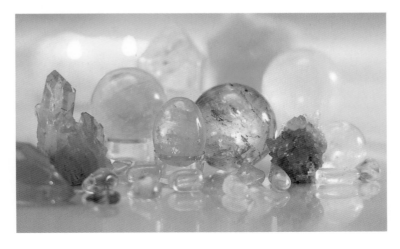

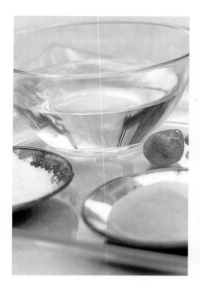

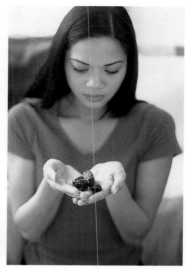

▲ CLEANSE CRYSTALS IN A BOWL OF SALT WATER BEFORE USE.

▲ ATTUNE YOUR ATTENTION TO CRYSTALS TO BENEFIT FROM THEIR ENERGY.

It also helps to promote feelings of inner peace and harmony. Quartz crystal also helps to calm vata and enhances intuition.

PITTA

Pearls (or mother-of-pearl), red coral and moonstone are all good for reducing excess pitta. All three stones have a soft and cooling energy vibration that can help to calm inflammatory conditions, such as angry emotions, skin rashes, all "-itises", and acid indigestion. Amethyst encourages compassion

and dignity and is also good for pitta imbalances.

KAPHA

Deep red stones, such as ruby or garnet, stimulate kapha energy and balance the effects of excess kapha conditions, including water retention, lethargy, depression, weight problems and sinus and respiratory disorders. The refined, subtle vibrations of lapis lazuli will also help to lift excess kapha from its slow, heavy nature to something more light and ethereal.

Aromas and massage

Our sense of smell is directly related to the balance of the doshas. Fragrant essential oils, extracted from hundreds of different plants and their components, can be used to balance the mind and heal the emotions.

Essential oils are inhaled and/or massaged into the skin. They should not be put directly on the skin or taken internally; some oils are contra-indicated in pregnancy or for some medical conditions.

AROMAS AND THE DOSHAS
Warm, sweet, calming and earthy aromas balance vata. These include camphor, eucalyptus, ginger, musk, sandalwood and jatamansi (a spikenard species from India). A blend of basil, orange, geranium, and cloves is good for harmonizing vata imbalance, and other useful fragrances include lavender, pine and frankincense.

Pitta is soothed by cooling, calming, sweet aromas such as honeysuckle, jasmine, sandalwood and rose. Rose geranium, lemongrass, fennel or mint are helpful.

Warm and stimulating or spicy, earthy fragrances are helpful for kapha. These include eucalyptus, cinnamon, myrrh, thyme, basil, musk, camphor, cloves, rosemary, ginger and sage. Juniper oil is especially useful for lymphatic drainage.

▼ LOOKING AT A ROSE AS WELL AS SMELLING ONE LIFTS THE SPIRITS AND PROMOTES FEELINGS OF WELL-BEING.

▼ ESSENTIAL OILS ARE APPLIED TO THE SKIN IN A "CARRIER" OIL, SUCH AS ALMOND OR WHEATGERM.

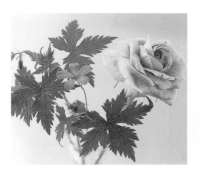

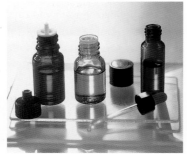

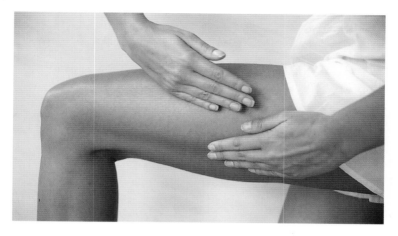

Massage and the doshas

To massage with essential oils, add 7–10 drops of the chosen essential oil to 25ml/1½ tbsp carrier oil.

Vatas enjoy gentle, soothing and relaxing massage. Use stroking movements and pay attention to areas of tight, dry skin. Pitta massage should be calming and relaxing. Use deep and varied movements and go easy wherever there is stiffness or soreness.

A vigorous massage stimulates the sluggish kapha metabolism. Use fast and strong movements, using very little oil or none at all (talcum powder may be used instead). To encourage lymphatic drainage, pay particular attention to the hip and groin area and around the armpits.

▲ PITTAS SHOULD HAVE A SLOW MASSAGE RHYTHM AND AVOID SUDDEN MOVEMENTS.

▼ A DAILY FOOT AND HAND MASSAGE WILL ACT AS A GROUNDING AND STABILIZING INFLUENCE FOR VATAS.

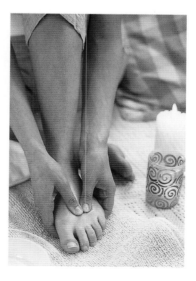

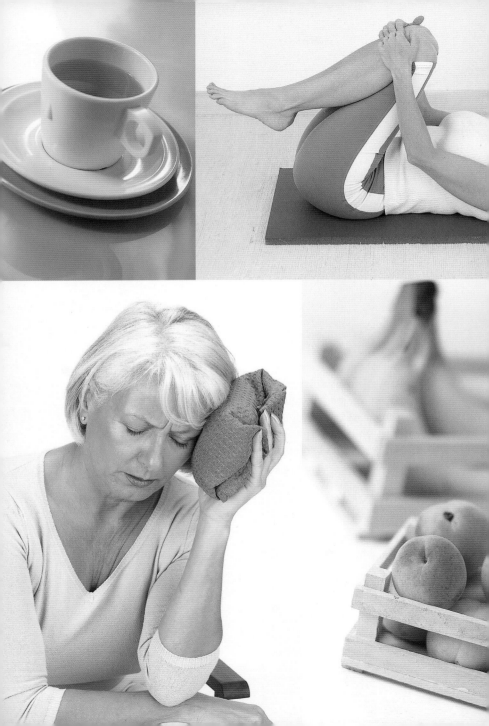

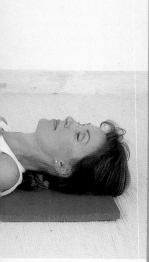

AYURVEDA
FOR COMMON AILMENTS

In Ayurveda, health problems are treated according to dosha. Some conditions may affect vata, pitta or kapha types, while others may be linked to one dosha. Diarrhoea, for example, is a pitta condition, while constipation is a vata one. When treating an ailment, you will need to determine the character of the symptoms, and follow the eating and lifestyle plan for that dosha to bring it back into balance.

Some of treatments in the following section recommend special Ayurvedic herbal remedies. These herbs are available from Ayurvedic Health suppliers and can be obtained via the internet. Always consult a qualified Ayurvedic or medical doctor if your symptoms fail to improve, or if you are unsure.

Digestive disorders

The gastro-intestinal tract is the most important part of the body, and the seat of the doshas. Our dosha type and lifestyle factors all influence the digestive system and each dosha is subject to particular disorders.

Regular bowel movements are a sign of a healthy gastro-intestinal tract (GI). Vata types are prone to irregular digestion and typical vata conditions include constipation, gas/flatulence, and tension (causing stomach cramps or spasms).

Constipation
Drinking a glass of hot water each morning will help to get things moving. Herbs include triphala and satisabgol (psyllium husks). Triphala is a special Ayurvedic combination of three herbal fruits. It should not

▼ Buy Ayurvedic herbs from a specialist stockist.

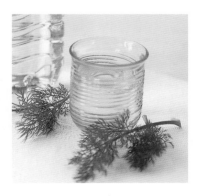

be used during pregnancy or if you suffer from ulcers of the GI. Satisabgol is gentle and soothing and a good "bulking" agent.

Gas, Bloating and colic
If undigested food stays in the system for too long it begins to ferment, causing a range of unpleasant symptoms. Ayurvedic medicine recommends hingvastak, a herbal mix that includes asafoetida, ginger, black pepper and cumin.

Pitta digestion tends to be too fast. These types easily "burn" up food in anger or frustration and typical pitta problems include acidity and heartburn and diarrhoea.

Acidity and heartburn
Sip aloe vera juice to cool an inflamed digestive system (but not if you are pregnant). Use herbal preparations of shatavari, licorice (not to be used with high blood pressure or oedema) and amalki to balance acidity.

Diarrhoea

Avoid hot spices and eat small meals. Drink nettle tea to balance the digestive system and add coriander (cilantro), saffron, fresh ginger and nutmeg to your diet. A simple diet of rice, split mung dhal and vegetables is recommended while symptoms last.

The kapha metabolism is slow and problems of the GI lead to obesity, nausea, a build-up of mucus and poor circulation. Herbs for kapha conditions include trikatu ("three hot things"), which contains ginger, pippali and black pepper. Hot spices in general, such as chilli peppers, garlic and ginger are helpful for invigorating and cleansing the system. Regular vigorous exercise will help to keep kapha people moving and avoid stagnation.

◀ IF YOU HAVE A STOMACH UPSET, TRY TAKING A TONIC OF NETTLE TEA. IT WILL HELP TO BALANCE THE DIGESTIVE SYSTEM AND ALLEVIATE PITTA CONDITIONS.

▼ HERBAL TEAS ARE POWERFUL TONICS THAT ARE USED IN AYURVEDA.

▼ CHILLIES ARE GOOD FOR THE KAPHA DIET: THE HEAT OFFSETS THE SLUGGISH NATURE.

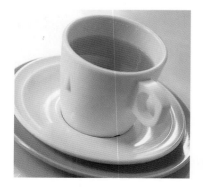

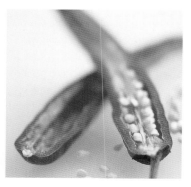

High blood pressure

Hypertension or high blood pressure is a potentially life-threatening condition and must be treated by a qualified medical practitioner. Ayurveda recommends steps that you can take which can help to bring it under control.

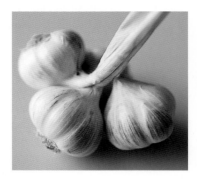

▲ EAT PLENTY OF GARLIC (RAW, FRESH IS BEST) AND TAKE REGULAR EXERCISE.

Lifestyle and diet play an important role in the prevention and treatment of hypertension. Physical and emotional stress cause the blood vessels to constrict and blood pressure to rise. Regular meditation and gentle yoga will help to counter this. A profound and simple way to relax is to lie in corpse pose for 10–15 minutes a day. Inverted postures (such as a headstand or a shoulderstand) and forward bending movements should be avoided.

Hypertension is often linked with high levels of cholesterol – increased lipids (fats) in the blood and fatty deposits on the artery walls, causing them to narrow. Stick to a kapha-reducing diet: avoiding dairy foods, especially hard cheeses, full-fat milk and sweet foods, salt, fried or cold food, cold drinks and red meat.

HONEY WATER

Add 5ml/1 tsp honey and 5–10 drops of apple cider vinegar or lime juice to a cup of hot water and drink a cup each morning. This helps to "scrape" fat from the system and lower cholesterol levels.

▼ LIMES ARE ACIDIC IN NATURE AND CAN HELP TO REDUCE CHOLESTEROL.

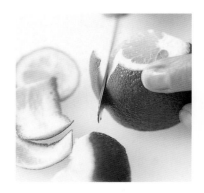

Emotional stress

Our health is a complex interplay between our mind and emotions and our physical body. Mental and emotional stress can lead to physical ill-health and vice versa. Each of the doshas is prone to particular negative emotional states.

VATA

Of all the doshas, vata is the most prone to suffer the effects of stress. Anxiety, fear, insecurity, nervousness, restlessness and confusion are associated with increased vata. Slow down, eat regular, healthy meals and meditate each day. Fresh ginger and lemon tea are good tonics. A lavender, chamomile or jasmine oil massage is calming.

PITTA

Anger, criticism, irritability, frustration, envy and hostility are all signs of aggravated pitta. To cool the temper eat plain foods and cool drinks; avoid tea, coffee and alcohol. Focus on your emotions when you meditate. Include the following herbs in your diet: chamomile, coriander (cilantro), cumin, fennel, tulsi and sandalwood.

KAPHA

Boredom and a "can't be bothered" feeling are signs of unbalanced kapha. This dosha is associated with greed, possessiveness and attachment, which leads to over-eating and to be "greedy" and smothering in relationships. Work with the kapha eating plan, and be sure to take plenty of vigorous exercise. Give the other more "space" in your relationships.

▼ A SOOTHING MASSAGE WON'T TAKE AWAY THE CAUSE OF YOUR EMOTIONAL STRESS BUT WILL HELP TO RELAX YOUR MIND AND BODY.

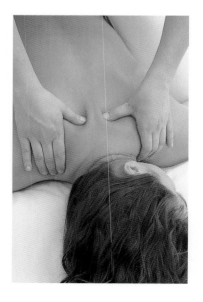

Premenstrual syndrome

Every month, many women experience unpleasant physical and emotional symptoms 7–10 days before their period. For some it is severely debilitating. Ayurveda classifies the symptoms of PMS according to dosha type.

Lower-back pain, lower abdominal pain and bloating, coupled with anxiety, fearfulness, insomnia and marked mood swings are associated with vata imbalance. Take 15ml/1 tbsp aloe vera gel mixed with a pinch of black pepper three times a day before meals. Include the following herbs in your diet: dashamula, kaishore guggulu or yogaraj guggulu.

Pitta-type symptoms include irritability, tender breasts, hives, raised body temperature (hot flushes, sweats) and cystitis. Make a herbal mix of two parts shatavari to one part each of brahmi and musta. Take 2.5ml/½ tsp with warm water, twice a day. Alternatively, add a pinch of cumin powder to 15ml/1 tbsp aloe vera gel and take three times daily.

One of the main features of kapha premenstrual syndrome (PMS) is water retention; the breasts become heavy and swollen, and the legs, feet and ankles may also swell. Emotionally, the woman feels weepy, depressed and lethargic. Add a pinch of trikatu to 15ml/1 tbsp of aloe vera gel and take three times daily. Other herbs to include in your diet are purnarnava, kutki and musta.

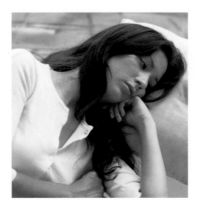

◄ FOR MANY WOMEN PMS CAN BE DIFFICULT AND DEBILITATING. MAKE A RECORD OF YOUR SYMPTOMS AND DO NOT IGNORE THEM.

TREATMENT TIPS
To treat vata and kapha PMS, eat ten cherries a day on an empty stomach a week or so before the period starts.

Low libido

Ayurveda acknowledges the importance of a healthy, fulfilling sex life. Our sex drive is affected by high stress levels, emotional factors and also by weakness or debility in the male or female reproductive organs.

Ayurveda suggests many foods that can strengthen the reproductive system. The following are equally suitable for both sexes.

ALMONDS
Soak ten almonds overnight. Peel them and eat before breakfast each day. Alternatively use them to make an almond milk drink. Blend them with a glass of warm milk, 5ml/1 tsp fructose, a pinch of nutmeg and a pinch of saffron.

DATES
Soak ten dates in ghee (a special form of clarified butter) with 1.5ml/¼ tsp of cardamon and a pinch of saffron. Cover and leave in a warm place for 2 weeks. Eat one date a day each morning; they taste delicious and will help with sexual debility and chronic fatigue.

ONIONS AND GINGER
Take 15ml/1 tbsp onion juice with 5ml/1 tsp of fresh ginger juice twice a day.

GARLIC MILK
Mix 250ml/8fl oz/1 cup milk, 50ml/2fl oz/¼ cup water and 1 chopped garlic clove. Boil to reduce the mixture. Drink at bedtime.

HERBAL TREATMENTS
Ayurvedic herbs to combat low libido include shatavari, ashwagandha, vidari, nutmeg and tagar.
For men Mix 5ml/1 tsp ashwagandha and 2.5ml/½ tsp vidari in a cup of warm milk and drink just before bedtime.
For women Substitute the ashwagandha with shatavari.

▼ TRY EATING THREE FIGS WITH 5ML/1 TSP OF HONEY AFTER BREAKFAST.

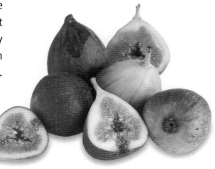

Headaches

This common problem occurs for many reasons; headaches may be stress related, caused by diet or be related to infections, poor eyesight or bad posture. Ayurveda classifies headaches into vata, pitta and kapha type.

Throbbing vata-type headaches are caused by tension and anxiety. Ease muscle tension by massaging the neck and shoulders with sesame oil; rubbing sesame oil on the top of the head and on the soles of the feet at bedtime is also said to control vata. Ayurvedic herbs to include in your diet are triphala to clear any congestion, jatamansi, brahmi and calamus.

Pitta headaches are associated with heat or burning sensations, flushed skin and visual sensitivity to light. They can be brought on by eating spicy food and by anger or frustration. A pitta headache may clear up if you eat something sweet; try some fruit. Cooling aloe vera juice can help: take 30ml/ 2 tbsp up to three times a day.

Kapha headaches are congested, dull and heavy, and often associated with sinus pain. Fresh air and plenty of exercise will help to alleviate congestion.

▼ IF YOU HAVE A HEADACHE, YOUR BLOOD SUGAR MAY BE LOW. COUNTER THIS WITH NATURAL SUGARS: A GLASS OF FRESHLY SQUEEZED FRUIT JUICE IS AN EXCELLENT CURE.

▼ IF YOU SUFFER FROM FREQUENT HEADACHES, YOUR DIET MAY BE THE CAUSE OF YOUR DISCOMFORT. KEEP A RECORD TO SEE IF ANY FOODS TRIGGER YOUR HEADACHES.

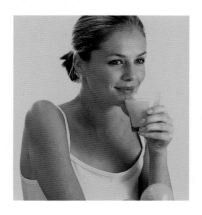

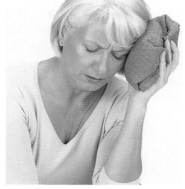

Insomnia

People in the West are likely to have a problem with excess vata as it relates to overactivity in the nervous system and leads to stress-related disorders. Insomnia is caused by an increase of vata in the mind.

Any vata-increasing influence can contribute to insomnia, including lots of travel, stress, an erratic lifestyle and the use of stimulants such as tea or coffee. Ayurvedic herbal treatment is with brahmi, jatamansi, ashwagandha and nutmeg. A foot massage with brahmi oil last thing at night may help.

Out-of-balance pitta can also contribute to insomnia when it is brought on by anger, jealousy, frustration, fever, or excess sun or heat. Herbs to include in your diet are brahmi, jatamansi, bhringaraj, shatavari and aloe vera juice. Massage brahmi oil into the head and feet.

INSOMNIA TREATMENT
As an aid to a good night's sleep, add 10ml/2 tsp fruit sugar and 2 pinches of grated nutmeg to a glass of tomato juice. Drink it late in the afternoon (16.00–17.00 hours) and follow it with an early dinner (18.00–19.00 hours).

▼ TEA, COFFEE, CHOCOLATE AND COLA CONTAIN CAFFEINE, WHICH KEEPS YOU AWAKE.

▼ SPEND TIME RELAXING BEFORE YOU PREPARE FOR BED. YOU COULD SCENT THE ROOM WITH SOOTHING ESSENTIAL OILS.

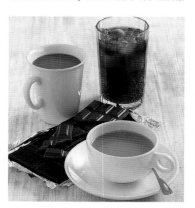

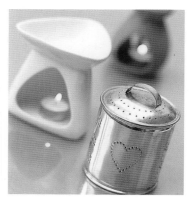

Colds and flu

The cold damp months of winter and early spring are the times of year when many people will get a cold. Symptoms typically include excess mucus production and feverishness, alternately feeling chilly or burning hot.

Kapha colds are thick and mucusy, with a heavy feeling in the head and/or body. Follow the kapha eating plan and eliminate dairy, nuts and heavy, oily food from the diet. Drink hot lemon spiced with ginger, cinnamon and cloves or cardamon, and use steam inhalations to help clear the sinuses.

The early stage of a cold is often marked by a dry, sore throat. Dryness in the body is a symptom of vata imbalance; helpful herbs include ginger, cumin, pippali, tulsi, cloves, peppermint, shatavari and ashwagandha.

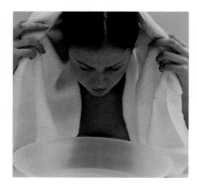

▲ A STEAM INHALATION, MADE USING GINGER ADDED TO A BOWL OF HOT WATER, HELPS RELIEVE A COLD.

When there is fever, a pitta imbalance may be indicated. Avoid hot, spicy food and use cooling herbal preparations; peppermint, spearmint, sandalwood, chrysanthemum and tulsi are all suitable.

GINGER
The best remedy for colds is ginger. It can be eaten raw, steeped in hot water and made into drinks. Its warming properties will invigorate the body and help with the elimination of toxins.

▼ MOST PEOPLE GET COLDS IN WINTER DURING THE KAPHA PHASE OF THE YEAR.

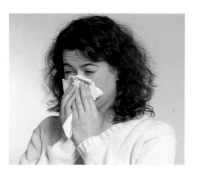

Coughs

Coughs are usually a by-product of colds and other respiratory infections. They fall into two broad categories: those that are dry and irritating, and those that are "wet" and congesting. Inflammation may be present in either type.

Vata coughs are dry and irritating with very little mucus. They may be accompanied by a dry mouth and sore throat. Herbs and spices include licorice (contra-indicated if you suffer hypertension), shatavari, ashwagandha and cardamon. A ripe banana mashed up with 5ml/1 tsp honey and a couple of pinches of black pepper is also effective; eat it two or three times a day.

Pitta coughs are usually associated with a lot of phlegm, which tends to stick on the chest. Fever or heat, combined with a burning sensation in the chest or throat may also be present. The best herbs for pitta coughs include peppermint, tulsi and sandalwood.

Kapha coughs are generally loose and productive. Keep warm and avoid damp, cold environments. A simple and effective treatment is to mix 2.5ml/½ tsp of black pepper with 5ml/1 tsp of honey and eat it on a full stomach. The heat of the black pepper will warm the body and help to drive out the cough. Ginger, lemons and cloves are also useful.

▼ TREAT A COUGH ACCORDING TO YOUR DOSHA TYPE.

▼ MAKE A WARMING LEMON DRINK TO SOOTHE A DRY COUGH.

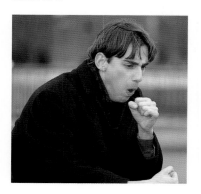

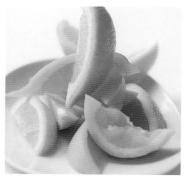

Skin problems

A glowing complexion and silky, "baby-soft" skin is a reality that many of us only dream about. Skin problems are extremely common and can range in severity from the occasional spot to chronic conditions such as psoriasis.

Vata skin problems will be dry and rough and include chapped lips, cracked heels, "sandpaper" hands and dandruff. Avoid letting the skin dry out and exposing it to cold and/or windy weather. Herbal remedies for vata skin are triphala and satisabgol (the latter is useful if you are also constipated).

Excess pitta causes skin problems that itch, burn or erupt into spots or rashes. The skin is usually red, swollen, raised or inflamed, often with a yellow head or pus discharge. Avoid sun, heat, hot baths or saunas, and increase your

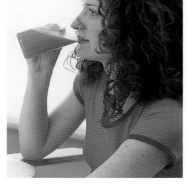

▲ Juices are good for the skin. Drink them when they are freshly made.

intake of water, salads, raw vegetables and fruits. Cooling spices are turmeric, coriander and saffron. Skincare products made with the fruit and seeds of the Neem tree are also useful.

Greasy, oily skin indicates a kapha imbalance. Increase your exercise and follow the kapha eating plan. Useful herbs include calamus, cinnamon, cloves, dry ginger, trikatu formula and turmeric.

TIPS FOR BEAUTIFUL SKIN

- Begin the day with a glass of hot water containing a squeeze of lemon.
- Take a daily capsule of turmeric.
- Enjoy regular massage.
- Use Neem or sandalwood soap for bathing.
- For some natural colour, drink fresh carrot juice and eat cooked beetroot (beet).

Urinary infections

Cystitis is one of the most common infections of the urinary tract, particularly in women. It is generally a bacterial infection and should always be treated straight away because of the risk of it spreading to the kidneys.

Cystitis is mainly a pitta condition because it burns and is inflamed and hot. Avoid hot foods and spices and use plenty of coriander (cilantro). Other remedies include aloe vera juice (contra-indicated in

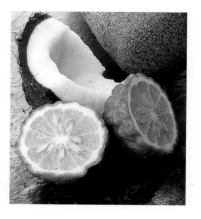

▲ COCONUT AND LIME ARE RECOMMENDED FOR PITTA CYSTITIS.

TIPS FOR TREATING CYSTITIS

- Avoid tea, coffee and alcoholic drinks.
- Personal hygiene is extremely important; always pull the toilet paper up and away from the body after defecation.
- Bathe with unperfumed oils and soaps until the infection has cleared.
- Coriander (cilantro), cumin and fennel tea is a good tonic. Use 1.5ml/¼ tsp of each herb per cup of boiling water.

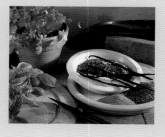

pregnancy), lime juice, coconut, pomegranate and sandalwood.

Kapha-type cystitis is accompanied by congestion and mucus in the urinary tract; the urine is often pale or clear. The treatments are cinnamon, trikatu combined with shilajit, gokshura and gokshuradi guggulu. Avoid salt, sugar and all dairy products.

In vata people, cystitis will tend to be less intense. Herbal remedies you can try include shilajit with bala, ashwagandha and shatavari.

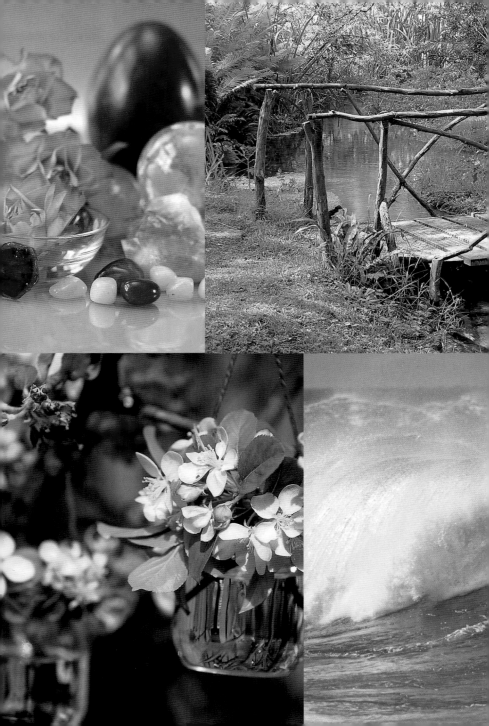

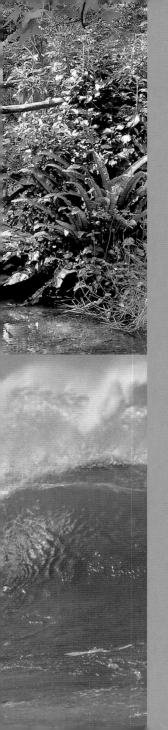

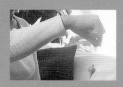

HEALING WITH
ENERGIES

The link between the Earth's natural energy and the human condition has been recognized by cultures across the world since time began. Indeed, humankind has strived to tap into this invisible life force, learning to harness the subtle vibrations of colour, light and sound, the energies of plants and minerals, and the cosmic power of the sun and moon.

This section explains how to diagnose and treat energy imbalances using both ancient and modern methods, from acupuncture and feng shui to Vega testing and radionics. It also describes how energy therapies can help with common health problems, including chronic fatigue, allergies and emotional stress, and with physical discomfort such as arthritis.

What is energy?

Energy is life. It is the invisible force that animates the human body and permeates everything in the natural world, including animals, plants, trees and rocks, as well as the earth, sun, moon and stars.

THE LIFE FORCE

Throughout the course of history, cultures all over the world have acknowledged the existence of a universal energy force flowing through everything in the world, including the human body. It has been given many names. In India it is referred to as "prana", in the Far East it is "chi" or "ki", while in some shamanist traditions it is

▾ A MASSIVE TREE STARTS LIFE AS A SEED THAT IS PULSING WITH LIFE FORCE ENERGY AS WELL AS THE POTENTIAL FOR GROWTH.

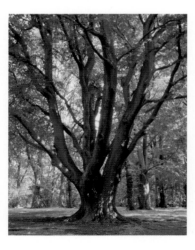

described as "chula" or "animu". Today, many people refer to it as "spirit" or the "life force".

Invisible like the air we breathe, the life force has a powerful influence on our health and well-being. It not only governs our physical health and survival, but also our mental and emotional well-being; it is the spark that fuels our ambitions, driving us to express our personal creativity and strive to fulfil our spiritual potential.

Good health is achieved when the life force is balanced and allowed to flow freely. When it is blocked or unbalanced, it leads to disturbances that will eventually manifest as "dis-ease" or a state of disharmony in the natural order. Energy healing is all about finding ways to strengthen, balance and free up this energy by using naturally occurring vibrations, such as light or colour, or the energies of natural forms such as plants and crystals.

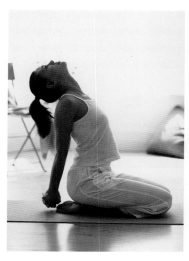

▲ WHEN THE LIFE FORCE IS IN HARMONY
YOU FEEL READY TO TAKE ON THE WORLD.

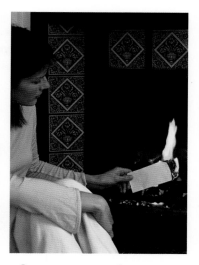

▲ BY TAPPING INTO NATURE'S HEALING
ENERGY WE ARE FILLED WITH WELL-BEING.

A UNIVERSE OF ENERGY

The life force connects us to the world we live in, weaving the fabric of life seamlessly together. Everything within the universe vibrates with energy and the world that we are part of is a vast web of energy patterns.

This idea has been verified by modern science. All matter, however dense it may appear, is made up of energy: it consists of atoms, protons, neutrons, electrons, waves and particles, all vibrating together at different frequencies. We live in the electromagnetic energy field of the earth, surrounded by wave forms, from low frequency radio waves at one end of the spectrum to high frequency cosmic rays at the other. Everything in the universe is made up of energy, which becomes more dense (and vibrates at a lower frequency) as it forms into matter. We are energetic phenomena and our world is dynamic. Like everything else in our lives, our health is influenced by the invisible energies that flow through us and swirl all around us.

Cosmic influences

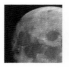

We are part of the cosmic web of life delicately connected and held in balance by subtle energy forces. Changes in any part of this energy system will have a "knock-on" effect on our health and vitality – for better or worse.

THE SUN

At the centre of our solar system, the sun is a fireball of light and heat, and is our most important energy source. It creates the conditions for life on earth and influences our health and vitality. When someone is sick, it is as though their "light" has dimmed. The word "influenza" comes from an Italian word meaning "to influence", and research indicates that all the major flu epidemics of the last 250 years (including the 1918 flu pandemic) have coincided with increased solar activity.

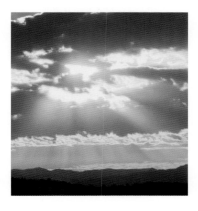

THE MOON

Lunar power controls the tides, affects weather, and influences human moods and behaviour. A woman's 28-day menstrual cycle follows the phases of the moon. The moon is also associated with psychological disturbances: the full moon is known as the time of lunacy or "moon madness", and its powerful energy can trigger such problems as epileptic fits, as well as increasing the potential for accidents.

BIORHYTHMS

The forces of the sun and the moon are often thought of as masculine and feminine energies respectively. The male solar energy is focused on action in the world outside, on ambition and achievement, while the female lunar energy is inwardly focused,

◀ BECAUSE THE SUN IS SO CRITICAL TO LIFE, IT WAS HELD IN AWE BY MANY EARLY CIVILIZATIONS AND REVERED AS A GOD. EVEN TODAY, PEOPLE DESCRIBE THEMSELVES AS "SUN-WORSHIPPERS".

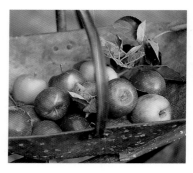

world", while at other times we feel lethargic and find it more difficult to get things done.

THE SEASONS

and more concerned with the intuitive world of feelings and emotion. According to the theory of biorhythms, we all have an internal male "solar" cycle and a female "lunar" cycle that affects us physically, emotionally and intellectually. These cycles produce a pattern of highs and lows, so that some days we may have lots of energy and feel "on top of the

The changing seasons also affect our energy levels and many illnesses are seasonal. Light deprivation is thought to be associated with seasonal affective disorder (SAD), which is a severe manifestation of the "winter blues". We suffer more colds and flu in winter, whereas early summer is the hayfever season.

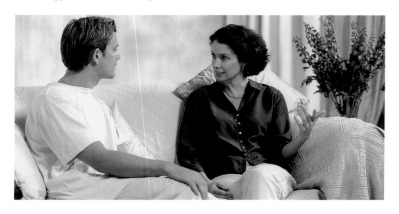

The human energy field

There is more to the human form than meets the eye. The vital force emanates around the body like a luminous sphere or "aura", entering through the chakras and running along energy pathways, or meridians.

THE AURA

The body's aura is subtle energy that vibrates at a different wavelength and frequency to the energy of the physical body. It is sometimes seen or depicted as a halo and may be felt when someone "enters your space". Auras vary in size, density and colour, but their overall size, shape and vibrancy is indicative of your state of health. The healthier you are, the larger and brighter your aura; when you are sick, your aura contracts as the body tries to conserve its vital energy. The size of the aura can also depend on mood and place.

SUBTLE ANATOMY

The energy pod around the human form can be visualized as seven layers of light, each vibrating at a higher frequency than the previous one. These layers are also known as the

THE SUBTLE BODIES

1 Etheric body: closest to the physical body; provides a blueprint for the physical body and its organs.
2 Emotional body: the seat of the emotions.
3 Mental body: mental activity, thoughts, ideas and day-to-day concerns.
4 Astral body: represents the personality.
5 Causal body: seat of willpower and gateway to higher consciousness; fulfilment of personal destiny.
6 Celestial soul body: spiritual essence, sometimes referred to as the "higher self".
7 Illuminated spiritual body: the highest and most refined level, where we become one with the source of love and healing, or the Divine.

▲ WE ARE MOST AWARE OF HUMAN ENERGY FIELDS WHEN WE SENSE THE MOOD OF SOMEONE CLOSE BY, OR FEEL OUR "SPACE" IS BEING INVADED WHEN ANOTHER PERSON COMES TOO NEAR TO US.

"subtle bodies", and each one has a particular function. The energy of these subtle bodies enters and leaves our system through the chakras, moving along energy channels known as "nadis" or "meridians".

Some people can discern auras around our physical body, and almost anyone can be taught to sense the different qualities within a person's auric field. Like the chakras, each level of the subtle bodies represents a certain frequency of personal energy.

The Indian philosophers and yogis of old described complex patterns in our "subtle bodies", and identified different energy systems beyond the physical:
• the etheric body is closest to the physical and provides the blueprint for the body and its organs. A disruption of harmony within the etheric almost always precedes physical illness;
• the emotional body contains our ever-changing patterns of emotions and feelings. As the least stable of the subtle bodies, it is therefore the easiest one to

modify with techniques such as crystal healing.
• the mental body contains the patterns in which we have organized our understanding of reality, with our beliefs and ideas, and everyday thinking;
• the finer subtle bodies are concerned with our spiritual identity and our connection with the universal or "collective unconscious". It is less easy to define these subtle areas of life, although, as you become more familiar with the practice of energy healing, you will learn to detect and balance them.

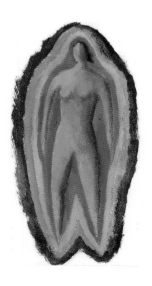

▶ THE SUBTLE BODIES ARE THE FINE, NON-PHYSICAL LEVELS OF OUR BEING.

Energy and health

Good health is achieved when our energy levels are in a state of balance. When they are depleted or out of balance, we become sick and unhappy. Living in balance and coping with change is the key to health.

Energy balancing

Chronic illnesses are on the increase, yet we tend to take our health for granted, paying attention only when something goes wrong. As we strive to meet the pressures of modern living, we push beyond our limits and "run on empty". We need to achieve a balance between the quality and quantity of the energy we give out and what we take in. This means balancing work and leisure, rest and exercise, by ensuring we have enough sleep and eating a balanced diet. If we take in too much of the "wrong" sort of energy, our systems become clogged up or blocked. This creates imbalance, first in the "subtle bodies" (layers of energy around the body), and eventually in the physical body.

The effects of stress

Many illnesses are stress-related, including digestive disorders such as irritable bowel syndrome (IBS), allergic conditions such as asthma, high blood pressure and "everyday" tension headaches. Stress is one of the biggest causes of energy imbalance; it affects us in many ways and at many levels. Negative mental and emotional states, such as anxiety, grief, fear, anger, worry and also depression, create turbulence in the subtle energy bodies and will lead to physical complaints if the imbalances are not corrected.

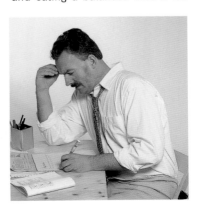

◄ Overwork can lead to mental and emotional stress, which affects relationships and causes health problems.

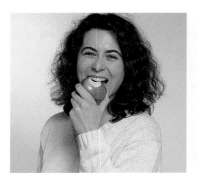

▲ WHEN YOU BITE INTO A FRESHLY PICKED ORGANIC APPLE, YOU CAN TELL THAT IT IS BURSTING WITH VITAL ENERGY.

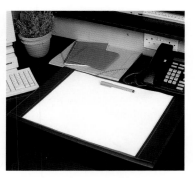

▲ KEEP A PLANT ON YOUR DESK TO HELP PROTECT YOU FROM THE NEGATIVE ENERGIES CREATED BY ELECTRONIC OFFICE EQUIPMENT.

We are also affected by "geopathic stress", which is related to the electromagnetic energy fields of the earth. One natural cause of variations in the earth's energy field are underground water courses or "black streams". These have been thought to cause ill health for centuries. Indeed, recent research has associated them with chronic fatigue syndrome (ME), although the energy waves of modern electrical appliances, such as televisions, microwave ovens, computers and mobile phones, are also disturbing the earth's energy field, and may, in fact, be contributing to "modern" illnesses, such as ME, in ways that we don't yet understand.

COPING WITH CHANGE

Any point of change, or transition, is a critical time in life. This can be anything from a change in your personal lifestyle (such as getting divorced or married, changing job, having children, or moving house) to the changing seasons of the year or climate changes when we go abroad.

At a time of transition we should try to take extra care of ourselves, as the immune system is under increased pressure while we are attempting to adjust to a new or difficult situation. If we pay insufficient attention to our energy levels and carry on as though we are invincible, we will eventually get sick.

Taking care of yourself

Your vital energy is your most precious commodity, and is worth looking after. For health and well-being, tune in to your energy field and learn to recognize the things that increase your energy levels and those that drain you.

ENERGY DRAINERS AND BOOSTERS
Take a good look at your lifestyle and use this guide to help you avoid the energy drainers and cultivate the energy boosters.

Key **x** = energy drainers
   ✓ = energy boosters
   • = tip

FOOD AND DRINK
At the most basic level, food and drink is the fuel our bodies need in order to function. The closer it is to its natural, unrefined state, the greater the energy boost.

x Refined, processed food, white flour, sugar, alcohol, caffeine, "ready" meals, microwaved food.

✓ Raw food, unsweetened fresh fruit and vegetable juices, sprouted grains and seeds, freshly picked salad, fruit, vegetables.

• Drink 6 to 8 glasses of still mineral water a day. This will help to keep your system free of toxins.

RELATIONSHIPS
The people in our lives can be our greatest source of pleasure, yet they can also be a major cause of energy depletion. Some relationships are unavoidable, but with others you can be more selective.

x People who don't listen, have no time for you, "take" but don't give, tell you what to do/put you down/criticize you.

✓ People who make you laugh and feel good, share the balance of power, listen, are appreciative and supportive.

• Have a satisfying sex life.

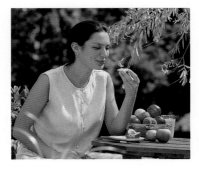

◄ MAKE SURE YOUR DIET INCLUDES PLENTY OF ENERGY-BOOSTING FOODS, SUCH AS FRESH FRUIT AND VEGETABLES.

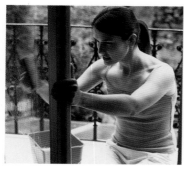

▲ Channelling energy into physical activities acts as a pressure valve.

Work

Since work is a major part of life, it's very important to find a way of working that suits you.

✗ Working long hours, not getting paid enough, "putting up with it", feeling forced to do it, lack of recognition.

✓ Enjoying what you do, getting a proper reward and recognition.

● Try to make your work fit around you and your needs; don't be a "wage slave".

Tip

Chronic illnesses are on the increase. Improve your resistance to disease by improving your energy levels. This will also help you to deal with any existing illness.

Lifestyle

Aim for balance in your activities and avoid going to extremes.

✗ Lack of sleep, exercise.

✓ Regular exercise and/or stress-reducing techniques, such as yoga, pilates, meditation, tai chi, working out.

● Make time for yourself each day.

Environment

Our surroundings have an instant effect on our energy levels.

✗ Packed city streets, busy shops, fluorescent lighting, clutter, lack of natural light and greenery.

✓ Nature, especially green leafy forests or windswept beaches, décor that makes you feel good, clear and tidy work spaces.

● Relax under a large leafy tree.

▼ Take regular exercise. Gentle stretching helps to release tension.

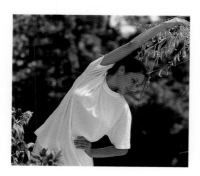

Technology and energy

Technological advances in the 20th century have made it possible to measure the electrical energy fields of the human body. Kirlian photography and Vega testing both monitor energy patterns, using them for diagnosis.

KIRLIAN PHOTOGRAPHY

In 1939, Semyon Kirlian, a Russian electrician, discovered a way of producing an image of the electromagnetic energy field that surrounds the human body. To take a Kirlian photograph, the body's electromagnetic field (usually via the hands and/or feet) is brought into contact with a high-voltage, high-frequency electric charge. A photograph is taken of the resulting "interference pattern". This pattern can then be used to detect the strength or weakness of the body's electrical energy field and shows where it is out of balance. A healthy body is indicated by a regular, bright field around the hand or foot, whereas a thin, patchy field indicates energy blocks or disturbances.

The pattern is affected by physical and emotional states. For instance, if you are in shock or exhausted, the energy pattern may not register, whereas if you are anxious or irritable, the image may have an erratic outer edge, with sharp points, rather than a smooth, even contour. The menstrual cycle, medication, as well as chronic or life-threatening illnesses such as cancer, also affect the energy pattern. Taking exercise, having acupuncture or other "energy-based medicines", meditating or doing yoga have all been shown to increase the radiance of the Kirlian image.

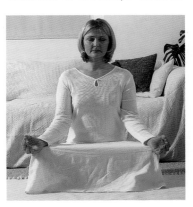

◀ KIRLIAN PHOTOGRAPHY IS ABLE TO DEMONSTRATE THAT THE AURA INCREASES IN SIZE AND RADIANCE DURING MEDITATION.

Vega testing

Research in Germany during the 1950s showed that acupuncture points on the body (where energy is concentrated and linked to specific organs) had electrical properties. Various electronic devices were then developed to measure and map these points, including the Vega machine, which was developed by Dr Helmut Schimmel in the 1970s.

Vega testing is used as a diagnostic technique, particularly to detect allergies or intolerances. During a Vega-testing consultation, an electronic probe or stylus is placed on certain points, usually on the feet and/or hands, while you hold an electrode in order to complete the circuit. The machine

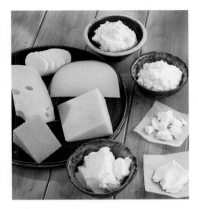

▲ Allergies, or over-sensitivity to certain foods, such as dairy products, are becoming increasingly common.

measures fluctuations in your energy field as the stylus is placed at different points, indicating which organs may be out of balance. Homeopathic dilutions of allergens, such as pollen, house dust, dairy produce, feathers or fur, can also be brought into the electronic circuit. An erratic reading is produced when your body is intolerant of a particular substance. The technique can also be used in order to verify which homeopathic remedies your body needs.

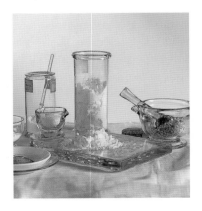

◀ It is possible to desensitize the body using homeopathic remedies of common allergens, such as dust or pollen.

Diagnosis by dowsing

Dowsing is an ancient art that can be used to diagnose energy imbalances and to detect invisible energy pathways. With a little practice, anyone can dowse. All you need is a simple pendulum and an open mind.

PRINCIPLES OF DOWSING

Dowsing is a method of divining or "tapping into" the intelligence of the life force to gain access to information. Holding a pendulum, the dowser will ask a clear, unambiguous "yes/no" question. The pendulum picks up on the energetic vibrations pertaining to the question and then moves in response. The direction of this movement indicates whether the response is positive or negative.

▼ A PENDULUM IS A POPULAR DOWSING TOOL. IT CAN BE MADE FROM METAL, WOOD, POLISHED STONE OR CRYSTAL, BUT IT'S UP TO YOU TO CHOOSE ONE THAT FEELS RIGHT.

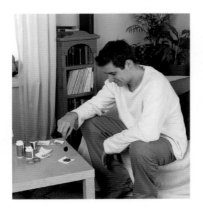

USING DOWSING

Dowsing is extremely useful as a diagnostic technique when you are working with healing with energies. For instance, you can dowse to check whether certain foods and vitamins are suitable for you, to detect allergies, to find out which colours, crystals or flower essences are helpful and even to find out where is the best place to live.

You can also dowse when giving healing, to find out where energy is blocked and to check when the energy is flowing again. The key to successful dowsing is asking the right question and remaining objective about the answer that comes back – it's rather like watching for the results of an internet search. Frame your questions clearly and hold the pendulum over the place or article in question. Reassess your findings at regular intervals to stay up-to-date with your changing needs.

Tuning in

Before you dowse you need to establish the particular pendulum motions that will mean "yes" and "no" for you. Once you are confident and also familiar with the responses, you are ready to start dowsing.

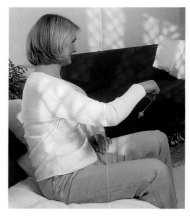

1 Sit upright and hold the pendulum over your lap. Allow it to swing back and forth. This is the "neutral" position.

2 Move the pendulum over your dominant-side knee. State clearly in your mind, "Please show me my 'yes' response." Pay close attention to what the pendulum does as this will be your signal for "yes".

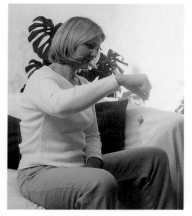

3 Return the pendulum to "neutral", then repeat step 2, moving to your non-dominant side to find the "no" response.

PENDULUM RESPONSES

The diagrams show classic pendulum dowsing responses. Dowsing responses are a very individual and personal thing, however, and you need not worry if yours are not the same as these. What is important is that you are clear which response means "yes", which means "no" and which is "neutral", and then you work with those.

ANTI-CLOCKWISE FOR "NO"
TOWARDS AND AWAY FOR "NEUTRAL"
CLOCKWISE FOR "YES"

Diagnosis by applied kinesiology

Applied kinesiology, or muscle testing, is a way of finding and correcting energy imbalances before they become serious health problems. It can also be used to find the underlying causes of long-standing illnesses.

MUSCLE TESTING

In the 1960s, George Goodheart, an American chiropractor, realized that muscles can tell us a great deal about our state of health. He found that the muscles could be strengthened by pressing, and by massaging other, seemingly unrelated, areas of the body. This is because the body is an integral whole, with all its major organs and systems connected by "energy circuits" or meridians. They power the system and link the muscles to different organs.

Excess or blocked energy in these channels can lead to weakness in the corresponding organ and can be detected in the relevant muscle. For example, the quadriceps in the thigh is linked to the small intestine; if you were sensitive to dairy products and drank a glass of milk, then the intolerance would register in the intestine, then in the quadriceps. By testing the strength of various muscles, a kinesiologist can work "backwards" to find out where the underlying problem resides.

▼ KINESIOLOGISTS ALSO USE MASSAGE TECHNIQUES TO BALANCE THE BODY AND TO STRENGTHEN AREAS OF WEAKNESS.

▼ DURING A CONSULTATION YOU WILL BE ASKED ABOUT YOUR MEDICAL HISTORY AND CURRENT MENTAL AND EMOTIONAL STATE.

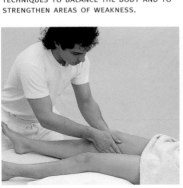

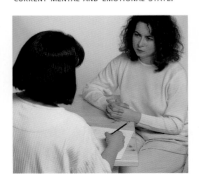

Kinesiology recognizes that there are three aspects to health – structural (or physical), mental and chemical – and that well-being relates to all three areas. A kinesiology session involves physical, chemical and/or mental "challenges" during which the patient is asked to resist pressure against an exerted limb. The muscle's energy circuit will "turn off" when an imbalance disrupts a particular pathway.

• Physical challenge: if your health problem is structural, pressure will be applied directly to the bones and muscles to find out where the problem is located.

• Chemical challenge: chemical substances, foods or homeopathic dilutions are placed directly on the tongue or skin, often in a glass phial. These tests are used for allergies.

• Mental challenge: you may be asked to focus on certain thoughts or feelings while the practitioner tests your muscle strength. In fact, many chronic illnesses have a strong emotional component, and you may find out more about the underlying cause of the complaint.

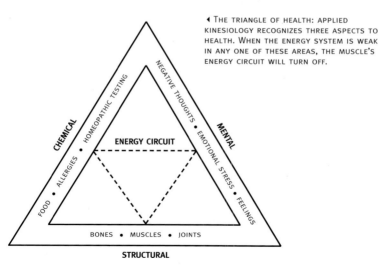

◄ THE TRIANGLE OF HEALTH: APPLIED KINESIOLOGY RECOGNIZES THREE ASPECTS TO HEALTH. WHEN THE ENERGY SYSTEM IS WEAK IN ANY ONE OF THESE AREAS, THE MUSCLE'S ENERGY CIRCUIT WILL TURN OFF.

Acupuncture

Acupuncture has been practised in China for thousands of years and is one of the oldest systems of healing. It involves inserting fine needles into specific points on the body to regulate the flow of energy through the meridians.

YIN AND YANG

In Chinese thought, the universe is characterized by opposing but complementary energies called "yin" and "yang". Together, they make up "chi" or the vital energy of the life force. Inner harmony is achieved when chi is balanced between these polarities and flows freely through the body, energizing and purifying the organs, tissues and blood. An excess or deficiency in either yin or yang, and/or blocks in the flow of chi, will lead to illness.

CHI AND THE MERIDIANS

The chi is the energy equivalent of the immune system; it supports, nourishes and defends the whole person against disease. Chi runs through the body along energy channels or meridians, which are the equivalent of the arteries and veins of the physical body.

There are 12 main meridians – of which six are yin and six yang – and many minor ones. Together they form an intricate network. Each meridian is named after an organ or function. The yin organs, such as the liver, are "solid", whereas the yang organs, such as the stomach, are "hollow". Along

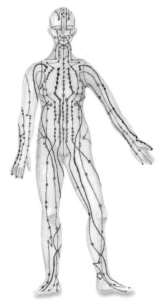

◀ FINE ENERGY CHANNELS, OR MERIDIANS, RUN THROUGH THE BODY, LINKING ITS SYSTEMS AND ORGANS. ACUPUNCTURE IS A TREATMENT THAT TAPS INTO THESE PATHWAYS AT SPECIFIC POINTS.

the meridians are approximately 365 acupuncture points where the chi is concentrated.

TREATMENT

During an acupuncture treatment, extremely fine needles are gently inserted into the skin at the relevant points to stimulate or reduce the flow of chi through the meridian. This may produce a pulling or tugging sensation, but it does not hurt like a normal needle or damage the skin. Needles are usually inserted to a depth of 6–12 mm ($^1/_4$–$^1/_2$ in) and left in position for anything from a few seconds to an hour. It is usual for between 6 to 12 needles to be used, at a combination of acupuncture points. It is common to experience a heaviness in the limbs and/or feelings of deep relaxation. If the imbalance is due

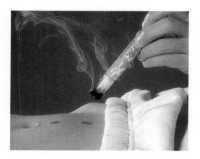

▲ MOXA STICKS ARE OFTEN USED IN AN ACUPUNCTURE TREATMENT TO BALANCE EXCESS YIN (COLD AND DAMP) IN THE BODY.

to a yang deficiency, then the herb moxa (or mugwort) may be burned to generate heat. Dried moxa is rolled into a stick, which is lit and held over the acupuncture point until it becomes too hot.

Acupuncture is a very effective method of pain relief. It has been used in place of anaesthetics during surgery, in dentistry and in childbirth, and is widely used to treat back pain, arthritis and other chronic conditions. Having acupuncture usually leads to an increase in energy, an improved appetite and better sleep, as well as an improved sense of well-being. It should only be carried out by a qualified practitioner.

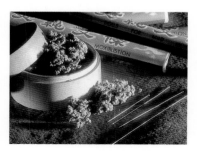

◀ MOXA IS USUALLY DRIED AND THEN ROLLED INTO CIGAR-LIKE STICKS.

Reiki healing

Reiki is a form of spiritual healing that originated in Japan. It works by drawing on "rei-ki" or universal-life energy, which is channelled to areas of need. Giving and receiving Reiki is a gentle and relaxing experience.

CHANNELLING THE POWER OF LOVE
The purpose of Reiki is to work for the "highest good". It connects with the force of unconditional love, which transcends time and space and promotes positive living and compassion for all. To learn Reiki it is usual to go through a special "attunement" with a qualified Reiki master, using ancient and secret symbols to attune the physical and subtle bodies to spiritual energies and opening up a healing channel for them. This channel remains active for life, although the more you use it, the more effective it will be. You can visualize the force as a beam of white light, entering your body and flowing out of your hands when you give healing.

REIKI TREATMENTS
A non-invasive form of healing, Reiki soothes away troubles and traumas in a peaceful way. Certain hand positions are used to dissolve energy blocks and re-balance the body. You can treat yourself with Reiki, as well as others, and you can also use it to treat sick plants and animals and in the environment to guard against negative energy.

◄ THE PERSON CHANNELLING REIKI IS NEVER DRAINED, AS THE ENERGY FLOWS NOT FROM BUT THROUGH THE HEALER, RATHER LIKE WATER THROUGH A PIPE, AND INTO THE PERSON OR OBJECT BEING HEALED.

Reiki refresher

A ten-minute Reiki treatment will refresh and energize you and fill you with positive, loving energy.

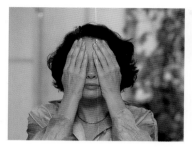

1 Place both hands over your eyes, close them and then relax. This helps to restore strained eyes and clear tension headaches. Move your hands to your temples to help clear an overactive or tired mind.

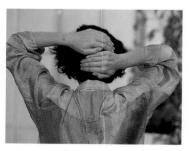

2 Move your hands round to the back of the head and neck area, dispelling tension and refreshing the brain.

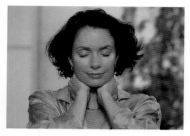

3 Put your hands on either side of your neck. This helps the thyroid gland and the area associated with communication.

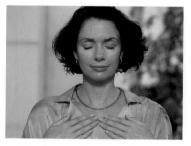

4 Place your hands above the breasts in order to help with lymph drainage and the clearing of toxins. This position may generate some warmth.

5 Finally, move your hands down to the sternum, fingers meeting at the heart chakra. This helps to restore emotional equilibrium. Finish with your hands below the navel to centre yourself.

reiki healing **313**

Homeopathy

Homeopathy is a system that stimulates the body to heal itself. Homeopathic remedies are prepared from plant, mineral and other extracts, but diluted to such an extent that only the "energy" of the original substance remains.

LIKE CURES LIKE

Homeopathy has been an established system for about 200 years. Discovered by Samuel Hahnemann, a German doctor, it is based on the "law of similars" or the principle that like cures like: the symptoms caused by too much of a substance can also be cured with a small dose of it. For instance, in a patient suffering from insomnia, a homeopath may prescribe the remedy coffea (coffee), which in normal doses would cause sleeplessness in a healthy person.

▼ HOMEOPATHIC REMEDIES ARE PREPARED FROM NUMEROUS DIFFERENT PLANT, ANIMAL AND MINERAL SOURCES. THE ORIGINAL SUBSTANCE IS DILUTED MANY TIMES.

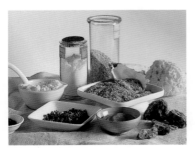

REMEDY PICTURES

Homeopathy is concerned not only with physical symptoms, but also with your mental and emotional state, and remedies are selected on the basis of matching your overall "picture" with a suitable remedy. While two people may suffer from the same illness, they will not necessarily be prescribed the same remedy, as each person is unique. You can use homeopathy to treat yourself for minor acute illnesses, but for chronic conditions you should seek professional advice.

ENERGY MEDICINE

Homeopathic remedies contain no chemical trace of the original substance. They are prepared through dilution and succussion (shaking) to leave only an energy "blueprint". This is then "broadcast" to your energy field, to stimulate the body's powers of healing on the mental, emotional and physical levels.

Light therapy

Light plays an important role in psychological and physical health, affecting our moods and immune system. Light therapy simulates natural daylight to treat a range of conditions, including skin problems and depression.

THE POWER OF LIGHT

Daylight is involved with the production of vitamin D, and sunlight also regulates the body's biological clock, affecting sleep patterns, appetite, temperature, sex drive and the production of hormones, including serotonin, the "happy hormone". Our biological clock is designed to be in tune with the natural rhythm of day and night, and seasonal change. Night work, long distance travel and extended periods of time indoors play havoc with our body chemistry, and light deprivation can lead to an impaired functioning of the immune system and depression.

TREATING DEPRESSION

Reduced daylight can cause severe depression. This is now officially recognized as a medical condition and referred to as SAD (seasonal affective disorder). It is often treated with light therapy.

TREATMENT

Light therapy involves lying under a fluorescent full-spectrum, or bright, white light. This has the same effect as daylight, but does not contain the harmful UV rays. Daylight averages about 5,000 lux, whereas normal artificial light averages between 500–1,000. At least 2,500 lux are needed for a therapeutic effect. Professional supervision is recommended.

▼ SOAKING UP THE SUN IS GOOD IN SMALL DOSES. SUNLIGHT CAN LIFT DEPRESSION AND HELP WITH MANY SKIN PROBLEMS.

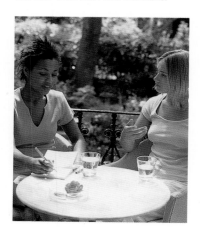

Colour vibrations

Each band of energy in the colour spectrum vibrates at a frequency that corresponds with one of the body's organs and energy systems. Colour therapy uses light of the appropriate colour to restore equilibrium in the body.

THE PSYCHOLOGY OF COLOUR

Instinctively we know that colours affect us in different ways. We speak of feeling blue, being in a black mood, being green with envy or red with anger. Every day and in countless ways we are influenced by the distinctive energy vibrations that each colour possesses, whether it is through the colour of our clothes, the food we eat, the rooms we live in or the scenery of the world outside. Colour is intrinsic to life.

▼ GREEN IS THE COLOUR OF FRESH GROWTH AND NATURAL HARMONY. IT SOOTHES SHOCK AND RELIEVES FATIGUE.

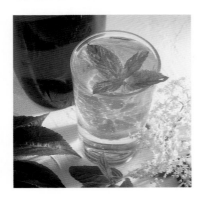

TUNING INTO COLOUR

It is not necessary to be able to see to have a sense of colour. Many blind people have, in fact, developed their sensitivity to the subtle vibrational energies of different colours in ways that we do not fully understand. For instance, the Aura-Soma colour system was developed in the 1980s by a British woman, Vicky Wall, after she lost her sight. The system uses colour essences in different combinations, which may be used in the bath or on the skin, to help balance emotional, spiritual and psychological states.

CHOOSING COLOURS

Use the colour vibration chart to help you select the colour that you feel is the most appropriate for you. If you are not sure which colour you need, use your intuition to choose the one that most attracts you. You can use dowsing with a pendulum to check your selection.

Colour vibrations
Choose colours according to your healing need or preference

colour	properties	healing uses
red	stimulating, energizing	low energy, sexual problems, blood disorders, lack of confidence
orange	cheering, enlivening	depression, mental disorders, asthma, rheumatism
yellow	inspiring, helping mental clarity and detachment	detoxifying, hormonal problems (menopause, menstrual difficulties)
green	fresh, vibrant, harmonious, idealistic	antiseptic, balancing, tonic, good for shock and fatigue, soothes headaches
blue	soothing, calming, promoting truth and inner reflection	insomnia, nervous disorders, throat problems, general healing
indigo	transforming, purifying	painkiller, sinus problems, migraine, eczema, inflammations, chest complaints, insomnia
violet/ purple	regal, dignifying	love of self, self-respect, psychological disorders and problems with the scalp (use sparingly, as purple is a "heavy" colour)
magenta	letting go	emotional hurts and upsets, accepting life's problems
black	absorbing, secretive	for when you need to hide (such as when grieving), or alternatively to convey an impression of power and control; self-discipline
white	reflecting, purity, innocence	a tonic; replaces all colours
gold	divine power, purity, the sun	depression and low energy, digestive disturbances, rheumatism, scars
silver	cosmic intelligence, the moon	hormonal and emotional balance, calms the nerves, for recovering equilibrium

Water therapies

Water is the elixir of life. It covers more than two-thirds of the earth's surface and our bodies are largely made from water. There are many ways of using water's cleansing and rejuvenating powers to increase health and vitality.

DETOX TREATMENTS

Hydrotherapy is based on improving elimination of waste products, and there are simple treatments you can build into your daily routine. Drinking plenty of water will help your body flush out toxins and increase energy levels. Sweating expels impurities through the skin: vigorous exercise, saunas or steam baths are ideal. Take plenty of showers to wash away the toxins.

▼ GET INTO THE WATER HABIT. DRINKING BETWEEN 6 AND 8 GLASSES A DAY WILL HELP TO KEEP YOUR ENERGY LEVELS HIGH.

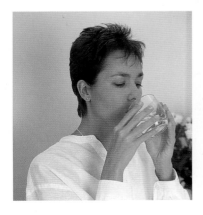

HOT AND COLD

Cold water has a stimulating effect, constricting the blood vessels and inhibiting biochemical reactions that cause inflammation. It helps to energize and cleanse the organs and subtle energy system. Taking a cold shower seals the body's aura, stopping energy from leaking out.

Warm or hot water dilates the blood vessels, increasing the flow of blood to the skin and reducing

▼ RAW FRUIT AND VEGETABLES HAVE A HIGH WATER CONTENT. INCLUDE PLENTY IN YOUR DIET TO HELP YOUR BODY DETOX.

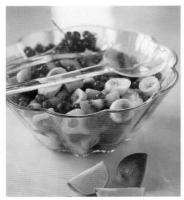

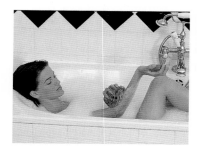

◄ WATER IS A POWERFUL CLEANSER. IT NOT ONLY CLEANS THE PHYSICAL BODY, BUT ALSO REMOVES PSYCHIC DIRT HELD IN THE AURA.

blood pressure. Warm water has a relaxing effect and can help to ease psychological and muscular tension by "drawing things" to the surface to be released.

FLOTATION THERAPY

Combining the benefits of water with meditation, flotation therapy involves "floating" in warm water in an environment that is free from external stimuli. Salts and minerals are dissolved in the water to enable the body to float without any effort.

Sessions normally last from 1 to 1½ hours and take place in a sound- and light-proof tank or bath a little larger than the body. The water is maintained at skin temperature (34.2°C/93.5°F) and you can switch on a light or open the tank at any time. The effect is profoundly relaxing for both body and mind. The brain releases endorphins (the body's natural painkillers) and many people experience feelings of euphoria. Flotation therapy has a deep-cleansing and balancing effect on the subtle bodies and is particularly useful for treating stress and anxiety. It also helps to relieve hypertension (high blood pressure), tension headaches, back pain and muscle fatigue, and is a good immunity booster.

HYDRATION

Some experts believe that dehydration underlies many health problems. Water helps to flush out toxins and keep the cells and organs healthy. Drinking 2–3 litres (3½–5½ pints) of water a day, cutting down on tea, coffee and alcohol – all of which are dehydrating – and eating more raw food (which has a high water content) is a good way to gain vitality. At first you may feel more tired, but after a few weeks you will notice that your energy levels increase and your skin will start to look fresher and clearer.

Feng shui

Dating back more than 1000 years, the Chinese art of feng shui is concerned with environmental influences on health and well-being. It offers practical suggestions of ways to balance the invisible energies in our surroundings.

CHI PATHS

According to ancient Chinese philosophy, our destiny is shaped by environmental forces, or the unseen energies that swirl all around us. Just as energy moves through the human body along the meridians, so it moves throughout the world around us, travelling along invisible energy pathways or "chi paths". Similarly, the energy in the environment is characterized in terms of the opposition between yin and yang. For instance, quiet and stillness are yin, noise and activity are yang. Round shapes, such as curves or circles, soft drapes and dark, absorbing colours enhance yin energy, whereas angular shapes and patterns, straight hangings and bright reflecting colours enhance yang energy.

BALANCING CHI

The purpose of feng shui is to create an environment in which chi flows smoothly and an even balance between yin and yang is maintained. This helps to create the right conditions for growth – no matter whether you are trying to create a happy home life, a successful business or a beautiful garden. Chi that is out of balance creates stagnant or excess energy pools, which in turn creates disharmony and disruption, as well as possible sickness and exhaustion.

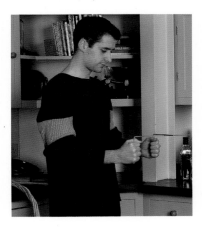

◄ FOR DETECTING CHI PATHS, L-SHAPED METAL RODS ARE EASIER TO WORK WITH THAN A PENDULUM. KEEP HIGH-USE AREAS ENERGETICALLY CLEAR AND WELL BALANCED.

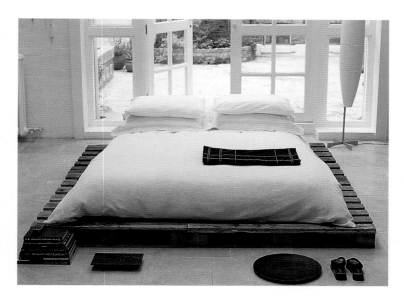

WORKING WITH FENG SHUI

Landscapes, buildings, rooms and everything in them vibrate with energy. Human beings function best when they are in the same range of vibrations as the earth. Using natural materials in your home will help to promote positive chi. Synthetic materials, chemicals, microwave ovens and electrical equipment all create negative chi. To help balance the effects of this chi, use crystals and/or plants near computers and television sets, and limit the time you spend using them.

▲ KEEPING YOUR SURROUNDINGS CLEAN AND CLUTTER-FREE HELPS CHI TO FLOW SMOOTHLY AND PROMOTES A CALM ATMOSPHERE.

DETECTING CHI PATHS

If you suffer from ill health or chronic tiredness, or your plans continually go awry, you may be exposed to negative chi paths. You can dowse to find the chi paths in your home and to indicate where chi is blocked or stagnant. Notice the health of any plants on the path and whether it runs under beds or chairs. It is best not to sleep or spend long periods directly in chi paths.

Healing sounds

Sound therapy is one of the oldest and most profound forms of energy healing. From the simple repetition of mystical words to complex rhythms and structures, sound waves can alter our mood and enhance well-being.

A UNIVERSE OF SOUNDS

Sound is our first experience of life. In the womb, a baby becomes familiar with the mother's heartbeat and voice. We feel most at ease with naturally occurring sound frequencies, such as the human voice, a running stream, birdsong, or rustling leaves. Constant exposure to discordant noises and high levels of background noise, such as from traffic, undermines the sensitivity

▼ THE POWERFUL HEALING VIBRATIONS OF A GONG CAN HELP "CLEAR THE AIR" OF NEGATIVE ENERGIES.

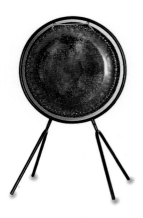

MANTRA

A mantra is a sacred sound that is used to "tune" the body's vibrational field and to raise levels of consciousness. In the Hindu tradition, the "om" mantra is believed to be the original sound from which the universe was born.

of our hearing and is a source of stress. Sound pollution weakens the immune system and has been linked to anxiety and depression.

VIBRATIONAL FIELDS

We pick up on sound waves not only through our ears, but also through our vibrational energy field. The subtle bodies, the chakras, and the physical body all vibrate at particular frequencies. When these vibrations are thrown out of balance, we are literally "out of tune", and become unwell. Sound therapy uses specific sound waves to retune these vibrations and restore harmony.

USING THE VOICE

The voice is an almost unlimited source of healing energy. Simple ways to work with it include chanting, toning and singing. Tones are pure sounds held on a single note, such as "aaaaa..." or "uuuuu...". Practised regularly, toning has a powerful effect on the body's cells and can raise energy levels, help to release emotional trauma and promote mental clarity. It can be combined with chanting, which involves the repetition of a mantra or short phrase. Chanting is one of the oldest singing techniques and has its roots in spiritual traditions.

▼ THE RHYTHMIC SOUND OF WAVES AS THEY CRASH ON THE SHORE CAN HAVE A CALMING EFFECT ON THE SPIRIT.

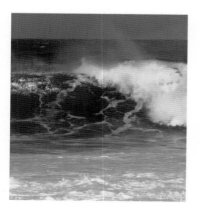

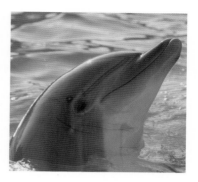

▲ MANY PEOPLE EXPERIENCE A SENSE OF EUPHORIA WHEN THEY HEAR THE HIGH FREQUENCY SOUNDS OF DOLPHINS.

MUSIC

Listening to music that is at the same frequency as alpha and theta brainwave patterns can promote relaxation and insight. Certain instruments, such as bells and gongs, generate particularly powerful healing sounds and their vibrations can be used to "clear the air" of negative energies.

BENEFITS

Healing sounds can dissolve tension, regulate heart rate and breathing, increase mental clarity and raise consciousness. Some high frequency sounds encourage the release of endorphins, and can produce feelings of bliss and euphoria.

Magnetotherapy

Magnets have been widely used in healing for thousands of years. A magnet generates an electromagnetic field (EMF) that can be used to influence the body's natural energy circuits to treat many common complaints.

USING MAGNETS

Magnets have the ability to speed up the flow of liquids and to prevent the clogging of channels. This gives them many benefits. For instance, they can be fitted to water pipes to reduce the build-up of scale; the magnets create a magnetic field that keeps the positively charged calcium ions (the ones that cause the scale) in suspension and away from the inner walls of the pipe.

▼ PLACING MAGNETS AT STRATEGIC POINTS ON THE BODY CAN RELIEVE MENSTRUAL PAIN AND OTHER EVERYDAY AILMENTS.

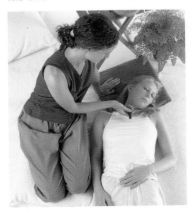

MAGNET THERAPY

Magnets can improve the flow of blood through the veins. They can help to clear blocked arteries, improve oxygen supply to the cells, stimulate the metabolism, and help with the elimination of waste. There is growing evidence that they ease muscle and joint pain and reduce inflammation. Magnets can be used to treat a variety of conditions, including arthritis, respiratory disorders, menstrual problems, headaches and insomnia.

Magnetic healthcare products include straps and wristbands, mattresses, car seat covers and shoe insoles, as well as special devices to fit to plumbing and heating systems. The magnet is worn or placed either at the site of pain, over lymph nodes (to encourage the drainage of toxins), or at specific acupuncture points. Many wearers report increased energy levels, improved mental clarity and general well-being.

Radionics

Radionics is a method of distant healing that uses specially designed instruments to analyse and treat energy imbalances. It was pioneered in the 1920s by Dr Albert Abrams, an American neurologist.

THE WITNESS

During the course of his work, Abrams devised a special machine, which became known as "the black box", with which to read the pattern of his patients' energy fields. This pattern is held in every cell of the body and can be witnessed in any of its parts, such as a drop of blood, a nail clipping or a lock of hair. Provided any small part can be given to the radionics practitioner as a "witness", it is not necessary for the patient to be present during diagnosis and treatment.

TREATMENT

You will be asked to complete a health-check questionnaire and send a hair or blood sample to the practitioner, to act as the witness, and to provide an "energetic link" between you. The witness is then placed on a black box and readings are taken to indicate your physical, mental and emotional state, your energy flow,

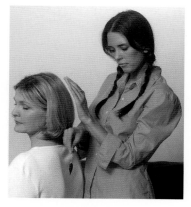

▲ A RADIONICS PRACTITIONER MAY ALSO USE DOWSING TO VERIFY HIS OR HER DIAGNOSIS AND TREATMENT PLAN.

any indications of major diseases and the cause of any existing health problem. Once a diagnosis has been made, the black box is used to "broadcast" healing energy to you. Some practitioners may also suggest homeopathic or Bach flower remedies, or colour therapy. Radionics aims to improve general health and well-being and is particularly helpful for diagnosing and treating allergies.

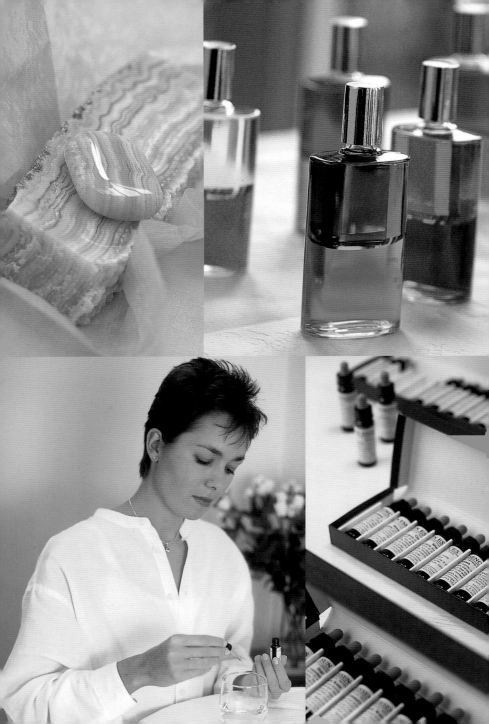

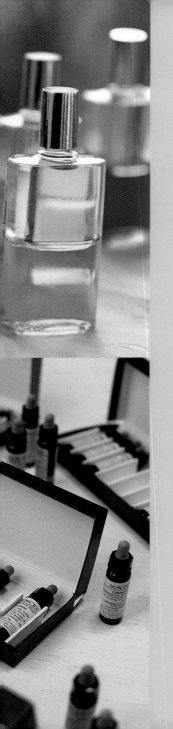

ENERGY
TREATMENTS

The therapies in this section aim to tap into the subtle energies of the Universe, and attune them to the human energy field, to restore balance and harmony, and help you return to optimum physical, mental and emotional health.

The treatments range from healing medicines, as used in homeopathy or flower and gemstone essences, to harnessing and directing the healing powers of magnets, water, light, sound and colour. Many of these techniques can be safely practised at home with just a few simple accessories, but some, such as acupuncture and radionics, should only be carried out by a qualified practitioner. Always seek advice if unsure.

Stress

A certain amount of stress is healthy, providing challenge and stimulation, but when faced with too much pressure the body responds by working harder until finally we get sick. Many common health problems are stress-related.

Financial pressures, problems in relationships, bereavement or divorce, moving house, getting married, noise and traffic are all common "stressors" that most of us cannot avoid.

Meditation, calming colours and healing sounds can all help to reduce stress levels. Kinesiology has specific techniques to help with the release of emotional stress, and will also check for any nutritional deficiencies. Ensuring that we are fully meeting our dietary needs is also an important part of the recovery process.

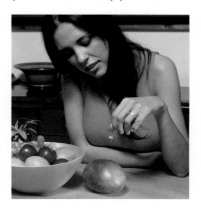

DOWSING FOR DIET

To check your nutritional needs, check your "yes" response to the question: "is the time right to dowse about my diet?" If "yes", use your pendulum to dowse in turn over the following key food groups: protein; fats and oils; carbohydrate; fibre; water; minerals; vitamins. You can then refine your quest to dowse over specific foods, checking to see if they are right for your body at this particular stressful time.

HOMEOPATHIC REMEDIES

These work to boost your "vital force" and are prescribed on an individual basis. However, some may be useful in acute situations:
- Ignatia 6c: soothes grief and disappointment
- Nux vomica 6c: helps with stress from overwork and irritability
- Sepia 6c: when you feel unable to cope, weepy and irritable.

◄ DOWSING FOR DIET WILL HELP YOU TO BOOST YOUR VITALITY IN TIMES OF STRESS.

Depression

Most people experience mood swings as well as the highs and lows of life. However, persistent worries, fears and tensions create energy blocks and we can get stuck on a "low" if we do not find a way to release the energy.

There are many triggers to negative mood states, including worries related to your state of health, finances, children or relationship problems. Physical illness or hormonal changes, such as those of menstruation, childbirth and menopause, may also be involved.

To encourage a more optimistic mood, use cheerful and enlivening colours, such as yellow or orange, with a touch of pink if you are feeling emotionally upset.

Avoid wearing black, grey and dark colours, and over-exposing yourself to "negative vibes" in the environment: this can include reading too much distressing news. Plenty of exposure to natural light, especially sunshine, is very helpful.

▼ WHEN YOUR SPIRITS ARE LOW, FLOWER REMEDIES CAN HELP RESTORE WELL-BEING.

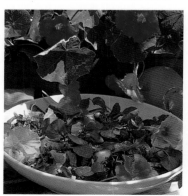

BACH FLOWERS
There are several Bach flower remedies that can help with depression. Select the one that most closely matches how you feel.
- Gorse: hopelessness and despair due to a setback
- Sweet chestnut: utter dejection and bleak outlook
- Mustard: gloom descends like a black cloud for no obvious reason
- Willow: introspective, pessimistic; self-pitying
- Honeysuckle: dwelling on the past, lack of interest in the present

MUSTARD   HONEYSUCKLE

Headaches and migraine

Most "everyday" headaches are caused by stress and tension. They can range from a dull throbbing to an intense stabbing pain. Migraines are even more disabling, and are often accompanied by nausea and vomiting.

Headaches can be triggered by a variety of factors, including toxic overload (from prescription drugs, caffeine, alcohol, or junk food), dehydration, low blood sugar, food intolerance, eyestrain, sinusitis, weather conditions and hormonal swings. Migraine triggers may include foodstuffs, such as red wine, chocolate or cheese, and attacks are exacerbated by stress.

Water is one of the best first-aid treatments for headaches and migraine, so drink a glass or two

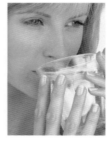

◀ IF YOU FEEL A HEADACHE COMING ON, TRY DRINKING A GLASS OR TWO OF MINERAL WATER. YOU MAY FIND THAT THE HEADACHE JUST DISAPPEARS OR IS AT LEAST LESS PAINFUL.

at the first sign of pain. Splashing your face with water and lying down at the onset of a migraine is also helpful. Tension headaches may be relieved by a bath, sauna or steam bath. Alternating hot and cold will improve circulation.

The colour green is restful on the eyes and may help you to relax, while amethysts can ease tension headaches. For pain relief, press between the thumb and forefinger of each hand, or press your thumbs into the hollow areas at the base of the skull on either side of the spine, and tilt your head back for a few moments, breathing deeply.

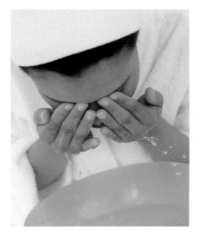

◀ RELIEVE TENSION HEADACHES BY SPLASHING COOL WATER OVER YOUR FACE.

Arthritis

There are two types of arthritis. Osteoarthritis is the more common and is marked by degeneration in the cartilage that protects the joints; in rheumatoid arthritis the joints become inflamed and painfully swollen.

According to the World Health Organization, acupuncture is an effective treatment for arthritis and it is increasingly recommended by conventional medicine. Regular acupuncture treatments can help to ease joint pain, stiffness and inflammation, and restore a greater range of movement to the joints.

Water treatments can also be effective; cold compresses can help to relieve pain and swelling, or alternate hot and cold will help to boost the circulation and ease stiffness. Check your diet using kinesiology, dowsing or Vega testing and make sure you are getting enough of the foods, vitamins and minerals that your body needs. Cut down on the energy-draining foods, particularly those that are acid-forming, such as dairy products, chocolate, wine, caffeine and sugar.

MAGNET THERAPY

Wearing a magnetic wristband is an increasingly popular self-help treatment for arthritis. It can improve the circulation and help to break down the toxic crystal deposits that have accumulated around the joints. The magnet should be worn on the inner wrist, next to the pulse point. Drinking plenty of water will help the body to flush out the toxins.

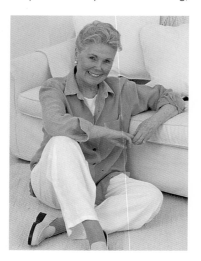

◄ ARTHRITIS CAN BE TREATED IN A NUMBER OF DIFFERENT WAYS TO ENSURE THAT YOUR LATER YEARS ARE ACTIVE AND LESS PAINFUL.

Colds and flu

Catching a cold or flu is a sign that your energy levels are depleted and your body's defences are weakened. Colds are often linked with seasonal changes in weather patterns, when the body needs extra support.

In the early "sore throat" stages of a cold, drink hot lemon and honey and eat light meals. In the later stages, eating raw foods and drinking fresh fruit and vegetable juices will have a cleansing and energy-boosting effect, and can help with clearing mucus. Avoid tea, coffee, sugar and dairy products. Resting and giving your body a chance to recover is also essential; carrying on regardless will drain your energy further and, in the long run, may mean that it takes even longer to get better.

▾ RED ONION IS USED TO MAKE THE HOMEOPATHIC REMEDY ALLIUM CEPA. THIS IS INDICATED FOR COLDS WITH PROFUSE SNEEZING AND "CRYING" EYES.

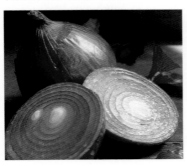

COLOUR TREATMENTS

To ease a sore throat, wrap a blue or green scarf around your neck to bring healing energy to your throat chakra. Alternatively, drink blue or green colour infusions.

HOMEOPATHY CURES

There are several homeopathic remedies for colds and flu.
- Allium cepa 6c: head colds characterized by sneezing
- Ferrum phos 6c: cold that comes on slowly, with a red swollen throat
- Nux vomica 6c: irritability, feeling chilly, watery eyes
- Kali bich 6c: blocked sinuses with yellow-green mucus
- Aconite 6c: sudden onset of flu, often at night, with chill and high fever
- Belladonna 6c: sudden onset of flu, with headache, fever
- Gelsemium 6c: "traditional" flu, with shivers, shakes, aching muscles, debility

FERRUM PHOS   KALI BICH

Chronic fatigue syndrome

Chronic fatigue is an extremely disabling condition for which there is no conventional medical treatment. It can be a symptom of a number of conditions, such as depression or anaemia, or may follow a viral infection, such as flu.

CFS is a complicated condition. Its symptoms are a sign that your energy is severely depleted and out of balance. This means that you need to be particularly wary of "energy drainers" and cultivate things that give you energy.

Start by assessing your diet and lifestyle. Find out if you have any food intolerances or allergies; kinesiology, Vega testing, dowsing and radionics can all be used to check for this. Then, consider the impact that electromagnetic energy fields may be having on your health. Is your home or workplace an energy haven or is it draining you? Metal conducts electricity, so don't position a bed near a radiator, or sleep in a brass bed next to a power point. Protect yourself from the electric fields of domestic appliances and make sure your computer screen has low-level radiation. Work with feng

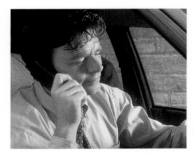

▲ TRY TO AVOID PROLONGED PERIODS WHEN YOU ARE EXPOSED TO STRESS AS THIS WILL DEPLETE YOUR ENERGY LEVELS.

shui to keep energy pathways clear, and use colours that enhance energy: purples and blues to boost the immune system, greens to lift depression, and yellows to promote a positive outlook.

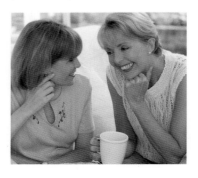

▶ SPENDING TIME WITH FRIENDS NOURISHES THE MENTAL AND EMOTIONAL BODIES AND CAN HELP TO TRIGGER THE BODY'S SELF-HEALING MECHANISMS.

Allergies and intolerances

True allergies are very rare, but over-sensitivity to certain foods or environmental factors is relatively common. These over-sensitivities or intolerances seem to be implicated in many common chronic health problems.

If you suspect that you may be suffering from an intolerance, the first step is to identify the key triggers that have a destabilizing effect on your immune system. Kinesiology, Vega testing and radionics will help you locate these. Use dowsing to check your response to common allergens. These include alcohol, caffeine, corn, dairy produce, soya, sugar, wheat, chocolate, tomatoes, moulds, pollen, house dust, animal hair, exhaust fumes, glues, paints, electro-magnetic radiation, fungicides and pesticides.

DESENSITIZATION STRATEGIES

The obvious strategy is to avoid contact with an allergen. This can mean making dietary changes and changing your washing detergent, for instance. Some allergens are unavoidable, however, in which case you need to reprogramme your immune system. Taking homeopathic dilutions of the offending substance, such as house dust or pollen, can help you to build up immunity. These remedies work rather like vaccinations, but on an energy level rather than a physical level.

▼ A USEFUL HOMEOPATHIC REMEDY FOR HAYFEVER IS EUPHRASIA (EYEBRIGHT), INDICATED WHEN EYES ARE RED AND SORE.

▼ IF YOU FIND YOU ARE INTOLERANT TO WHEAT PRODUCTS, IT WILL MEAN ELIMINATING CERTAIN TYPES OF BREAD FROM YOUR DIET.

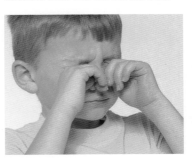

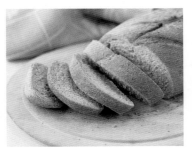

Digestive problems

A healthy digestive system is crucial for health and well-being. Any digestive disorder, no matter how trivial it may seem, is a sign of an energy imbalance that needs to be taken seriously and treated accordingly.

Many digestive problems are linked to poor eating habits, food intolerance and emotional stress. If you suffer from frequent digestive problems, test for food allergens and eliminate any triggers from your diet. Many people are intolerant of wheat, corn and dairy products without realizing it. Eat a diet that is rich in energy-building foods, and avoid irritants such as tea, coffee, strong spices and alcohol. If your digestion is weak, raw food and elaborate meals with rich sauces are best avoided; instead, follow a plain diet that includes lightly steamed vegetables, chicken, fish, tofu and wholegrain rice. Drink plenty of water.

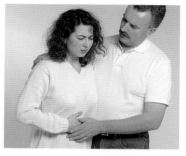

▲ MANY DIGESTIVE PROBLEMS ARE LINKED TO EMOTIONAL UPSETS.

BACH FLOWERS

When the problem is stress-related, taking Bach flower remedies can help to balance the mental and emotional bodies.
• Walnut: helps with a change in circumstances, such as a new job, moving house or divorce
• Scleranthus: constant dilemmas, unable to make decisions
• Vervain: wired up, unable to relax, chasing perfection
• Impatiens: impatient and also irritable, always in a hurry
• Crab apple: when revolted by food as well as eating; cleansing and detoxifying

---

TIP

A quick treatment for nausea and vomiting is to apply finger pressure to the acupuncture point that is situated about 3 cm (1¼ in) above the wrist on the inside arm.

Skin problems

The state of our health and well-being shows in the skin. Skin disorders can indicate problems with digestion or circulation or inadequate removal of toxins from the body. They may also be a visible sign of stress.

If your skin problem is stress-related, you need to find ways to release tension. Aerobic exercise will boost your energy and encourage the body to unwind. It also helps the body to release toxins. Drinking plenty of water helps to flush the toxins out of your system; starting the day with a glass of warm water will also encourage a sluggish digestive system to work more efficiently.

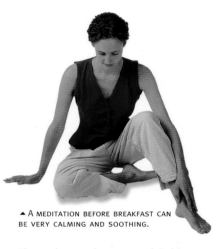

▲ A MEDITATION BEFORE BREAKFAST CAN BE VERY CALMING AND SOOTHING.

▼ IF YOU HAVE PROBLEM SKIN, TRY STARTING THE DAY WITH A GLASS OF WARM WATER RATHER THAN A CUP OF TEA OR COFFEE.

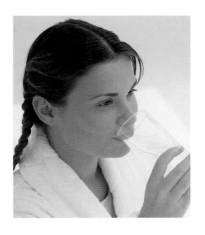

The redness, dryness and itching of many skin problems indicates excess heat. A cold shower will help to redress the balance, bringing the energy back inside the body and closing the pores.

COLOUR MEDITATION
A short meditation will set you up for the day; tune in and visualize which colours you need. Green, pale pink or blue are often helpful for aggravated skin conditions such as eczema or dermatitis.

PMS and menstrual cramps

Many women experience problems with menstruation. Fluctuating hormone levels, emotional stress and physical tension can unbalance the system, producing symptoms from extreme mood swings to severe physical pain.

Magnets can help to ease period pain by improving the flow of blood to the area. Apply the magnet midway between the pubic bone and the navel and leave in position for up to ten minutes. This should help to relieve the cramp. Alternatively use a Reiki hand treatment. Place one hand on the lower stomach and the other on the lower back; visualize healing Reiki energy flowing through your hand, dissolving any tension and bringing peace and well-being.

MOONTIME

The menstrual cycle mirrors the 28-day cycle of the moon. Your "moontime" is a time when your energy levels are low, and ideally you should spend more time relaxing so as to build your energy in preparation for the coming period. If you want to tune in to the cycles of the moon, moonstone is the ideal stone to work with. Moonstone helps to balance and relax emotional states. It can also have beneficial effects on all the body's fluid systems and ease tension in the abdominal area.

Apply moonstones to your body in a pattern that amplifies their potential for relaxing and healing. Place one stone at the top of your head, one on the front of each shoulder and one on each hip. Close your eyes and relax.

▼ To treat period pains, channel healing energy through your hands with a relaxing Reiki treatment.

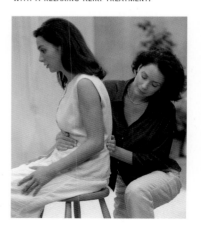

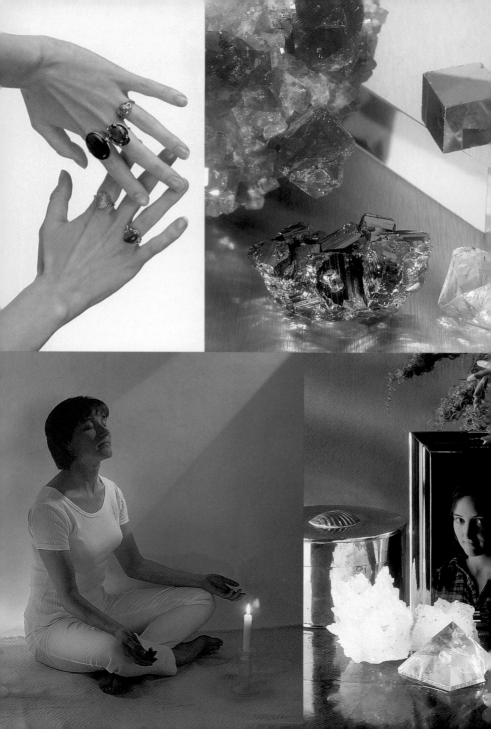

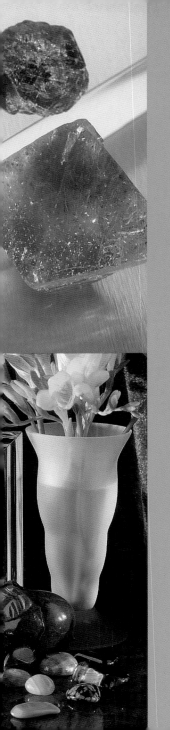

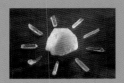

HEALING WITH
CRYSTALS

The stabilizing power of crystals has made them a natural instrument of holistic healing, thanks to their orderly atomic structure. By placing a crystal against an aching muscle, for example, healing energies are directed to the source of the complaint – often a tense and congested area – and the pain alleviated.

Crystals appear in many forms, each with its own healing properties, and can be used in conjunction with chakra healing to treat specific parts of the anatomy. Harnessing the potent and mysterious powers of these gemstones can be easily achieved at home, either with a particular layout for, or simple contact with, the body, through crystal essences or with a simple crystal lightbox.

How a crystal is born

Our word "crystal" is derived from the ancient Greek term "krystallos", meaning "ice". The Greeks thought rock crystal was water that had frozen so completely that it could never melt again.

The Greeks were not entirely mistaken, of course, because ice is indeed the crystal form of water, and we call ice crystals snowflakes, and recognize their six-sided forms. Every substance, from water to carbon, or blood, will form crystalline structures given the correct circumstances of temperature and pressure.

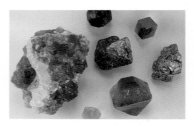

▲ THE INTERNAL LATTICE STRUCTURE OF A CRYSTAL IS REVEALED IN ITS EXTERNAL GEOMETRY OF FLAT PLANES AND ANGLES.

Deep within the Earth's crust superheated gases and mineral-rich solutions find their way towards the surface along cracks and fissures at very high temperatures. As they cool, the atoms of the boiling gases and liquids begin to arrange themselves in regular patterns. These repeating three-dimensional patterns of atoms are known as crystal lattices. All crystals have their own characteristic microscopic lattice forms.

As the mineral solutions near the Earth's surface cool and the pressure drops, atoms from different minerals often combine to create more complex crystals. Usually harder minerals, such as diamond, emerald and quartz, form at a higher pressure and temperature, and have a dense lattice structure. Softer minerals, such as calcite and turquoise crystallize at lower temperatures and have a more open lattice.

The structure of the Earth is continually changing, but the essential quality of all crystals is their very stable atomic structure. Whatever the outside force – whether heat, pressure, electricity or light – crystals always make minute adjustments to restore their internal stability and lattice form.

This unique orderliness and stability makes crystals valuable in modern technology. They are used in watches and lasers, and as switching and regulating devices in engines powering all manner of things from cars to space shuttles.

No one is really certain how crystals help in healing, but it may be that the very nature of crystals increases the levels of harmony in their immediate environment. Crystals are known to be the most orderly matter in the universe. Because coherence is a stronger natural force than chaos, introducing order into a disorganized state – for example, by placing a crystal on an aching muscle – can increase the chances of the imbalance or disharmony returning to stability and order.

Whether the imbalance in us is a physical illness or emotional or mental upset, our energy pattern has lost its order. The simple, powerful resonance of a crystal, with its locked-in power of ancient fire and unique purity of form, may help us reinstate our own balance and harmony.

▼ WHETHER NATURAL OR CARVED, THE INTERNAL ORDERLINESS OF A CRYSTAL'S ATOMS CAN INFLUENCE ITS SURROUNDINGS.

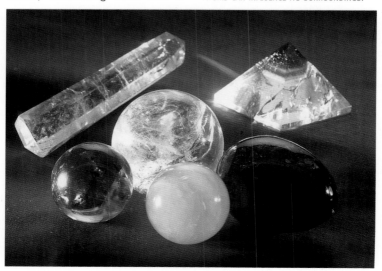

Crystal variations

Crystals come in all manner of colours, shapes and sizes. They consist of many different ingredients, determined by conditions, such as location, temperature and pressure. Here are some of their many types and forms.

GEODE

If a mineral solution crystallizes in a hollow rock cavity, and the rock then erodes, geode crystals are formed. Geodes can be of many shapes and colours, according to the type of original rock and minerals.

PHANTOM CRYSTAL

These stones are so named because within the body of a phantom are smaller outlines of the crystal form. During formation, where a crystal stops growing and then begins again, a few particles of other minerals may settle on the faces, clearly showing the stages of growth. These are fascinating and beautiful crystals to look at and make good personal meditation crystals.

FLUORITE CRYSTAL

This gemstone forms around a cubic lattice structure making interlocking cubes, octahedral and pyramid crystals. It comes in a wide variety of colours, though violet is one of the commonest.

CELESTITE

This is soft stone, which is most often formed by the evaporation of water from mineral deposits, leaving a clear and delicate blue crystal.

AMETRINE

As the name suggests, this is a mix of amethyst, giving the violet colour, and citrine, which adds the golden yellow. Both are varieties of the common mineral, quartz.

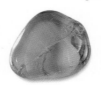

Rock Crystal Wands

Crystals can be microscopic in size or very large indeed, growing to several metres in length. Long, thin prisms of crystal can be effective healing tools.

Iron Pyrites

This ore of iron and sulphur is a common mineral in the Earth's crust. It can form perfect single cubes, sparkly masses resembling gold and flat, disc-like clusters of crystal.

Citrine

A form of quartz that occurs when violet amethyst is subjected to heat, either naturally or artificially.

Opal

Is a member of the quartz family with a high water content, creating the colourful play of light. It is microcrystalline with no regular geometry visible.

Rutilated Quartz

A clear or smoky crystal, rutilated quartz contains fine threads of golden or orange rutile (titanium oxide) crystals.

Amethyst

This is another form of quartz, whose purple or violet colour comes from iron particles in the crystal.

Blue Lace Agate

From the chalcedony family of crystals blue lace agate is made up of tiny blue and white quartz crystals, in swirls or lines.

Amber

A fossil pine tree resin, amber is found in rich yellows, orange brown and deep reds and greens, often with trapped foliage or even insects embedded within.

The chakra system

Knowledge of the chakra system comes from ancient Indian texts. These describe energy centres or chakras in the body, with seven major points arranged along the spinal column. These chakras are used in crystal healing.

THE SEVEN CHAKRAS

In Indian philosophy the chakras are the areas of energy near the spine where particular internal organs and systems are focused. Seven points are counted along the spinal column from the crown of the head down to the base of the spine. Each chakra is linked with a physical function and also a mental or emotional state; and each has come to be represented by a particular colour. By matching the appropriate crystals with the relevant chakra centres, it is possible to help restore natural functioning of the body at many different levels.

▼ CHAKRA IS AN ANCIENT INDIAN WORD FOR "WHEEL". WHEREVER DIFFERENT STREAMS OF ENERGY CONVERGE, A SPIRALLING DYNAMIC FUNCTION IS CREATED.

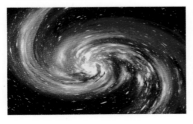

CHAKRA FUNCTIONS

• the first or base chakra at the base of the spine is red in colour, and concerns physical survival, and energy distribution in the body;

• the second or sacral chakra, apart from its control of the reproductive system, is concerned with creativity and pleasure-seeking; its colour is orange;

• the third or solar plexus chakra, is located between the bottom of the ribcage and the navel. Yellow in colour, it connects with confidence, personal power and gut instinct;

• the fourth or heart chakra is at the centre of the chest, is green and deals with relationships and personal development;

• the fifth or throat chakra controls the power of speech and communication, including learning, and is a blue colour;

• the sixth, third eye or brow chakra is in the centre of the forehead, its colour is indigo and it supervises mental powers, memory and psychic abilities;

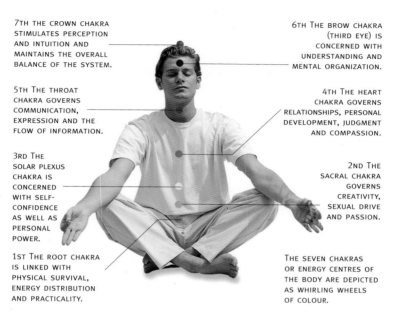

7TH THE CROWN CHAKRA STIMULATES PERCEPTION AND INTUITION AND MAINTAINS THE OVERALL BALANCE OF THE SYSTEM.

6TH THE BROW CHAKRA (THIRD EYE) IS CONCERNED WITH UNDERSTANDING AND MENTAL ORGANIZATION.

5TH THE THROAT CHAKRA GOVERNS COMMUNICATION, EXPRESSION AND THE FLOW OF INFORMATION.

4TH THE HEART CHAKRA GOVERNS RELATIONSHIPS, PERSONAL DEVELOPMENT, JUDGMENT AND COMPASSION.

3RD THE SOLAR PLEXUS CHAKRA IS CONCERNED WITH SELF-CONFIDENCE AS WELL AS PERSONAL POWER.

2ND THE SACRAL CHAKRA GOVERNS CREATIVITY, SEXUAL DRIVE AND PASSION.

1ST THE ROOT CHAKRA IS LINKED WITH PHYSICAL SURVIVAL, ENERGY DISTRIBUTION AND PRACTICALITY.

THE SEVEN CHAKRAS OR ENERGY CENTRES OF THE BODY ARE DEPICTED AS WHIRLING WHEELS OF COLOUR.

• the seventh or crown chakra is located at the top of the head, its colour is violet, and it oversees the balance of the chakra system and higher spiritual growth.

THE SUBTLE BODIES

Health problems can arise when energy in the subtle bodies or chakras becomes congested or is under- or over-stimulated. The root chakra, for example, can become "muddied" by eating the wrong foods, and through lack of exercise. Or when it is not linked properly to the physical body, you are likely to experience low energy and persistent tiredness. Problems in one body or chakra can also have a knock-on effect on the others. Crystal healing aims to bring the subtle bodies and the chakras into alignment. During any healing process, health and balance is understood to return to the subtle bodies first. Once the vibrational pattern is restored, the physical body then returns to health at its own slightly slower pace.

Crystal colours

The simplest methods of crystal healing combine the colour of stones with the appropriate chakra. The colour of a crystal will always indicate its main energy function, so it is useful to learn the basic properties of each colour.

RED (BASE CHAKRA)

This colour stimulates, activates and energizes, but also grounds and focuses. Associated crystals are garnet, jasper and ruby.

GARNET

ORANGE (SACRAL CHAKRA)

A mix of red and yellow, orange combines their activating and organizing roles in boosting energy flows or treating blockages. Related crystals include dark citrine, orange calcite, carnelian, topaz and copper.

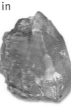

ORANGE CALCITE

YELLOW (SOLAR PLEXUS)

The vibrant colour yellow is concerned with strengthening and preserving the body's systems (e.g. nervous, digestive and

AMBER

immune). The associated crystals are amber, rutilated quartz, tiger's eye, citrine quartz and iron pyrites.

GREEN (HEART CHAKRA)

As the mid-spectrum colour, green acts to balance our emotions and relationships, encouraging growth in all areas of life.

MALACHITE

Heart stones include bloodstone, green aventurine, malachite, amazonite, moss agate, peridot and emerald.

BLUE (THROAT CHAKRA)

The blue chakra relates principally to communication, both within ourselves and from us to the outside world. Related stones are celestite, blue lace agate, turquoise and aquamarine.

AQUAMARINE

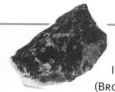
LAPIS LAZULI

INDIGO
(BROW CHAKRA)
Dark blue, or indigo, governs perception, understanding and intuition. Associated with this centre are lapis lazuli, sodalite, kyanite, azurite and sapphire.

VIOLET (CROWN CHAKRA)
The traditional colour of spiritual illumination and service, violet also represents the mind's control of the body and the self. Related stones include amethyst, fluorite, sugilite and iolite.

AMETHYST

WHITE
With qualities of universality and clarity, white is also connected to the crown chakra. White light contains and reflects all other colours, symbolizing the potential to cleanse or purify energy. Clear quartz, herkimer diamond, Iceland spa, moonstone and selenite are favoured white crystals.

MOONSTONE

TOURMALINE

BLACK
The colour black absorbs light as much as white reflects it. Black reveals the hidden potential of a person or condition. It holds its energies in reserve, grounds and anchors energy. Related crystals are smoky quartz, obsidian, tourmaline and haematite.

ROSE QUARTZ
PINK
A blend of both red and white, pink is associated with the base and heart chakras, and works to restore underlying balance. Pink stones include rose quartz, rhodonite and rhodocrosite.

MULTICOLOURED
These are various, and their actions reflect their colour combinations. Rainbow inclusions can be found in many transparent crystals including quartz. Other stones are azurite-malachite, hawk's eye, opal, labradorite and ametrine.

AMETRINE

Choosing and cleansing crystals

All the crystals described in this book are relatively easy to find at a reasonable price. When building up a personal collection, aim for quality rather than quantity. Purchase stones that attract you and that you feel happy with.

CHOOSING YOUR CRYSTALS

When selecting suitable crystals, remember that you will be placing stones on a relaxed, prone body, whether yours or somebody else's. So avoid stones that are too heavy or too small. Flatter stones stay in place better than round ones. Try to acquire at least two stones per spectrum colour.

Small natural crystals of clear quartz are often needed, so try to find about a dozen, each of around 2–3 cm (¾–1¼ in) in length. Small crystals of smoky quartz, amethyst and citrine have many uses.

A small, hand-sized crystal cluster of clear quartz or amethyst is useful for cleansing and charging your stones.

Larger single stones and tumbled stones are good to hold and as meditation aids.

▼ HANDLE YOUR CRYSTALS CAREFULLY, SINCE SOME ARE SOFT AND CAN SCRATCH, WHILE OTHERS ARE HARD AND BRITTLE.

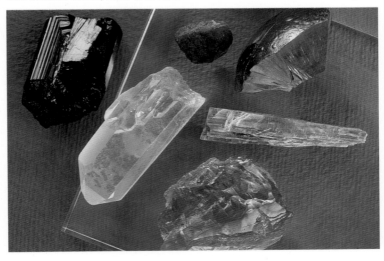

CLEANSING YOUR CRYSTALS

New stones should be cleansed before you begin using them. Cleansing removes unwanted energy from the crystals and restores them to their original clarity. Cleanse your crystals every time you use them for healing. Try the following methods:

• Sun and water: hold the stones under running water for a minute and place them in the sun to dry.

• Incense or smudge stick: hold the crystal within the smoke; herbs such as sandalwood, sage, cedar and frankincense are good purifiers.

• Sound: the vibrations of a bell, gong or tuning fork can energetically clean a crystal.

• Sea salt: put dry sea salt (avoid salt water as it can corrode crystals)

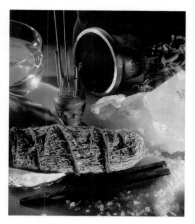

▲ MATERIALS FOR CLEANSING CRYSTALS INCLUDE SALT, WATER, A TUNING FORK, INCENSE AND SMUDGE STICKS.

in a small container and bury your crystal in the salt crystals for approximately 24 hours.

▼ CLEAN STONES ON A CRYSTAL CLUSTER (BELOW LEFT) OR SURROUND ONE STONE WITH CLEAR QUARTZ POINTS FOR 24 HOURS (BELOW).

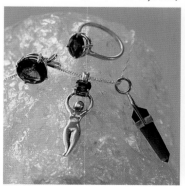

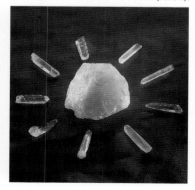

choosing and cleansing crystals **349**

Techniques: know your stones

When you acquire a new crystal, spend some time getting familiar with it and developing a sensitivity to its subtle energy field. Try these simple techniques, being aware of how you feel at each step.

SENSING YOUR CRYSTALS

1 Examine your crystal from all angles, then close your eyes and feel it as you hold it in your hands for a minute or two.

2 Open your eyes and gaze at the crystal. Then close your eyes once more. Does the crystal feel the same as before?

3 Hold the crystal in one hand, then the other. Also try holding it in both hands.

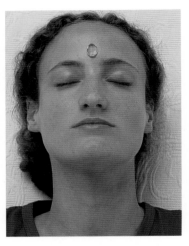

▲ LIE DOWN, CLOSE YOUR EYES AND RELAX AND SENSE THE EFFECT OF YOUR CHOSEN CRYSTAL ON A CHAKRA POINT.

4 Now lie back and place the crystal on your chakra centres. The solar plexus, heart and brow are often good places to try.

5 Still lying down, place the crystal close to your body, noting how it feels on the right and left sides, near your head and feet.

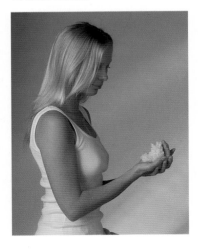

◄ DEVELOP A SENSITIVITY TO A NEW CRYSTAL BY HOLDING IT.

A VISUALIZATION EXERCISE
This exercise is best done with a crystal you already know and feel comfortable with.

1 Sit comfortably and hold the crystal in both hands. Relax and focus on it.

2 Slowly let your awareness float down into the crystal and come to rest there.

3 Think how the crystal feels — warm or damp, cool or dry, smooth or rough? Take a minute or two to explore its inner energy.

4 Relax again, and attune yourself to the crystal's inner vibration or sound — is it a tone, a pulse or a tune, high or low, simple or complex? Listen for a few minutes, then relax again.

5 Take some deep breaths, then imagine you are breathing in the crystal's energy. Does it have a taste or smell?

6 Relax again, and open your inner eyes to imagine the lattice structure of the crystal, its inner light and landscape. Don't analyze anything you see, just let it come and go.

7 Now become aware again of the crystal's taste, smell, sounds and touch. Gradually bring your awareness out of the crystal and back into your own body. Make notes so that you will be able to remember your experiences better.

▼ HOLD THE CRYSTAL NEAR YOUR SOLAR PLEXUS AND IMAGINE YOUR BREATH IS ENTERING YOUR BODY THROUGH THE STONE.

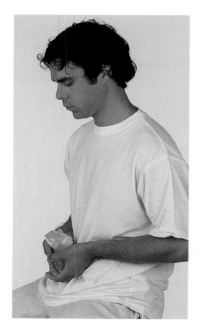

Meditating with crystals

Clear quartz can be a wonderful aid to meditation and contemplation. Just think, you are looking into solid matter of extraordinary stability and subtlety. Its constant harmony may help you increase or regain your own.

If you are upset or stressed, gaze deeply into your favourite quartz crystal, and allow your mind to quieten down. When the body and mind begins to settle, it is easier to find solutions and balance.

Sit quietly with your quartz crystal and look closely at it. Then relax and shut your eyes. Pay attention to how you feel and think. Are your thoughts calm or busy, happy or sad? Note any sensations in your body.

After a few minutes, repeat the process using other quartz crystals and compare your experiences. Take deep, slow, breaths before you get up.

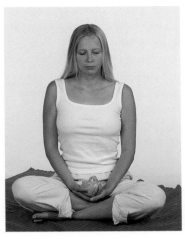

▲ SIT IN A COMFORTABLE POSITION TO MEDITATE WITH YOUR CRYSTALS.

Sit comfortably with a smoky quartz in your left hand and a clear quartz in your right. After a few moments swap them around. Do you feel any difference? Once you find a combination that suits you, try to spend a few minutes every day, preferably at the same time, sitting and meditating with your favourite crystals.

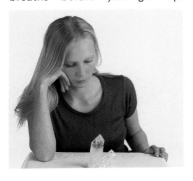

◀ GAZE INTO THE DEPTHS OF YOUR CRYSTAL AND CLOSE YOUR EYES.

In another form of crystal meditation, place the crystal in a position in front of you that lets you gaze into its depths. Don't try to control your thoughts or worry about "doing it right". Just relax and enjoy the stone's company. Then close your eyes, feel calm, take some deep breaths and follow your thoughts. Open or close your eyes as you wish, but take the crystal's energy with you as you meditate.

If you find it difficult to relax and meditate with one crystal, you can make a pattern or mandala with your stones. This "active contemplation" may suit you better.

▼ MAKING A PATTERN OR A MANDALA OF YOUR STONES CAN CALM AN AGITATED MIND

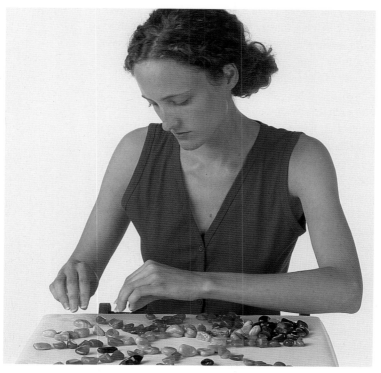

Hand-held crystal healing

We are all aware that positive thoughts are healing and negative thoughts are harmful. Using a quartz crystal in combination with directed positive thought can release a flow of healing energy, towards ourselves or to others.

A quartz crystal will direct the energy either towards or away from your body, depending on where the point is facing. An additional crystal can be held in the "absorbing" or "receiving" hand. This helps us to feel the quartz's healing energy clearly in our awareness.

ENERGY CHANNELLING

If you have an area of over-excited energy, you may feel congested, hot, tense, irritated or frustrated. Place the palm of your left hand over that area. Hold the quartz crystal in your right hand, with its point away from you and towards the ground. Breathe deeply and evenly, imagining all the excess energy releasing from your body. Let it pass out through the crystal into the earth and away from you.

If you need to recharge depleted energy or want extra healing energy, the process is reversed. Hold the quartz in your right hand, pointing it towards the area concerned. Hold your left hand away from your body, with the palm facing upwards. Breathe deeply and evenly, imagining healing energies from the universe passing from your upturned hand, through the crystal and into you.

▸ TO RELEASE EXCESS ENERGY INTO THE EARTH HOLD A QUARTZ CRYSTAL IN YOUR RIGHT HAND POINTING AWAY FROM YOU AND TOWARDS THE GROUND.

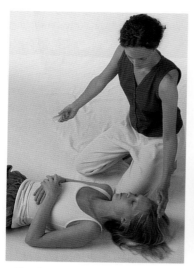 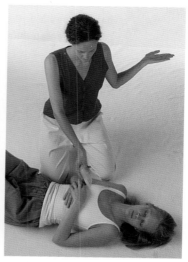

1 To clear away unwanted energy, release tensions and help relaxation, hold your "receiving" hand close to your partner. With your "directing" hand, hold the quartz and allow the excess energy to drain away into the earth. Try moving the quartz in circles to aid the process.

2 When you finish, revitalize the other person's aura by holding the crystal in the "directing" hand, with the point towards the body. Hold the "receiving" hand palm upwards and allow the universal energy to flow through the crystal into the newly cleansed area or chakra.

Try these exercises with opposite hands to see how it feels. Right-handed people often find their left hand more absorbing or "receiving", and the right hand directs the outward flow of energy. Left-handed people may find the opposite is true for them.

Grounding and centring

When you feel solidly anchored in the present, with a sense of inner calm and clarity, that is the experience of being grounded. Being ungrounded is a state of feeling confused and unfocused.

GETTING GROUNDED

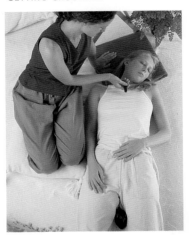

▲ ADOPT THIS LAYOUT TO CENTRE AND GROUND YOUR ENERGIES IN JUST A COUPLE OF MINUTES.

Holding a grounding stone can help us focus chaotic energy and restore everyday awareness. A simple grounding exercise is to sit or stand with your feet firmly on the floor, then imagine roots growing from your feet into the earth. With each breath, allow the roots to spread deeper and wider until you feel anchored and secure.

A GROUNDING LAYOUT

Lie down on your back and relax. Place one smoky quartz crystal point downwards at the base of the throat and another between the legs or close to the base of the spine. In most crystal healing patterns it helps to use a grounding stone close to the base chakra or between the feet and legs. Any changes created by the healing can then be more easily integrated into daily life.

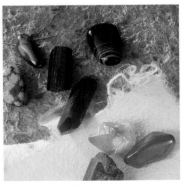

▲ MANY OF THE CRYSTALS THAT HELP IN GROUNDING ARE DARK OR RED. TOP, LEFT TO RIGHT: SNOWFLAKE OBSIDIAN, HAEMATITE, DARK TOURMALINE, SMOKY QUARTZ, ONYX. BOTTOM, LEFT TO RIGHT: STAUROLITE, CITRINE, JASPER.

CENTRING YOURSELF

Feeling centred means being in a state of mental, emotional and physical balance. You know your boundaries and feel in control of your energies. Centring can be achieved by techniques that focus your attention within your body.

1 Sit quietly, and be aware of your breathing. Feel yourself breathing in from your feet and back out through your feet into the earth.

2 Be aware of your midline — an imaginary line extending from above the top of your head to below your feet, situated just in

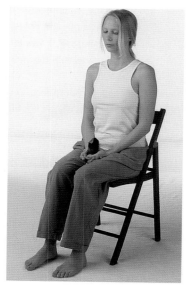

▲ RESTORE YOUR FOCUS WITH A BLACK GROUNDING STONE.

front of your spine. Pull your breath into this midline from above and breathe out through the line into the ground. Repeat until you feel calm and focused.

3 Strike a bell, gong or tuning fork, and listen for as long as the sound remains.

4 Slowly and consciously bring your fingertips together and hold them for a minute or two. Take deep breaths in.

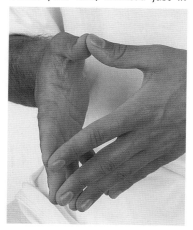

▲ BRING YOUR FINGERTIPS TOGETHER SLOWLY TO FOCUS YOUR ATTENTION.

Pendulum healing

Many people will be familiar with the idea of using a pendulum for dowsing. A pendulum made from a natural crystal can, however, be used as a healing tool in its own right, even if the individual has no experience with dowsing.

Using a crystal pendulum for healing is effective in removing energy imbalances from the body's finer energy sytems.

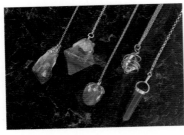

▲ THERE ARE MANY STYLES OF PENDULUM, SO CHOOSE ONE THAT FEELS RIGHT FOR YOU.

The healer has a clear intent that the pendulum will only move away from a neutral swing (back and forth) when it finds an energy imbalance that can be corrected quickly and safely. The crystal will move in a pattern that allows the imbalance to be cleared and will then return to the neutral swing. It is not necessary to know the nature of the imbalances – they may be on many levels from the physical, emotional, mental or spiritual bodies. Nor does the physical location of an imbalance necessarily indicate that it is where the source of a problem lies. The movement of a crystal's energy field through the aura simply helps to break up any build-up of unhelpful patterns, and releases them safely.

Whilst dowsing for assessment, any sort of pendulum, wood, metal, plastic, glass or stone can be used. Healing techniques using pendulums, however, will best employ a natural crystal. Because every crystal has its own range of properties the best crystal pendulums to use are ones that have a broad, generalized energy. These will respond to and balance many different types of energy imbalance. Clear quartz, amethyst and smoky quartz all make useful healing pendulums. Other clear and transparent crystals also work with broad ranges of energy.

As it is a healing tool, a crystal pendulum needs to be cleansed regularly before and after use.

REMOVING ENERGY IMBALANCES

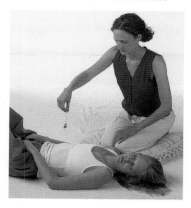

▲ HOLD THE PENDULUM LIGHTLY AND FIRMLY
BETWEEN THE THUMB AND FOREFINGER.

1 Grip the pendulum. Allow the wrist to relax and hold your arm in a comfortable position.

2 Start the pendulum moving in a line, to and fro, in what is known as a neutral swing.

3 Slowly move up the centre of the body, beginning beneath the feet. Wherever the pendulum swings away from the neutral, simply stay at that point until the neutral swing returns.

4 When you reach the top of the head, go back to the feet and begin again. Now hold the pendulum nearer to one side of the body and again slowly move upwards. Repeat for the other side.

5 If the pendulum goes on moving over an imbalance for a long time, put another crystal on that spot and move on. Later check the area again. An appropriate choice of stone will have balanced the energies so that the pendulum remains in a neutral swing.

Although some methods place importance on the way a pendulum moves, in this technique any movement away from neutral simply indicates an imbalance that the crystal is able to correct.

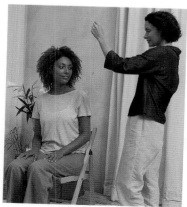

▲ CRYSTAL PENDULUMS CAN HELP TO
BALANCE THE SUBTLE BODIES.

Balancing the chakras

One of the easiest ways to balance the chakra system is to place a stone of the appropriate colour on each area. This will give each chakra a boost of its own vibration without altering its energies or the system's overall harmony.

SEVEN COLOUR CHAKRA LAYOUT

For this exercise use small stones, such as polished or tumbled crystals. Make sure that they have been energetically cleansed before beginning. If working on yourself, lay the stones near to where you will be lying so that they are easy to find and position. Even though you might sense little change, allow yourself a few moments to recover after having the stones in place for five or six minutes.

1 It is a helpful start to place a grounding stone, such as smoky quartz, between your legs to act as an anchor.

2 For the base chakra, place a red stone at the bottom of the spine or two stones of the same sort at the top of each leg.

3 For the second or sacral chakra, position an orange-coloured stone on the lower abdomen.

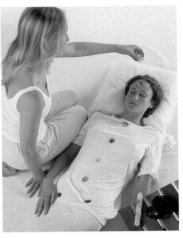

▲ REST THE CROWN CHAKRA STONE AT THE TOP OF THE HEAD. CHOOSE CLEAR QUARTZ IF YOU HAVE USED AN AMETHYST FOR THE BROW.

4 At the solar plexus use a yellow stone, positioned between the navel and ribcage. If there is tension here, put an energy-shifting stone, such as tiger's eye or clear quartz, on the diaphragm.

5 Place a green stone in the centre of the chest to balance the heart chakra. Add a pink stone for emotional clearing.

6 For the throat chakra use a light blue stone, placing it near the base of the throat, at the top of the breastbone.

7 An indigo or dark blue stone positioned in the centre of the forehead is used to balance the brow or third eye chakra. Amethyst or another purple stone may also be tried.

8 The crystal for the crown chakra should rest just above the top of your partner's head. If you choose an amethyst for the brow chakra, use a clear quartz crystal for the crown; if you used a dark blue stone for the brow, choose a violet crystal or gemstone to position at the crown chakra. It is always important to cleanse your stones at the end of a treatment.

INTUITIVE HEALING LAYOUTS

Once you become more confident in crystal healing or know the energies of the person you are treating better, allow yourself to be more intuitive in choosing suitable crystals for them.

1 Lay your crystals on the table. Then, after grounding your energies for a minute or two, and with the person's needs in mind, pick up the stones that attract your attention. Don't think of colours or even of chakras.

2 Place the stones where you feel they need to be on the body. Ask your partner how they feel, and make adjustments accordingly. After about five minutes remove the crystals and ground the energies with a smoky quartz.

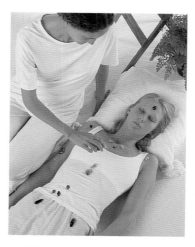

▲ WHEN POSITIONING YOUR CHOSEN STONES TRY TO DO SO QUICKLY AND WITHOUT THINKING TOO HARD ABOUT IT.

The crown chakra

Located just above the top of the head, the crown chakra has a violet and purple colour or aura. It supervises and balances the chakra system as a whole and channels universal life energy into the system.

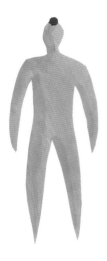

Healing at this chakra will have an energizing effect on the whole body, though the effects may be slow to appear, because this most subtle of chakras works to clarify and harmonize the whole system. The crown chakra maintains our links to the rest of creation, feeding us much as the base chakra does.

Imbalances at the crown chakra can take the form of apathy and indifference, narrow-mindedness, loneliness

This is the centre at which imagination, inspiration, empathy and selfless service to others are nourished. Its colour is violet and purple, vestments of which are frequently chosen by secular and religious leaders to remind others of their power and authority. White, gold and magenta also relate to the crown chakra.

▶ TRY USING A CRYSTAL APPROPRIATE FOR THE CROWN CHAKRA DURING TIMES OF SELF-DOUBT, STRESS OR PROLONGED APATHY.

and lack of faith or belief. Sleep problems, stress and problems associated with learning may also be encountered.

CRYSTALS FOR THE CROWN CHAKRA
• AMETHYST is perhaps the most useful all-purpose stone used by crystal healers, and is especially popular as an aid to meditation. Amethyst acts to quieten the mind and will allow finer perceptions to manifest within us.

• FLUORITE exists in a variety of colours, often in the violet range, and it helps integrate subtle energies with normal consciousness, as well as aiding co-ordination, both physical and mental.

• SUGILITE can be useful in group situations, bringing greater collective harmony and coherence, and assisting those who dislike their circumstances and feel that they don't fit in.

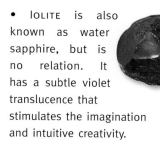

• IOLITE is also known as water sapphire, but is no relation. It has a subtle violet translucence that stimulates the imagination and intuitive creativity.

• KUNZITE is pale pink and violet with a striated crystalline structure, and is good at removing emotional debris and helping in self-expression.

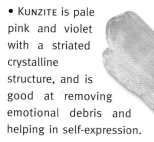

• CHAROITE AND ROCK CRYSTAL can also be used at the crown centre.

The brow chakra

The sixth chakra is located below the centre of the forehead, just above and between the brows and is our "inner eye". Its colour is indigo and, like the crown chakra, has been linked with both the pineal and pituitary glands.

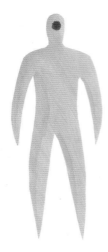

This chakra is often referred to as the third eye, the single eye that looks deep within to see and understand as contrasted with the two physical eyes, which look outwards and receive optical data from the world of the senses.

The brow chakra is the "inner eye" of the imagination, creativity and dreaming. It "sees" hidden patterns and groups and grasps spiritual essences. This is a psychic place at the threshold of the inner and outer worlds, and is a natural seat of knowledge. It is no accident that when we think hard we often put our hand to this point to make our focus deeper.

Healing at this chakra can benefit many conditions linked to headaches and migraines, recurrent nightmares and bad sleep, depression and stress. The eyes, nose and ears can also gain much from treatments here, with eye strain, clogged sinuses and earache being eased with a

▸ TO CLEAR A BLOCKED NOSE MASSAGE BETWEEN THE BROWS WITH LEPIDOLITE.

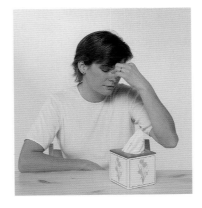

gentle application of an amethyst, purple fluorite or lapis lazuli. Poor concentration and memory can also be improved by using these stones regularly.

CRYSTALS FOR THE BROW CHAKRA
Indigo or midnight blue is the colour of the third eye chakra, and among the stones which have been found to work best are:

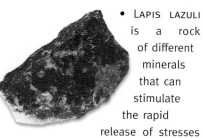

- LAPIS LAZULI is a rock of different minerals that can stimulate the rapid release of stresses and energize the mind.

- SAPPHIRE, which can relax and bring peace to the mind and balance all aspects of the self by releasing tension.

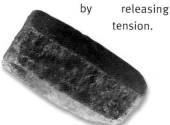

- SODALITE is similar to but less vivid a blue than lapis lazuli, and works to calm and open the mind to receiving new information and messages.

- KYANITE has a "fan-like" appearance and is favoured for moving on blocked energies and rapidly restoring the body's basic equilibrium.

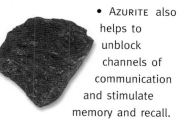

- AZURITE also helps to unblock channels of communication and stimulate memory and recall.

- LEPIDOLITE and PURPLE FLUORITE are also often used to good effect at this centre.

The throat chakra

The throat chakra is concerned with the free flow of communication at all levels. It allows self-expression and personal creativity, enabling us to hear, learn and teach. Its colour and related crystals are light blue.

On the physical level this chakra governs the proper functioning of the throat area, which under stress can mean conditions such as tight shoulders, tonsillitis, laryngitis or sore throats. Crystals can help lighten these blockages.

More generally this is the centre of self-expression, which often reflects our self-image. Any difficulty in communicating, whether caused by emotional or physical problems, can be eased by balancing the energies of the throat chakra. Attention given to this chakra may be of considerable value.

Unblocking the subtle energies at the throat centre will allow us to say our piece and be heard. Emotions can also become blocked here as desires rise from the heart chakra and are unable to be expressed because of external restrictions, such as social values and family expectations. Working at this chakra can allow creativity to flow again.

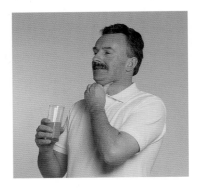

▸ Throat complaints can be treated by working this chakra.

When stressed, we can often feel pressure on our neck and shoulders. A light blue crystal placed near the throat can quickly alleviate symptoms. This centre can often feel restricted in a healing session as stress is released. An appropriate stone will help to ease the flow and promote a relaxed sense of peace and openness.

CRYSTALS FOR THE THROAT CHAKRA

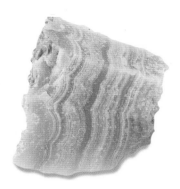

• TURQUOISE has been valued since ancient times as a supportive and protective stone, which can strengthen the subtle bodies and the fine communication systems within the body.

• AQUAMARINE is a blue variety of beryl and a stimulator of the body's own healing systems; it also supports efforts to stand our ground and be honest with our feelings.

• BLUE LACE AGATE is a banded form of blue quartz that will calm and soothe, while at the same time lighten our thoughts.

• CELESTITE forms a delicate blue crystal that is "dreamy" in quality. It helps to lift heavy moods and to express spiritual needs. It is also useful for throat problems.

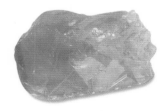

• SAPPHIRE and SODALITE, also used for the brow chakra, can be valuable alternative crystals to try out at the throat centre.

The heart chakra

Located midway in the chakra system, the heart centre is associated with the colour green – the middle of the spectrum of light. The heart chakra is thus a place of balance, harmony and equilibrium at all levels.

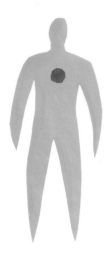

have seriously life-damaging effects on the majority of animals, including humans. Restriction, even if it is only imaginary, depletes the immune system allowing disease and illness to take hold. Balancing the energies of the heart chakra can quickly restore life-energy throughout the body, creating a sense of calm, relaxation and the confidence to be able to make positive changes. Love is the open, expansive expression of the heart chakra when balanced.

The heart is nowadays associated with the emotions, but in the past it was thought to be the seat of the mind and the soul. This chakra balances our internal reality with the outside world, so is concerned with relationships of all kinds, especially how personal desires and growth can find an outlet via interactions with others.

Feelings of being trapped, the inability to escape from life circumstances and a loss of hope

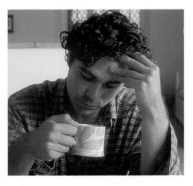

▲ BALANCING THE HEART CHAKRA WILL HELP TO RESOLVE EMOTIONAL ISSUES AND CLARIFY DIRECTION IN LIFE.

CRYSTALS FOR THE HEART CHAKRA

• GREEN AVENTURINE is
an excellent heart
balancer and
encourages easy
expression of the
emotions.

• MALACHITE helps
dig out deep feelings and hurts,
and can break
unwanted ties
and patterns
of behaviour.

• AMAZONITE
calms and
balances the
emotions and
helps with throat
and lung problems.

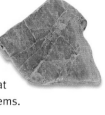

• MOSS AGATE is an ideal
crystal for supporting
the lungs and
easing breathing
difficulties, and
feelings of being
emotionally
stifled.

• BLOODSTONE is a green quartz
flecked with red jasper, giving it
an active balance of energy and
calm. It stimulates emotional
growth while also aiding circulation
of the blood.

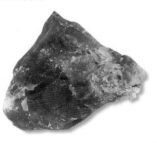

• PERIDOT is a vivid light green
crystal and a good cleanser of the
subtle bodies, enabling us to
initiate necessary
change in our lives
and encouraging
personal growth.

• EMERALD is a green type of the
mineral beryl and is useful in
guiding us to a personal direction
for growth, bringing
clarity to the heart
and emotions.

The solar plexus chakra

The solar plexus chakra establishes us in our own sense of personal power. It is the power station of the body, physically related to the nervous, digestive and immune systems. The governing colour is yellow.

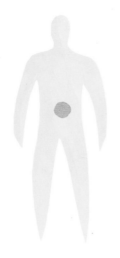

Major nerve centres are also found within the solar plexus. The ability to recognize and deal appropriately with energy of all kinds is the function of the solar plexus chakra. Information and control are the sources of all power. So an efficiently functioning solar plexus chakra imbues the individual with a sense of personal confidence, courage, optimism and ability to make the right decisions in any situation.

Since life in most modern societies is complex and demanding, as well as subject to many polluting influences, the solar plexus chakra can become overwhelmed and unbalanced. The result is an accumulation of stress and anxiety, the inability to resist infections, an intolerance to foods, additives and chemicals creating allergies, apathy and a loss of enthusiasm and humour. Mental clarity, memory and the ability to focus clearly and study will also be affected.

The solar plexus chakra and its related minor energy centres occupy the area below the ribcage and above the navel. Physically, this area of the body contains the digestive system enabling us to break down and assimilate nutrients from our food. Important organs such as the spleen are found here that sustain our immune system, protecting the body from dangerous micro-organisms in the outside world.

CRYSTALS FOR THE SOLAR PLEXUS CHAKRA

• AMBER is among the best-known of yellow crystals. Actually a pine resin, it varies in colour from pale yellow to a rich orange brown. It is beneficial for the nervous system and in self-healing processes.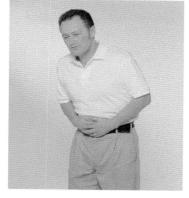

▲ STRESS IS A WELL-KNOWN CAUSE OF MANY DIGESTIVE PROBLEMS. YELLOW STONES WILL HELP TENSE MUSCLES TO RELAX.

• RUTILATED QUARTZ is clear or smoky, and contains fine threads of golden or orange rutile crystals. It can move healing energy and works well with broken or damaged tissues.

• TIGER'S EYE is a yellow and brown banded form of shiny quartz, and is used to speed up energy flow and anchor subtle changes into the physical body.

• CITRINE QUARTZ can be bright and clear yellow in colour, and is used to keep the mind focused.

• IRON PYRITES, also known as "fool's gold" because of its yellow colour, is able to cleanse and strengthen, particularly in the digestive system.

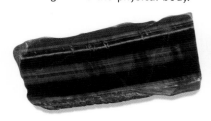

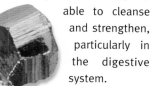

the solar plexus chakra **371**

The sacral chakra

The sacral chakra is located between the navel and the front of the pelvis, the pubic bones. Physically it is related to the reproductive organs and excretory systems. Orange stones naturally balance this chakra.

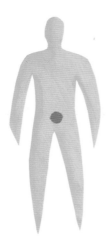

The energy of the sacral chakra focuses on sensation, feeling and movement. The exploration of the world and its pleasures and pains are the motivating energy of this centre. All types of creativity begin here. Flow is essential – the flow of curiosity, feelings and information, the fluid that feeds our cells and chemical processes, and the release of toxins from our system – all come under the influence of the sacral chakra. The

sacral chakra, when balanced, encourages change and the moving to new adventures. Any form of restriction and rigidity can be helped with orange stones that will restore the natural qualities of the sacral chakra. Blocks of energy anywhere in the body can affect the physical organs and create problems. Infertility and impotence on any level can often be helped by releasing emotional blocks. Stiffness of joints, constipation,

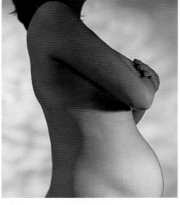

▲ THE SACRAL CHAKRA IS THE WOMB OF ALL CREATIVITY AND THE BIRTH OF EVERY IDEA.

water retention and menstrual difficulties all originate from restricted energy flow. Likewise boredom, indifference or creative blocks indicate that the sacral chakra needs some attention.

CRYSTALS FOR THE SACRAL CHAKRA

• CARNELIAN is a popular orange crystal, and has a sense of warmth and gentle healing energy.

• ORANGE CALCITE offers delicate encouragement of potential, and with its soft and watery feel it can help melt away our problems.

• DARK CITRINE is a balanced and browny-orange stimulator and brings out practical creative skills, as well as being supporting and grounding.

• TOPAZ has elongated crystals and parallel striations, and is a clearing stone that will direct energy around the body.

• COPPER is used, in both nugget and in bracelet forms, to release any stagnation or a lack of flow in our physical and subtle body systems.

Other crystals used at the sacral chakra include ORANGE JASPER, TIGER'S EYE and SUNSTONE.

The base chakra

Esoterically, this first chakra is the red-coloured root of the lotus, whose thousand petals bloom at the crown. It is the basis and support of our complex physical, mental and subtle system, the source of our primal energy.

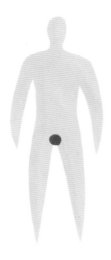

the body, especially the bones. Problems with physical movement, strained ligaments, pulled muscles and misaligned bones can be improved when the base chakra is balanced, as can be complaints affecting the colon, such as diarrhoea or constipation. Lack of

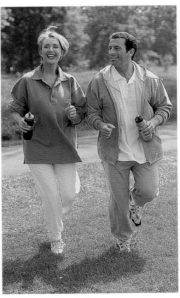

▲ KEEPING THE BODY'S ENERGIES MOVING FREELY AND EFFICIENTLY IS THE TASK OF THE BASE CHAKRA.

The base chakra is situated at the base of the spine and its main functions are to support consciousness within the physical body. All issues to do with survival and protection are focused at this point. The base chakra is concerned with practical skills, the reality of the present moment and the immediate needs of the individual. At a physical level the base chakra relates to all structural systems of energy, fatigue and exhaustion, a loss of interest in life or an excessive interest in spirituality to the detriment of one's well-being, all indicate the need to enhance the life-energy of the base chakra through the use of red stones.

The base chakra is represented in Indian tradition by Ganesha, the elephant god, who guards a person's material wealth and good fortune. Ganesha is also venerated as overseeing the initiation of new projects or new directions in life, especially when taken on the basis of a secure material foundation.

Grounding, motivation and new starts are hence some of the keynotes of the body's first and base chakra. If the base chakra's energy is deep-rooted and strong, the entire chakra system rising from it can also be powerful and effective. It is a two-way conduit of energy in all its forms, both physical and subtle.

Crystals can be placed so that they rest on the ground between the legs, close to the base of the spine. Alternatively, stones can be placed on the top of the legs near to the groin area.

CRYSTALS FOR THE BASE CHAKRA

Among the stones often used at this chakra are:

• GARNET, in its red forms, is an efficient energizer. It can increase energy wherever it is placed and will also activate other stones placed nearby.

• JASPER is a reddish form of quartz, and helps to ground and gently activate the whole body when placed near to the base chakra.

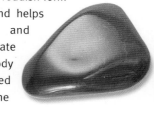

• RUBY is a red variety of carborundum and combines well with energies of the heart centre as well as gently energizing the subtle bodies.

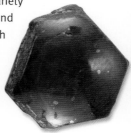

Brown and black crystals can also stabilize and balance the energies of the base chakra.

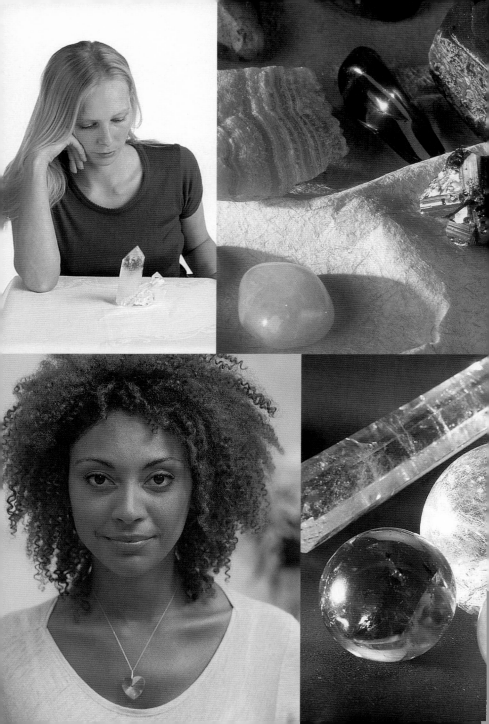

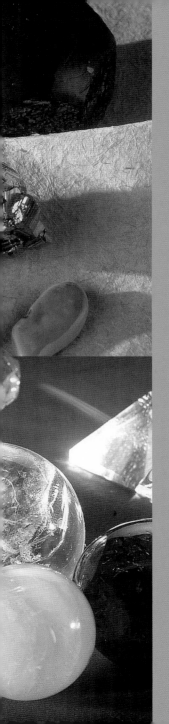

CRYSTAL
TREATMENTS

The therapeutic powers of crystals can be directed through the body to help balance the physical and emotional states, and to heal everyday complaints and ailments ranging from headaches, migraine and menstrual cramps to stress, insomnia and inability to concentrate. The following pages will help you to identify healing crystals and select the appropriate source to ease tension, calm body and mind or boost energy levels.

You will learn how to make gem essences so that you can benefit from a concentrated form of the stone's power. You will also discover how to enhance your surroundings, simply by placing crystals in the appropriate place in your home or work environment.

Relieving pain

Crystal healing is by its nature calming and relaxing. Painful conditions often seem to make the body tense itself. This can often prevent the proper flow of healing energy, blood, oxygen and nutrients to where they are needed.

The placement of crystals naturally begins to ease the imbalances that create pain. By releasing blockages within our subtle bodies, crystals can help stimulate the body's own healing mechanisms to work at a site of tension or pain.

BACKACHE RELIEF
Lodestone is an old name for magnetic iron ore, which was once used for navigational purposes. Placing one piece near the top of the neck and another at the base of the spine can help to relieve back tensions and stimulate spinal energies.

Help ease back pain with a small, clear quartz at the brow chakra. Imagine a beam of healing white light passing deep into your head with each in-breath.

CLEAR QUARTZ

▼ TO REALIGN THE BODY'S ENERGIES, USE EIGHT PIECES OF TOURMALINE. PLACE TWO AT THE CROWN, TWO MIDWAY ON EACH SIDE, AND TWO AT THE FEET. LIE DOWN AND REST INSIDE THIS CROSS-SHAPED ENERGY PATTERN.

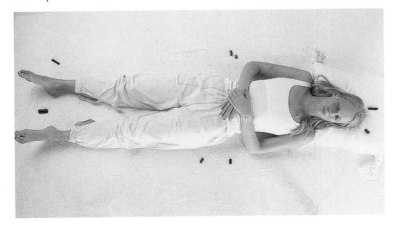

EASING TENSE MUSCLES

Black or green tourmaline crystals (called also schorl and verdelite) have been found useful where structural adjustment is needed. Knotted muscles can be relieved by placing a piece near them. Neck, jaw or head tension can be eased by wearing earrings made of this stone.

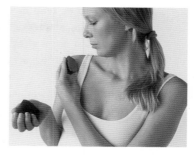

▲ TURQUOISE CAN BE USED WHENEVER THERE IS A NEED FOR CALM, HEALING ENERGY.

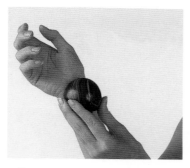

▲ MALACHITE, A SOFT MINERAL FORM OF COPPER, IS GOOD AT CALMING PAINFUL AREAS AND DRAWING OUT IMBALANCES.

Malachite is a copper ore that forms in concentric bands of light and dark green. It can calm painful areas and draw out imbalances, but because it absorbs negativity it needs regular cleansing.

Copper can help to reduce inflammations

COPPER

and swellings, either in bracelet form or carried as a natural nugget in the pocket.

Turquoise can be placed on the body wherever there is pain, while carnelian is a powerful healer of the etheric body.

TURQUOISE

Among pink stones, rose quartz helps to calm aggravated areas and reduce the fears that accompany injury and pain. Placing pink stones at the solar plexus and sacral chakras can help to soothe both mind and body.

ROSE QUARTZ

Soothing headaches

Headaches tend to occur when there is an imbalance or blockage of energy to the head. Amethyst, with its long tradition as an effective healing stone, can be very useful in soothing headaches.

All cool-coloured stones (blue, indigo and violet) are useful where there is an energy imbalance resulting in restriction of energy flow and experience of pain. Headaches are notoriously individual in cause and cure. Amethyst, combining the colours of red and blue, is a good crystal to try as it naturally tends to bring balance in any extreme situation.

HEADACHE RELIEF

If a headache can be caught in its early stages it can be a lot easier to reduce the symptoms with crystal healing. First of all, try a simple chakra layout using the appropriate colour stone at each chakra. This will help to stabilize all energy levels in the body.

▼ AMETHYST IS AN ESSENTIAL PART OF YOUR HEALING CRYSTAL COLLECTION.

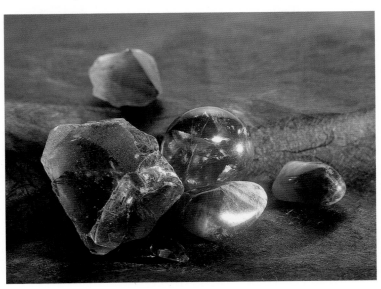

HEAD-SOOTHING CRYSTAL LAYOUT

Place one amethyst point on either side of the base of the neck, just above the collar bones, pointing upwards. Place a third stone, also pointing upwards, on the centre of the forehead. A fourth may be added if desired at the top of the head. This placing brings the throat, brow and crown chakras into powerful harmony.

Another common cause of headaches is an imbalance between the head energy and that at the solar plexus, often the result of stress or unsuitable food. If you have a headache and an upset stomach, for example, use a stone that will also balance the solar plexus, such as ametrine.

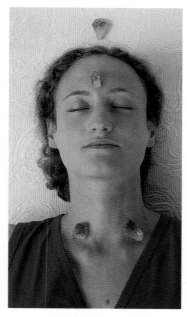

▲ A FOUR-STONE AMETHYST LAYOUT TO SOOTHE HEADACHES.

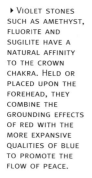

▶ VIOLET STONES SUCH AS AMETHYST, FLUORITE AND SUGILITE HAVE A NATURAL AFFINITY TO THE CROWN CHAKRA. HELD OR PLACED UPON THE FOREHEAD, THEY COMBINE THE GROUNDING EFFECTS OF RED WITH THE MORE EXPANSIVE QUALITIES OF BLUE TO PROMOTE THE FLOW OF PEACE.

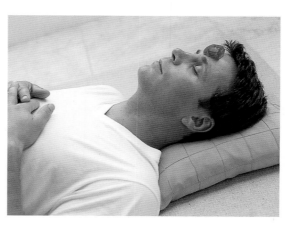

Easing PMS and menstrual cramps

 Period pains and menstrual cramps are often made worse by physical and emotional tensions, which restrict the body's natural energy flows. Moonstones and opal are among the stones recommended for easing these tensions.

CALMING THE EMOTIONS

Moonstone helps in balancing and relaxing emotional states, and also works beneficially on all fluid systems of the body, relieving pain in the abdominal area. Traditional Ayurvedic texts in India state that moonstone is the ideal stone for women to wear, and indeed, it can be made into charming jewellery.

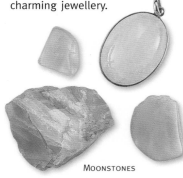

MOONSTONES

RELIEVING STOMACH CRAMPS

Dark opal is similar in properties to moonstone, acting powerfully at the first and second chakras to ease menstrual cramps in a short time. Place a small piece in a hip or trouser pocket.

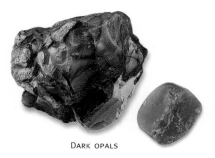

DARK OPALS

To reinforce chakra healing for PMS, carry with you a dark opal or an orange stone, such as carnelian, associated with the sacral chakra. When you have the chance, rub the stone lightly across your lower abdomen, from just below the navel, making a large circle to the left, and allowing it to spiral towards the middle. Feel the warmth of the crystal's energy flowing into you from the stone and the easing of tension that this brings.

CARNELIAN

Five-moonstone pattern

A healing pattern of five moonstones amplifies the relaxing and therapeutic potential of the stone to ease physical and emotional tensions. Lying down comfortably, position one stone at the top of your head, one near each armpit and one on each hip.

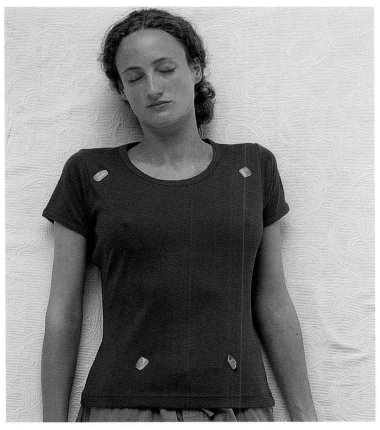

▲ Find a comfortable position in which to lie down, close your eyes and allow the five-moonstone pattern to ease away any menstrual tensions within your body.

Energizing crystals

Sometimes poor energy is simply caused by a temporary imbalance in the chakra system, especially the base and solar plexus. Redistribution of natural energy reserves can help to revitalize depleted areas, and restore vitality.

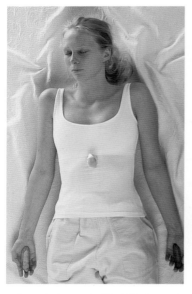

Red, orange and yellow stones, such as garnet, amber and topaz, can promote increased energy. Yellow citrine makes a wonderful substitute for summer sun on a dull winter's day.

More earthy tones, such as tiger's eye, dark citrine and jasper, can help you focus on practical action to be taken.

▲ FOR A QUICK ENERGY BOOST TO THE WHOLE SYSTEM, HOLD A CLEAR QUARTZ CRYSTAL, POINT UPWARDS, IN EACH HAND, AND PLACE A LARGE CITRINE STONE AT THE SOLAR PLEXUS.

GARNET

AMBER

TOPAZ

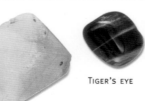

TIGER'S EYE

JASPER

CITRINE

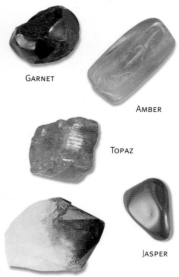

DARK CITRINE

Aiding concentration

The natural, organized structure of a crystal lattice automatically increases the clarity and orderliness of a study area or workplace. A beautiful clear crystal such as quartz can bring stillness and focus to the mind.

Yellow is known to stimulate the logical functions of the mind, so a bright yellow amber, citrine or fluorite will assist your memory and recall. Fluorite is particularly good as it helps balance the working of the brain hemispheres.

Deep blue stones, such as kyanite, sodalite and sapphire, will encourage your communication skills and a better understanding of ideas and concepts.

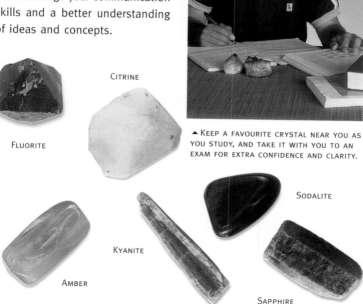

CITRINE

FLUORITE

▲ KEEP A FAVOURITE CRYSTAL NEAR YOU AS YOU STUDY, AND TAKE IT WITH YOU TO AN EXAM FOR EXTRA CONFIDENCE AND CLARITY.

SODALITE

KYANITE

AMBER

SAPPHIRE

Releasing stress

A shock, accident or loss may leave you shaken and vulnerable. Look out for stress symptoms, such as tensing of muscles, recurrent mental replays of events and sudden welling up of emotions.

CALMING LAYOUT

The effects of stress can be released by this layout. Continue regularly until the stress eases.

1 Place a rose quartz at the heart chakra, with four quartz points facing outwards, positioned diagonally around it.

2 At the sacral chakra, below the navel, place a tiger's eye, and surround it with another four quartz points, facing inwards and also placed diagonally around it.

3 The stones at the heart release emotional tension, while those on the abdomen balance the chakras above and give grounded energy and stability.

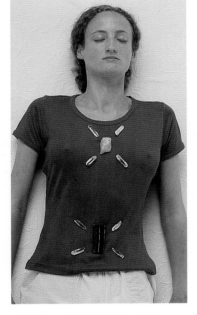

▲ YOU WILL NEED EIGHT SMALL, CLEAR QUARTZ CRYSTALS, A ROSE QUARTZ AND A TIGER'S EYE.

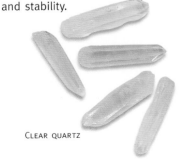

CLEAR QUARTZ

ROSE QUARTZ

TIGER'S EYE

Calming crystals

Here is a calming crystal layout to help during times of emotional stress to restore calm and equilibrium. Signs of stress being released include muscle twitches, deep breaths or sighs, yawning and watery eyes.

SOOTHING CRYSTAL LAYOUT

1 Place a rose quartz at the heart chakra, surrounded by four quartz points in a cross formation. Points should be facing outwards to remove emotional imbalances; or set points facing inwards to stabilize an over-emotional state.

2 Position a citrine stone at the solar plexus chakra, with its darker point facing downwards. This increases the sense of security and feeling of safety.

3 Place an amethyst on the third eye chakra to calm the mind. If the release is found to be too strong, remove stones from the heart area and place a hand over the solar plexus.

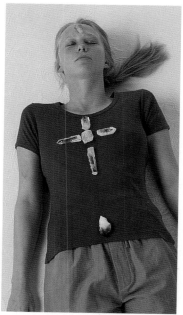

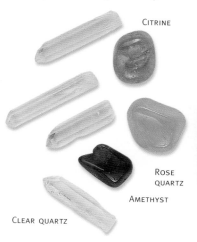

CITRINE

ROSE QUARTZ

AMETHYST

CLEAR QUARTZ

▲ FOR A CALMING LAYOUT USE FOUR CLEAR QUARTZ CRYSTALS, A ROSE QUARTZ, A CITRINE AND AN AMETHYST.

Aiding restful sleep

Taking crystals to bed is an easy and comforting way of dealing with insomnia. Experiment with different crystals for different types of sleeplessness. Hold the stones, put them on or under your pillow or near to you as you settle.

DEALING WITH SLEEPLESS NIGHTS
Chrysoprase, an apple green form of chalcedony quartz, has been found in many cases to encourage peaceful sleep. Place a stone under your pillow or by your bedside table.

If tension or worry is the cause of restlessness, try amethyst, rose quartz or citrine.

If something you have eaten is disturbing your sleep pattern, a digestive calmer such as ametrine, moonstone or iron pyrites may work for you.

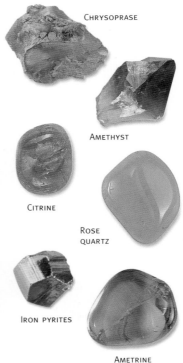

CHRYSOPRASE

AMETHYST

CITRINE

ROSE QUARTZ

IRON PYRITES

AMETRINE

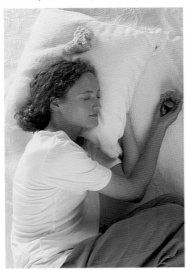

▲ HOLD THE APPROPRIATE STONES OR HAVE THEM NEARBY AS YOU SLEEP.

388 crystal treatments

Banishing bad dreams

Where there is fear, particularly related to bad dreams, place a grounding and protecting stone, such as tourmaline, staurolite or smoky quartz at the bottom of the bed. Labradorite can also help chase away unwelcome thoughts or feelings.

A stronger energy might be needed to counter nightmares: place a large, smooth moss agate or tektite by the bed where you can touch it and feel its reassuring solidity.

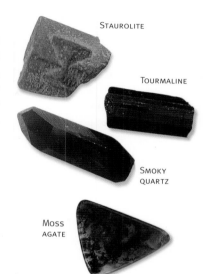

STAUROLITE

TOURMALINE

SMOKY QUARTZ

MOSS AGATE

▼ If tension and worry are the causes of restlessness try placing rose quartz, amethyst or citrine by your pillow.

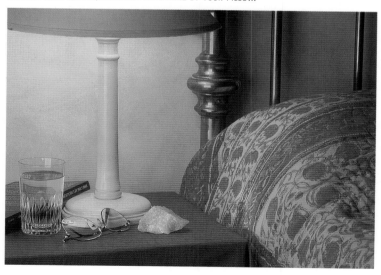

Crystal essences

You can benefit from the healing properties of gems by making your own crystal essences. These are vibrational preparations made by immersing gemstones in spring water and exposing to direct sunlight.

Gem essences are believed to work by allowing the energy pattern of a chosen stone to be imprinted on the water. Sunlight is best for this process, but leaving a stone in water by your bedside overnight and drinking the water first thing in the morning can also be beneficial. Remove the stone before using the essence.

The charged water can be drunk on the spot or bottled for later use in helping the healing processes of the body. It is not necessary to ingest a gem essence in order for it to be effective. Rubbing a few drops on pulse points or around a chakra area, or close to an area of imbalance can work just as well. Keep crystal essence bottles in the fridge and try to drink them within one week. You should not freeze them. Fresh-made essence is usually best. You can also spray indoor plants or add the essence water to your bath.

Caution: some stones are toxic or dissolve in water (crystals of salt, for example). Gem water made from the quartz family is safe. Try citrine, amethyst or tiger's eye.

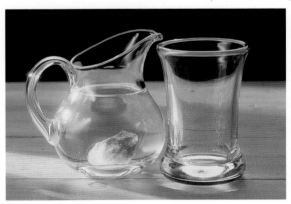

◀ DRINKING A HOME-MADE CRYSTAL ESSENCE, SUCH AS THIS ONE MADE BY PLACING AN AMETHYST IN CLEAR SPRING WATER, GIVES YOU A CONCENTRATED FORM OF YOUR STONE'S HEALING POWER.

MAKING A MOONSTONE ESSENCE

A moonstone essence has the ability to calm our emotions. Moonstone is soft and cooling, because of its feminine orientation.

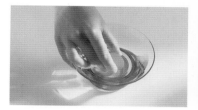

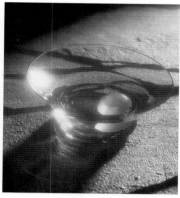

1 Take a cleansed gemstone and place it into a clear glass bowl. Fill the bowl with fresh spring water until the stone is covered.

2 Leave the bowl outside under the light of a full moon for three hours, or overnight if the night is calm and clear.

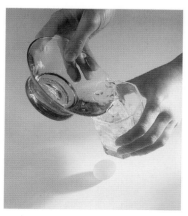

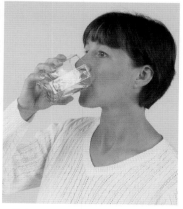

3 Remove the moonstone, remembering to cleanse it after use, and pour the liquid into a clear glass.

4 Take a drink of the moonstone infusion first thing in the morning in order to prepare yourself for a harmonious day.

Enhancing your home

Crystals can make attractive decorations for the home and they can also enhance the surroundings by bringing a balancing and cleansing influence on many levels, helping to neutralize emotional debris and pollution.

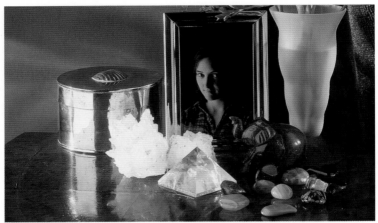

▲ ADDING CRYSTALS TO A SACRED SPACE KEEPS THE ENERGIES FRESH AND POSITIVE.

Crystals can create a sacred space in your home, as a simple quiet place in which to rest or as an elaborate altar with sacred images. Honour an anniversary or guest with a temporary special space or set aside a permanent meditative area in your home or garden.

Make a crystal lightbox by placing a large transparent or translucent stone in front of a light source. Change the mood by using a yellow crystal for relaxation, red for energy and violet for mystery.

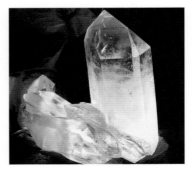

▶ CRYSTALS WITH INTERNAL FRACTURES OR RAINBOWS, SUCH AS RUTILATED QUARTZ OR MOSS AGATE, CAN MAKE BEAUTIFUL LIGHTS.

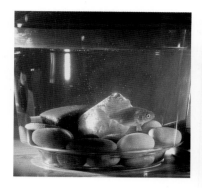

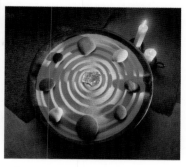

◄ CRYSTALS IN AN AQUARIUM REVEAL THEIR VIVID COLOURS, AND ALSO ENERGIZE THE SURROUNDINGS.

▲ CREATE A MINI ZEN GARDEN BY FILLING A FLAT BOWL WITH CLEAN SAND OR DRY GRAVEL. ARRANGE INTERESTING STONES AND CRYSTALS ON IT, AND USE A COMB OR FORK TO DRAW PATTERNS IN THE SAND.

Pets can be treated with gems and crystals, both to maintain health and when they are unwell. Use a crystal pendulum to balance the energy in four-footed animals, or place crystals safely around a sleeping area. Energizing water can be dropped on your fingers and then stroked through the fur of a cat or dog. A small gemstone can be attached to a dog or cat collar. Sick animals may find the presence of a crystal in their basket or hutch comforting.

A quiet corner of the garden is a good place for reflection, and crystals placed near the plants keep them healthy too. House plants benefit from crystals placed in their soil, quartz and emerald (gem quality is not necessary) are popular. Aquamarine and jade are also said to enhance plant energies, while turquoise can help plants recover from damage and disease.

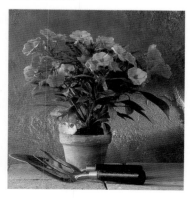

▲ A QUARTZ CRYSTAL WILL ENHANCE A HOUSE PLANT'S OVERALL HEALTH.

Crystals in the workplace

Whether you work at home or in the office, crystals can be used to enhance your working area in simple, effective ways. Consider the factors you would most like to improve and select the types of colour and crystal that might help.

If you work in an office or factory, there is much you can do to make your personal space a pleasing place to be:

• Keep natural stones or crystals as paperweights or as dividers in a file or bookcase.

• Use carved stone pots or bowls on the desk as containers in which to store pens or paperclips.

• Place stones on the soil of potted plants in your work area.

• Have a favourite crystal as a "worry stone" for your pocket. The telephone and computer can be particular causes of tension and stress, demanding our attention and raising the body's adrenaline levels when emotions are triggered.

▶ KEEP A SMALL BOWL OF STONES NEAR THE PHONE AS A FOCUS FOR YOUR ATTENTION. IT WILL ALSO HELP AVOID UNNECESSARY DEPLETION OF YOUR ENERGY BY BECOMING OVERLY INVOLVED IN OTHER PEOPLE'S PROBLEMS.

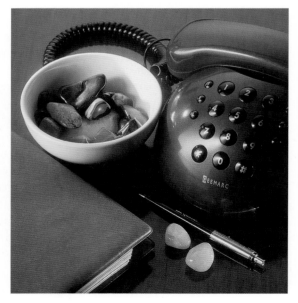

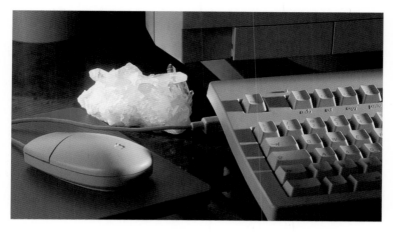

Moonstone helps to foster understanding of our colleagues' points of view and, as such, is an excellent aid to communication. It also acts to balance our emotional states and clear away tensions, and restores the balance of the body's fluid systems.

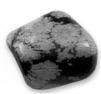

Obsidian is a form of black volcanic glass, often with white flecks (snowflake obsidian), patches of dark red (mahogany

SNOWFLAKE OBSIDIAN

obsidian) or a smoky translucence (Apache tears). It is known as a good aid to concentration, working patiently to bring imbalances to the surface and reveal hidden factors

▲ OFFSET THE STRONG ELECTROMAGNETIC FIELDS CREATED BY COMPUTER SCREENS BY PUTTING A CRYSTAL ON THE MONITOR OR NEAR IT. CLEAR QUARTZ IS RECOMMENDED, BUT IT MUST BE CLEANSED FREQUENTLY.

surrounding a situation. Other stones can then assist by clearing away this clutter, leaving the mind clear and focused.

Fluorite is also found in a variety of colours, with violet or mauve among the most frequent. Its presence can help in a work environment through its capacity to release dynamic or inspirational ideas, as it is associated with the crown chakra and acts as a link between subtle and practical aspects of consciousness.

FLUORITE

Crystal colours directory

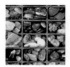

We have seen how coloured crystals are associated with the chakra system, and how they work in many different types of healing. This directory looks briefly at the most commonly used crystals according to their colours.

DIRECTORY OF COLOURED CRYSTALS

Note that some crystals are listed below under several colours. The colour categories are rarely exact in practice, and good stones can be a little or widely different from the suggested match.

This variety and individuality, however, is part of the attraction of choosing crystals. Finding a stone that resonates to your own vibration is the beginning of your healing experience.

RED	garnet, jasper, ruby, red tiger's eye, carnelian.
ORANGE	carnelian, orange calcite, dark citrine, topaz, copper, sunstone.
YELLOW	amber, rutilated quartz, tiger's eye, citrine quartz, iron pyrites, yellow topaz.
GREEN	green aventurine, malachite, bloodstone, amazonite, moss agate, peridot, emerald, jade.
BLUE	aquamarine, turquoise, blue lace agate, celestite, sapphire, sodalite.
INDIGO	lapis lazuli, sodalite, kyanite, azurite, sapphire.
VIOLET	amethyst, fluorite, sugilite, iolite, kunzite, charoite.
WHITE	clear quartz, herkimer diamond, Iceland spa, moonstone, selenite.
BLACK	smoky quartz, obsidian, tourmaline, haematite.
PINK	rose quartz, rhodonite, kunzite, rhodocrosite.
MULTICOLOURED	opal, azurite-malachite, labradorite, hawk's eye, ametrine.

QUARTZ: THE FAMILY THAT HAS EVERYTHING

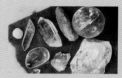

There is one remarkable family of crystals that on its own encompasses most of the colours and healing opportunities of the spectrum. As such, it deserves a special mention in any study of crystals.

QUARTZ is probably one of the commonest minerals on Earth, being composed of the abundant elements silica and oxygen. Stones in the quartz family may be bright, clear and simple or dark, dense and complex, depending on the heat and pressure involved in their formation. Colours and forms vary widely because the crystal lattice allows other atoms to enter at a microscopic level. These often alter the way that light passes through them, changing the visible colour.

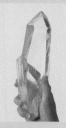

CLEAR QUARTZ is colourless and shiny; MILKY QUARTZ is white, as is OPAL (the high water content creating a display of flashing colour); ROSE QUARTZ is pink and translucent, while CARNELIAN is orange and JASPER is often red, but also yellow, green and blue; RUTILATED QUARTZ is golden yellow and CITRINE ranges from yellow to orange-brown; CHRYSOPRASE is bright apple-green and AVENTURINE is green or blue, with tiny sparks of mica or pyrites; in the blue range are the delicate BLUE LACE AGATE

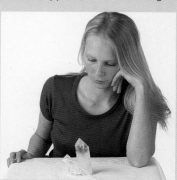

and dreamy purple AMETHYST; among the mixed colours are the agates, with wavy parallel coloured bands, including MOSS AGATE and BANDED AGATE, and TIGER'S EYE, with subtle browns, yellows, blue and red; at the darkest end of the spectrum are SMOKY QUARTZ, BLOODSTONE, or HELIOTROPE, in a dark, shiny green, TOURMALINE QUARTZ, embedded with fine black needles and onyx, with its straight lines of white on black.

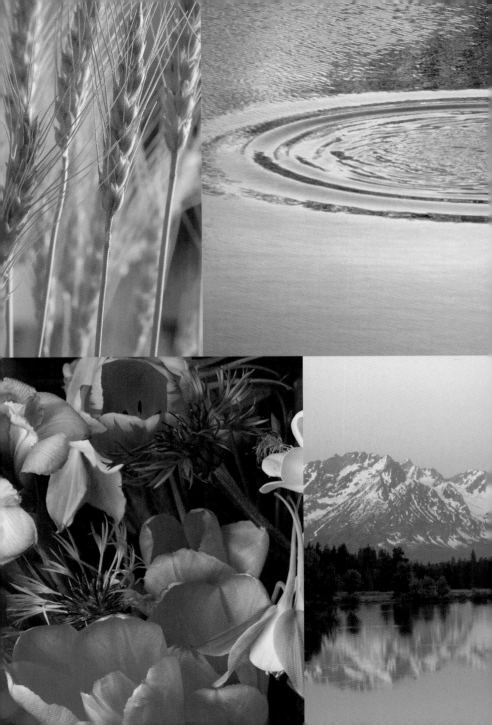

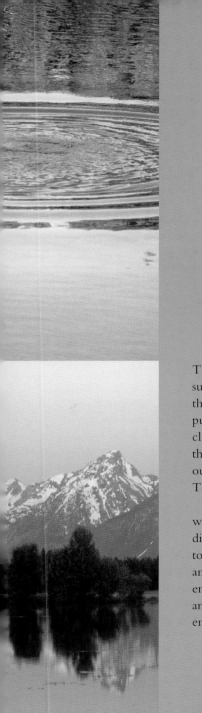

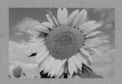

HEALING WITH
COLOUR

The vast majority of us spend our lives
surrounded by colour, but few of us pause to
think about its impact on our psyche. On a
purely instinctive level, the colour of the
clothes we wear, the foods we eat or
the paints and furnishings we use to decorate
our home reflect our mood and emotions.
This is colour healing in its simplest form.

By exploring the subject a little further,
we can also use colour healing to cure
discomfort, or to create a specific atmosphere
to actually enhance the purpose of a room,
and make it a playground for a range of
emotions. So, go ahead – follow your instinct
and find out how simple colour appreciation
enables you to optimize well-being.

Life in colour

You are swamped with colour from the moment you are born: it is an aspect of everything you eat, drink, touch and are surrounded by. You can use colours to depict your health, attitudes, emotions – even psychic experiences.

Nearly everyone takes colour for granted most of the time, but it is impossible to be indifferent to it. Colour affects every environment: at home, at work, at school, in the city or in the countryside. The colours of the clothes you wear affects your mood and reflects your personality, which in turn influences other people's perception of you and so affects your relationships.

Colour helps you to determine when fruits are ripe. Your skin changes colour with shock, shyness or excitement. Too much

yellow light can cause arguments between people, and blue light can quieten them. Colour constantly enriches your life, whether it is the green of grass or trees, deep blue sky, a purple and gold sunset, or a beautiful rainbow.

Without light there is no life, and no growth. A plant deprived of light will soon wither and die and living beings are continually reacting to the wide range of stimuli called light. From light come all the colours, each with its own impact upon living systems. Light is energy, and all energy acts upon everything with which it comes into contact. What you see as colour is simply the brain's way of recognizing the different energy qualities of light.

Many healing needs can be met by the use of colour to bring about harmony and balance within the psyche and the body. The invisible vibrations of colour

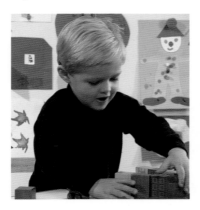

◀ CHILDREN ARE ATTRACTED BY THE STRENGTH OF BRIGHT COLOURS.

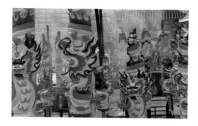

▲ Colour enriches your life. Many cultures use bright colours when celebrating special occasions.

can either relax or stimulate, according to the colours chosen for healing. Its power is both transcendent and intuitive, and there are several ways of harnessing it for health and well-being. Colour does more than just please the eye. You can eat it, drink it, and wear appropriately coloured clothes or jewellery, absorbing the colour through your skin as well as your eyes. Your home can be a haven of health and peace when you furnish it in colours appropriate to your needs and aspirations.

Disease is often regarded as an enemy, but think of it as your friend. It is telling you the truth about yourself, and the ways in which you are out of harmony with the "real" you. Working with colour and understanding the connection between yourself and colour offers a key to good health and vitality.

Although colour healing can be very effective, it should not replace any medical treatment. If the symptoms persist or worsen, consult a health professional.

▼ The beautiful colours of the sunset are joyous and calming.

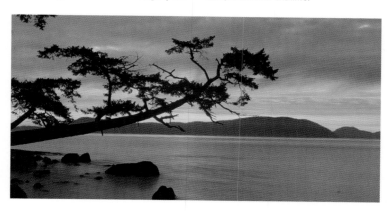

The evolution of colour healing

Ancient cultures worshipped the sun – whence all light, and all colour, comes – and were aware of its healing powers. The therapeutic use of colour can be traced in the teachings attributed to the Egyptian god Thoth.

EARLY COLOUR THERAPY

Following the ancient teachings, Egyptian and Greek physicians – including Hippocrates, the father of Western medicine – used different coloured ointments and salves as remedies, and practised in treatment rooms painted in healing shades. In 1st-century Rome, the physician Aulus Cornelius Celsus wrote about the therapeutic use of colour, but with the coming of Christianity such ancient wisdom came to be associated with pagan beliefs and was disallowed by the Church.

In the 9th century the Arab physician Avicenna systematized the teachings of Hippocrates. He wrote about colour as a symptom of disease and as a treatment, suggesting, for example, that red would act as a stimulant on blood flow while yellow could reduce pain and inflammation. However, by the 18th century philosophers and scientists were more concerned with the material world, and insisted on visible proof of scientific theories.

▼ THE ANCIENT EGYPTIANS KNEW ABOUT THE HEALING PROPERTIES OF COLOURS.

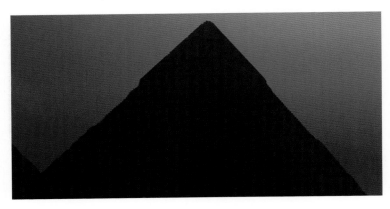

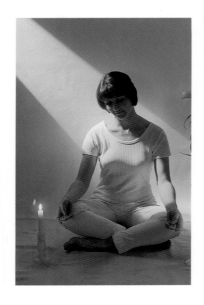

establishment's continued scepticism, therapists have since developed the use of colour in both psychological testing and physical diagnosis. The Lüscher Colour Test is based on the theory that colours stimulate different parts of the autonomic nervous system, affecting metabolic rate and glandular secretions, and studies in the 1950s showed that yellow and red light raised blood pressure while blue light tended to lower it. The use of blue light to treat neonatal jaundice is now common practice, and it has also been effective as pain relief in cases of rheumatoid arthritis.

Advances in medicine focused on surgery and drugs, and less quantifiable healing techniques that dealt with spiritual and mental well-being were rejected.

COLOUR THERAPY REDISCOVERED

In 1878 Edwin Babbitt published *The Principles of Light and Colour* and achieved world renown with his comprehensive theory, prescribing colours for a range of conditions. Despite the medical

▶ GREEN, TURQUOISE AND BLUE OBJECTS HAVE A TRANQUIL AIR.

Natural colour

From forests to cities, people adapt to the unique qualities of their surroundings. Colour creates the ambience of a place because the vibrational energy of colour operates directly on your energy levels and emotions.

THE CALM OF NATURE

Most people experience a lifting of mood on a woodland walk as the green of nature fills their vision. The effects of colour can be felt when relaxing by the sea in summer, the predominant colours being the blues of the sea and sky, which generate a feeling of expansiveness and peace.

Turquoise is an important colour that tempers the deeper blues with an extra sense of calmness and comfort. The golden yellow of sand and sunlight energizes and balances the body's systems, reducing anxiety and stress levels.

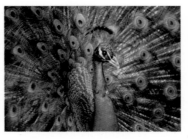

▲ THE STRIKING COLOURS OF THE PEACOCK'S TAIL FEATHERS ACT AS A TERRITORIAL WARNING SIGNAL TO ITS COMPETITORS.

THE SEEING WORLD

Full colour vision is a rare development in the animal world; it occurs in the higher vertebrates – including humans – as well as a few unexpected animals, such as the tortoise and the octopus.

Striking colour displays are used by many animals, such as the peacock, to attract mates or to deter enemies. Using colour as camouflage is also common. The squid has a complex language of expression, sending waves of colours across its body.

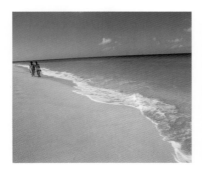

◄ THE BLUE OF THE SEA IS ONE OF THE MOST SOOTHING COLOURS OF ALL.

Colours in different cultures

Colour is an intrinsic part of human life, and although the physical effects of colour are biologically constant, its psychological interpretation and symbolism can vary when it forms part of a cultural language.

Red

In Tibetan and some pagan traditions, red is the colour of the female sun, white the male moon. The two symbolize the union of opposites: the power of creation. Red can also be associated with the male, for example Santa Claus, who also retains the symbolism of the Arctic shaman bringing healing and gifts to his people.

Green

In the Western tradition, green is associated with wild nature, the power of growth and uncultivated space inhabited by spirits, elves

▾ In Tibet, red is a colour associated with creativity, prayer and healing.

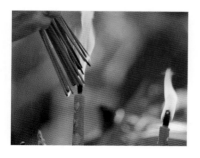

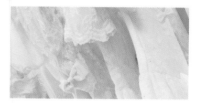

▴ White can be symbolic of purity and innocence, and so it is often chosen as the colour for bridal wear.

and fairies. In the world of Islam, the colour green is sacred. In a landscape dominated by arid wilderness, green represents the oasis, the sign of life, water and shelter: the symbol of paradise.

Black and white

In much of Europe death has been associated with black. In China, however, white is seen as the colour of winter, when all things return to a dormant state, so mourners wear white. Chinese people tend to avoid wearing white in everyday life because it reminds them of a shroud, whereas in the West white is associated simply with purity.

Colour at home

Colour is a sensation that enriches the world: there is no better way to use it than by harnessing its strength and benefits to enhance your home. Blending colours successfully can help to create a harmonious atmosphere.

WELCOMING THE SUN

When you are creating your home environment, take into consideration the amount of sunlight in each room. It is important that the glow from the sun's beams is received into your psyche, for its purifying effect. Allowing sunlight to flood into dark corners also rids a room of its staleness and kills some bacteria.

When you are decorating, think about the effects of colour, how the room will be used, and also about the people who will use it: do they have any problems that could be alleviated or worsened by your colour choices? What are their ambitions and aims?

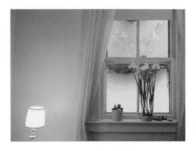

COLOUR AND SIZE

Take into consideration the size and shape of each room: the stronger the colour, the smaller a room will seem. Small rooms tend to look more spacious decorated in single pale colours. Colours become more intense in larger areas, and a strong colour can enclose a room, causing claustrophobia. Dark narrow rooms need light, clear colours.

Check how much daylight the space gets before using white, as a bright white room can be tiring for the eyes and cause frustration. Deep colours may look good with the sun on them; they become several shades duller at night in artificial light, but can look cosy if firelight or candlelight are used. If you are painting only one wall in a different colour, do not choose a wall where there is a door or window as this dissipates the colour energy.

◀ AN ORANGE ROOM WILL INSTIL CHEERFULNESS INTO ITS OCCUPANTS.

ROOM-BY-ROOM GUIDE TO COLOUR

The colours of your home should suit not only the function of each room, but should also be used to create harmony. Use coloured flowers or ornaments for particular occasions to influence the atmosphere.

Entrance hall: To welcome your guests include warm colours, such as the range of reds.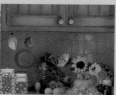
Or to create a sense of space choose softer pastel shades.

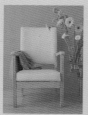 Living room: Yellow puts people in a good humour; add brown to give a sense of security.

Dining room: Include a hint of silver at a dinner party. It aids digestion and is uplifting – adding sparkle to guests' conversations.

Kitchen: Too much green may slow you down just when you need to be active, but a touch of yellow inspires efficiency.

Bedroom: Calming blue is a perfect colour for the bedroom. A touch of indigo can also help if 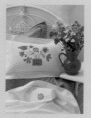 you suffer from headaches or insomnia. Stimulating red may cause sleeplessness, so avoid.

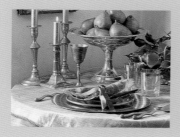

Bathroom: Hints of pale green will soothe and feed a tired nervous system.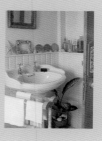

Colour at work

Until quite recently, coloured decor for offices was almost unthinkable. Sterile white, grey or drab browns were the norm. Today, the trend is to make the most of the effect that colour has on people and the ambience it can create.

THE EFFECT OF COLOUR

Promoting the effective use of colour in the office is important both for the comfort of the employees and the productivity of the business. If thoughtlessly applied, colour can interfere and distract from work. If only white is used it can cause frustration. Blue creates an atmosphere of calm and is good for creativity. Brown creates tiredness and lethargy and grey induces depression and melancholy. If you use beige, add green or rose pink to alleviate the negative slackness that it can bring to the room.

Don't forget details such as company stationery, as it also makes a colour statement. You could change from white paper to a shade that may better reflect your company's image.

THE CITY OFFICE

Offices in which activity is high, in areas such as sales and banking, should use red upholstery. This definitely puts workers in the hot seat and adds impetus and drive to their performance. Add green walls, to counteract the red and reduce headaches that are brought on by the pressure of work.

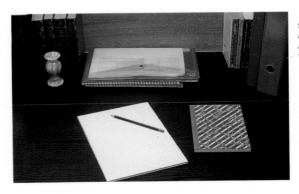

◀ BLUE IN THE STUDY AREA CREATES A SENSE OF CALM AND CAN INSPIRE THE WRITER.

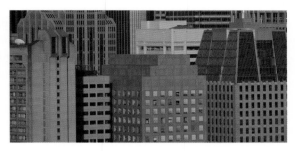

THE EXECUTIVE OFFICE

When you are the boss you need an office where employees and directors can talk to you and be reminded that you lead the way. A purple carpet gives an impression of big ideas and creativity along with luxury and authority. Touches of gold encourage feelings of trust and loyalty, but don't forget to add healthy green plants to represent money and to balance power and character.

THE OPEN-PLAN OFFICE

When choosing colours for a large office, you would be well advised to make the overall decor a basic cream and introduce touches of brighter colours, such as orange, emerald green, rose and rich blue. If only one accent colour can be used, choose a bright turquoise as this will help to give a greater sense of privacy.

THE HOME OFFICE

An office at home can encourage the workaholic. An effective combination would be a royal blue carpet with yellow curtains and pale blue or primrose yellow walls: this should succeed in keeping the business in the office only, and not allow work to penetrate into your personal life.

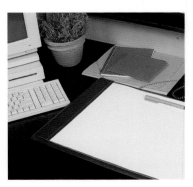

Light waves and colour

Visible light is a small portion of the electromagnetic spectrum, which also includes ultraviolet and infrared light. These last two are just beyond the vision of humans, but can still have an effect on our health.

LIGHT WAVES

The distance between the two crests of a wave (the wavelength) determines what type of wave it is. Radio waves are very long; cosmic rays are very short. Around the middle of the spectrum is the tiny portion we experience as visible light. Within this, further gradations produce different colours. The longest waves are at the red end of the spectrum, and the shortest waves are at the purple end, with those of the other colours falling in between. Colour therapists often refer to pure colours as "rays".

◀ WHITE LIGHT REFRACTED THROUGH A PRISM REVEALS ITS COMPONENT COLOURS – THE FULL RAINBOW SPECTRUM.

WHAT IS COLOUR?

A coloured surface absorbs or reflects certain wavelengths of light. A red flower absorbs all light striking it except the red end of the spectrum, which is reflected. A white surface reflects all light that hits it, while a black surface absorbs it all.

The emotional and physiological response of humans to colour is profound: even people without sight will identify warm and cool colours. The stimulating effects of reds and oranges and the calming qualities of blues and violets, for example, are linked to the biological triggers of daylight and nightfall, and these [responses] are harnessed in colour healing.

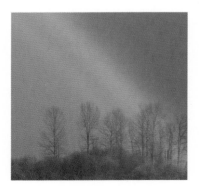

◀ A RAINBOW IS WHITE LIGHT REFRACTED OR SEPARATED INTO ITS COMPONENT COLOURS.

Sense of sight

Colour has been shown to initiate profound changes in the nervous system. The eyes allow the light energy of colour to be carried to the centre of the brain, influencing cellular function, physical activity, emotional and mental states.

THE EYE

The human eye is a sophisticated sensing device. Light passes through the transparent lens and stimulates the specialized light-sensitive cells in the retina at the back of the eyeball. These send electrical impulses via the optic nerve into the brain to be interpreted. The process of vision is primarily a function of the brain, for the eyes "see" only a small area at any one time. The eyeballs move very rapidly across the field of vision, 50–70 times a second, and the visual part of the brain makes sense of all the information.

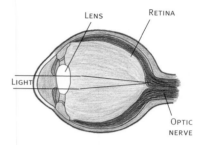

LENS   RETINA

LIGHT

OPTIC NERVE

▲ LIGHT ENTERS THE EYE, TRIGGERING THE NERVES IN THE LIGHT-SENSITIVE CELLS IN THE RETINA, WHICH THEN LINK UP TO THE BRAIN.

COLOUR AND THE BRAIN

Nerves go directly from the retina to the hypothalamus and pituitary gland (both are parts of the brain), which control most of the body's life-sustaining functions, and modify behaviour patterns and regulate energy levels. Thus the application of light can directly influence the body.

In addition, specialist cells within the skin have a sensitivity to light and so this is a second area in which your body can be directly influenced by colour.

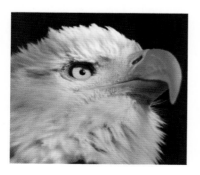

◂ SOME CREATURES CAN SEE A WIDER SPECTRUM OF COLOURS THAN HUMANS.

The psychology of colour

Colour can affect your personality whether this is due to cultural conditioning or personal associations. If you were wearing blue on a very happy occasion, for example, the colour may continue to remind you of that experience.

COLOUR AND MOOD

There are psychological associations with each colour, and colours can be linked with moods. Reds, oranges and yellows are warm and expansive and give a feeling of energy, excitement and joy. Blues, indigos and purples are calming and cool. They quieten the temperament and induce relaxation. The psychology of colour is a language that you can learn, just as you can learn to read and write. When you understand the basic meanings of colours you can choose the colours in your life according to your needs.

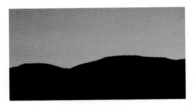

▲ THE SUNSET COLOURS, PINK AND GOLD, ARE NURTURING AND EXCELLENT FOR HEALING EMOTIONAL TRAUMA.

RESTORING BALANCE

Each colour vibrates at a distinctive rate that corresponds with a part of the body. When you are well you may like most colours, but illness will bring out preferences for specific colours. It is these that are needed for healing. When you are exhausted you may be drawn to reds. Some-one who is over-excited would benefit from blues, but depression needs yellows and golds.

The following guide will help you to explore how you feel, and help you to choose colours to enhance your well-being.

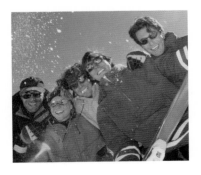

◄ RED IS THE COLOUR ASSOCIATED WITH ADVENTURE SPORTS SUCH AS SKI-ING.

Chakras and colour

Ancient texts describe seven energy centres, or chakras, arranged along the spinal column. Each one focuses energy, and each is associated with a colour. They are forever changing and balancing to preserve your well-being.

WORKING WITH CHAKRAS

Every individual has a particular chakra pattern, some being more dominant than others. This can lead to an energy imbalance, so you will need to determine which chakras need balancing. In this way you will be able to maintain a harmonious and healthy state.

Colour therapy is a technique that can work directly with chakras. Shining coloured light on the chakra, over the whole body or through the eyes all create

▾ THE POSITION AND COLOUR OF CHAKRAS (ENERGY CENTRES) ON THE BODY.

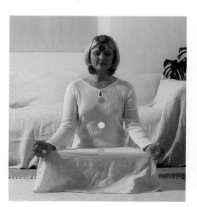

physical, emotional and mental changes which re-balance the chakras. If coloured light is not easily available, visualizing the necessary colours can also work.

THE SEVEN CHAKRAS

CROWN CHAKRA: purple
Overall balance, intuition.
Linked to pineal gland.

BROW CHAKRA: indigo
Understanding, perception.
Linked to pituitary gland.

THROAT CHAKRA: blue
Communication, expression.
Linked to thyroid glands.

HEART CHAKRA: green
Relationships, development.
Linked to heart and thymus.

SOLAR PLEXUS CHAKRA: yellow
Sense of identity, confidence.
Linked to pancreas and spleen.

SACRAL CHAKRA: orange
Creativity, feelings, sex drive.
Linked to adrenal glands.

BASE CHAKRA: red
Survival, stability, practicality.
Linked to gonads.

The energy of brilliance

Brilliance represents the universal intelligence and its source is the sun. Created when all rays of colour come together in perfect balance, it is the light from which all colours spring: the light seen in near-death experiences.

THE CHARACTER OF BRILLIANCE

Brilliance itself is not a colour: it is the original or cosmic light. Add a touch of brilliance to any colour and it will become brighter. Without brilliance there can be no vision. Brilliance cuts directly through to the truth. It is the hard light that exposes all flaws and

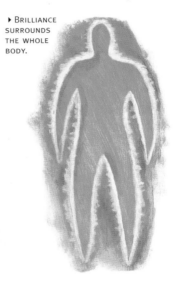

▸ BRILLIANCE SURROUNDS THE WHOLE BODY.

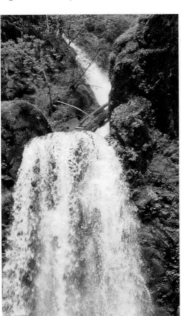

corruption. It contains the essence of all qualities, both positive and negative, sparkling in the brilliance of perfection. It clears the way for necessary actions. Brilliance clears any cloudiness in a person or over-dominance of any one colour. To recharge yourself at any time simply visualize pure brilliant

◂ BATHING IN A WATERFALL IS LIKE STANDING IN A CASCADE OF BRILLIANT LIGHT.

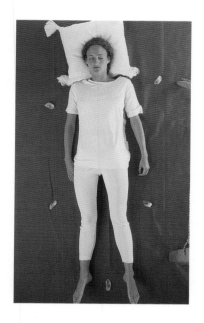

▸ This arrangement of six clear crystals is called the Seal of Solomon. It will quieten your mind and inspire brilliant insights.

light. When you say that someone is "brilliant", you are really acknowledging his or her purity of vision and action.

Brilliance and the body

The lymphatic system and the tissues that filter out the debris from the body relate to brilliance. Crystal clear water is pure liquid brilliance: bathing in a waterfall is the equivalent of standing under a cascade of clear light. Another

When brilliance can help

• Brilliance will bring a ray of hope to your life when all seems lost. • It can also bring change, and allows the delusions of your life to dissolve. You will see situations clearly and it will allow you to wipe the slate clean. • Applying brilliance may bring about a move to a new home, a change of job, or a subtle inner transformation. You will find that old patterns fall away and are replaced with new ones, full of joy and an uplifting of the spirit.

way to apply brilliance to yourself is to stand in front of an open window, or to go outside and take a brief sunshine bath: you can renew yourself time and time again.

▸ Brilliance captured in clear crystals inspires clear thoughts.

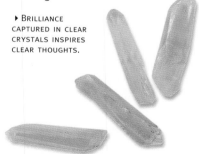

The energy of red

Red is the nearest visible light to infrared. It is a fiery force: the spirit of physical life, full of power and drive. It signifies courage and liberation, passion and excitement. Too much red burns, but at the right level it supports life.

THE CHARACTER OF RED

When the influence of red is managed well within the system, its energy can be harnessed to motivate people. These are the innovators and entrepreneurs who are full of ideas. They prefer to move from one project to another, getting things started and then moving on.

People under the influence of red are often renowned for their daring exploits and can be somewhat extrovert and boastful about their skills. An overload of red causes restlessness and impatience in those nearby. It can result in selfishness, making people focus on their own needs and survival above everything else. Sometimes this drive to survive is what fuels

◀ FOR AN EXCITING DAY, DRESS YOUR CHILD IN RED CLOTHES.

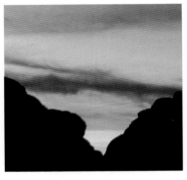

▲ A BRIGHT RED SKY AT SUNRISE CAN SIGNIFY THE APPROACH OF A CHANGEABLE AND STORMY WEATHER SYSTEM.

impulsive actions and rash comments. Red at its worst is tyrannical, seeking advancement no matter who or what suffers.

At its best, red will ensure a satisfying and passionate love life. Red brings focus to the physicality of life, to the process of living.

CAUTION
Do not use red lighting in chromotherapy above the waist for heart conditions. Medical advice should be taken regarding any heart problem.

The colour red is symbolic of what you need to survive. Life should be grabbed and lived with a sense of immediacy. Without red you may become listless and out of touch with reality.

RED AND THE BODY

Primarily, red is associated with the genitals and reproductive organs. Another area of red focus is the blood and circulation, as it increases the body's ability to absorb iron. Red also prompts adrenalin to release into the bloodstream – hence its link with aggression.

WHEN RED CAN HELP

• Use red to help circulatory problems, such as cold hands and feet, hardening of the arteries, anaemia and exhaustion. • Red can also be used to treat infertility and is especially good for stiff muscles and joints, particularly in the legs and feet.
• Red is useful in cases of paralysis, and works excellently if also combined with physiotherapy (physical therapy). • Red counteracts shyness and enables you to put your life back into action.

Red is a colour charged with energy and vitality. After an illness, when the body has been weakened, red is excellent for stimulating renewed strengths and encouraging recovery.

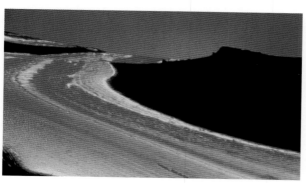

◀ THE LAVA FLOW FROM VOLCANOES IS RED. IT IS NATURE'S WARNING SIGNAL FOR DANGER.

the energy of red **417**

The energy of orange

As a mixture of red and yellow, orange blends the properties of both colours. Orange energy displays some sense of direction and purpose – it moves along those pathways that fuel its own existence.

THE CHARACTER OF ORANGE

Orange has a persistent nature and can be summed up by one word: opportunity. Always one jump ahead, orange has the courage to grasp opportunities as soon as they occur. Orange is a strong colour that dares to trust intuition, tapping into creative resources and allowing skills to develop. The orange personality loves to experiment with new and exciting recipes in the kitchen. They are physical and will be drawn to sports of any kind.

▾ THE FLAMES OF A FIRE SHOW THE MANY DIFFERENT SHADES OF ORANGE.

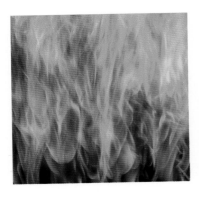

▸ THIS GINGER KITTEN WILL GROW UP TO BE BRAVE, FRIENDLY AND FULL OF FUN.

Curiosity is one of the driving characteristics of the orange vibration and this brings with it exploration and creativity, particularly on practical physical levels. It tests, then accepts or rejects. It has impetus, self-reliance and practical knowledge.

Orange strength is subtle – it stimulates gently. It broadens life and is very purposeful. Orange breaks down barriers and gives the courage to make changes and face the consequences, good or bad. Because the orange energy is purposeful and has an instinct for moving on, it can creatively remove those blocks that cause restriction and stagnation.

The orange personality is genial, optimistic, tolerant, benign and warm-hearted, believing in friendship and community. The unkind practical joker is negative

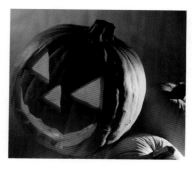

▲ BOOST A PARTY ATMOSPHERE BY ADDING ORANGE DECORATIONS TO ENHANCE COMMUNICATION BETWEEN GUESTS.

▶ ORANGE IS THE COLOUR OF THE SACRAL CHAKRA AND GOVERNS THE GUT INSTINCTS.

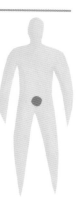

It governs the gut instincts and it enables you to become aware of the needs of your physical body.

orange. A balance of orange energy brings a willingness to get involved; it gives you the ability to fill your time creatively.

ORANGE AND THE BODY

The lower back, lower intestines, the kidneys, adrenal glands and abdomen are all linked to orange.

▼ IN THE FLOWER WORLD, ORANGE REPRESENTS THE DOCTOR.

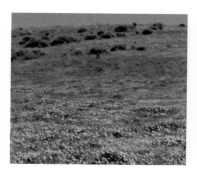

WHEN ORANGE CAN HELP

• Grief, bereavement and loss can all be treated with orange. Orange vibrations will bring you through the shock of deep outrage and will give added strength where it is needed to pull through adversity. • It can also be useful when there is an inability to let go of the past. Orange removes the inhibitions and psychological paralysis that occur when people are afraid of moving forwards in their life. • Orange can help with the fear of enjoying sensual pleasure, it can relieve over-seriousness, a feeling of bleakness and boredom, or a lack of interest in the world outside.
• Orange can be used to treat asthma, bronchitis, epilepsy, mental disorders, rheumatism, torn ligaments, aching and broken bones.

The energy of yellow

Yellow is the brightest colour of the spectrum. Its sunny hue brings clarity of thought, warmth and vitality. Yellow pinpoints issues and leaves no stone unturned in its search for understanding.

THE CHARACTER OF YELLOW

The yellow vibration is concerned with discrimination and decision-making, both skills which are constantly needed for physical and mental well-being. Yellow is the colour of the scientist. It unravels problems and focuses the attention, loves new ideas and is flexible and highly adaptable. Yellow has no hesitation; it decides quickly and acts at once. It smartens the reflexes.

Yellow is the great communicator and a favourite pastime is networking. It has financial

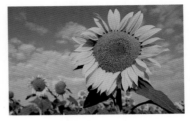

▲ YELLOW REPRESENTS MENTAL VIGOUR AND CAN GIVE YOU ENERGY WHEN YOU NEED IT.

ambition – though holding on to money may be difficult. Yellow has the ability to get things done. It has self-control, style and plenty of sophistication.

▼ YELLOW SWEEPS AWAY CONFUSION AND HELPS YOU THINK CLEARLY.

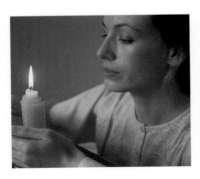

SHADES OF YELLOW

As with all colours, different hues of yellow will create markedly different responses. Pale primrose yellow is associated with great spirituality, questioning the world beyond, whereas a clean, clear yellow empties the mind and keeps it alert. Acid yellow can promote feelings of suspicion and negative criticism, and a tendency to bear grudges and resentment.

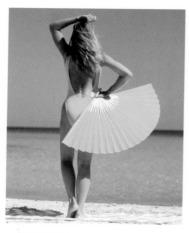

▴ SURROUNDING YOURSELF WITH YELLOW CAN HELP TO ENHANCE YOUR SENSE OF SELF-ESTEEM AND SELF-WORTH.

• Use yellow when you need to enliven a sluggish system: it will help to clear away toxins and stimulate the flow of gastric juices so improving nutrient digestion. • It can also be used to treat menopausal flushes, menstrual difficulties and other hormonal problems.

• Yellow is the great eliminator that clears toxins from your system. So apply if you are suffering from frequent minor illnesses, intolerances and allergies or constipation.

• Feelings of lethargy and depression brought on by dull weather respond well to a dose of yellow light, which can also help improve a poor memory or an inability to study. • Yellow can help to improve self-esteem, and reduce negativity and anxiety.

• In cases of diabetes, rheumatism and anorexia nervosa, yellow can sometimes help to relieve the symptoms associated with the illness.

Yellow broadcasts a feeling of well-being and self-confidence. People feel good around those under the yellow ray. They are sunny and willing, unless they are upset, when they can be acid and sharp-tongued.

YELLOW AND THE BODY

The colour yellow is connected to the pancreas, liver, skin, solar plexus, spleen, gall bladder, stomach

◀ YELLOW IS THE COLOUR OF THE SOLAR PLEXUS CHAKRA, AND GOVERNS THE STOMACH.

and nervous system. Both the immune system and the digestive system rely on yellow to keep the gastric juices flowing. This colour helps to clear blockages of all kinds.

The energy of green

The colour green is found midway in the spectrum. It is made up of two colours: yellow and blue. Yellow brings wisdom and clarity while blue promotes peace. Green's basic qualities are balance and harmony.

THE CHARACTER OF GREEN

Whereas reds, oranges and yellows are warm, and blues, indigo and violets are cool, green can be either. Green aids the memory, which makes it an important healing colour. Most physical and mental illnesses result from events in the past. Green can release these traumas.

Green is the colour of the plant kingdom. It stands for growth and therefore change, since life is a process of transformation from one

▼ THE GREEN OF FRESH HERBS CAN PROMOTE A SENSE OF HARMONY.

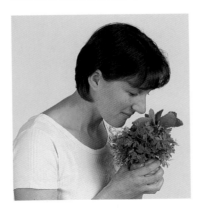

state to another. Growth needs balance and order for it to be sustainable, with each stage acting as a foundation for the next.

Green energy has to do with the pushing back of boundaries, of growing beyond what is known. Because green is connected to the heart it must develop relationships with the things around it, but it also needs a degree of control and power, which may be supportive or destructive. Positive green is the giver: sensible, socially aware, helpful and selfless. Green is about finding self-awareness which helps to bring self-acceptance.

Green is the vibration of relationships, of understanding the needs of others. In a positive, caring relationship, both lives are enriched and expanded and your interaction with the world is broadened. When a relationship is negative or manipulative, your own potential for understanding the world is curtailed and restricted.

The green personality is prosperous and loves to share what it accumulates. Green may have a conflict of ideas but it always strives to maintain the status quo. Green has the ability to discriminate. Used in a positive manner this can promote tolerance.

GREEN AND THE BODY

The colour green is connected to the shoulders, chest, lower lungs, thymus gland and heart.

▼ PARKS ARE A HAVEN FOR CITY DWELLERS, HELPING THEM APPLY GREEN IN THEIR LIVES.

WHEN GREEN CAN HELP

• Problems with personal relationships, especially when there is a difficulty with over-dominance or subservience, can be helped by green, as can feelings such as envy, jealousy and greed. The desire to dominate or possess is a negative tendency which green can help.

• Claustrophobia or feelings of restriction caused by being housebound or confined, or feelings of being trapped by other people's rules and regulations can be counter-acted by the green vibration.

• Green can restore stability to any situation. It helps to counteract biliousness and a feeling of nausea.

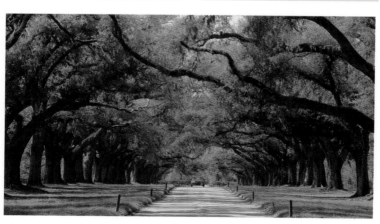

The energy of blue

The colour blue has a stillness about it. It values honour, integrity and sincerity. Blue thinks before acting and proceeds steadily and with caution. It is tranquil and avoids drawing attention to itself.

THE CHARACTER OF BLUE

There are two aspects of blue. One is the process of communication and the flow of energy, and the other is the experience of rest and peacefulness.

Blue is the spirit of truth and higher intelligence. It is spiritually calming, the colour of the writer, poet, and philosopher. The head and the heart speak directly through the blue throat when there is a need to communicate clearly. Honesty and integrity are key blue qualities, and so if blue is lacking, attempts at self-

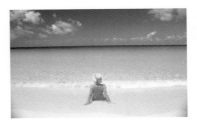

▲ GAZE AT THE SEA OR THE SKY FOR A NATURAL DOSE OF BLUE. IT WILL INSTIL A SENSE OF PEACE AND TRANQUILLITY.

expression can lead to frustration and disappointment. However, a blue personality that is out of balance can be subtly (or even unconsciously) manipulative. It dislikes upsets and arguments, but may cause them indirectly.

Blue is a cool vibration; it is the tranquil spirit, the colour of contemplation, and it brings rest. It can help to heal inflammations in the body by cooling the area down, and can also help to counteract infection.

This quality of peace gives blue a sense of detachment from emotional turmoil. It is not over-whelmed by closeness or

▼ DIVING IS THE PERFECT PASTIME FOR PEOPLE WITH AN ON-GOING NEED FOR BLUE.

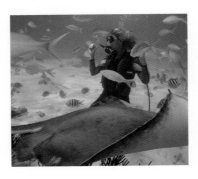

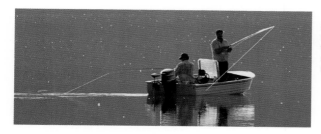

◀ ON A CLEAR SUNNY DAY, BEING ON WATER WILL FILL YOU WITH BLUE ENERGY.

detail, having the possibility of greater perspectives. The blue personality brings a wisdom to love. Blue is also linked to loyalty. This is the quality that can lead you towards the source of devotion.

The sky blue hue encourages a freedom of spirit. It brings solace where cruelty and brutality

have occurred. It is a universal healing colour as it constantly creates – and maintains – calm, while overcoming obstacles with no apparent effort.

BLUE AND THE BODY

The colour blue is concerned with the throat area, upper lungs and arms, and the base of the skull. It relates to weight gain. The connected glands are the thyroid and parathyroids. Infections in the throat area are often psychologically related to not speaking out. Since the blue personality hates arguments, it may even resort to coughing and spluttering to avoid any form of confrontation.

WHEN BLUE CAN HELP
• Coughs, sore throats, vocal problems, teething and ear infections can all be treated with blue. A stiff neck, which can represent the fear of moving forwards, also responds. • Blue is particularly useful in reducing the temperature of a fever in adults and children. • Blue can help to calm those who are over-excited or agitated. When used for people with terminal illnesses it can bring a tremendous feeling of peace.

▶ BLUE IS THE COLOUR OF THE THROAT CHAKRA, AND RELATES TO PERSONAL EXPRESSION.

The energy of indigo

Indigo has a strong belief in law and order and a great love of tradition. However, it can also be a transformer, a defender of people's rights, and it has an affinity with a deep inner world.

THE CHARACTER OF INDIGO

The indigo vibration is related to subtle perceptions, such as clairvoyance and other psychic skills. The deep, directionless depths of indigo can heighten our awareness of what is not immediately apparent.

The indigo personality loves structure and hates untidyness. It may ally itself with the Establishment, often upholding the social order in a positive, constructive way. However, a weak indigo personality may become bossy (and over-controlling), or a slave to rigid ideas.

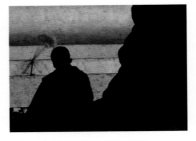

▲ INDIGO PEOPLE WILL OFTEN SEEK SOLITUDE TO DEEPEN THEIR EXPERIENCE OF THE SPIRITUAL OR MYSTICAL REALMS.

When in tune with its inner qualities, the indigo personality can be self-reliant, stepping aside from the world to come up with new ways of thinking. Indigo is an ideal colour for contemplative and spiritual pursuits, such as solitary meditation and visualization, where the inner senses are the most important. Indigo is a stronger philosopher than blue.

The indigo personality may aspire to be a spiritual master, an inspired preacher or writer. Indigo can reconcile science and religion.

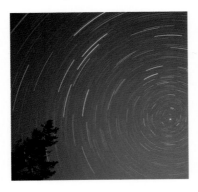

◀ GAZE INTO THE INDIGO OF THE MIDNIGHT SKY TO PREPARE FOR THE NEXT STEP IN LIFE.

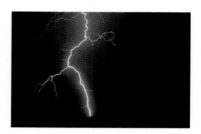

▶ LIKE A BOLT OF LIGHTNING, INTUITIVE INDIGO REALIZATIONS OFTEN OCCUR ALMOST INSTANTANEOUSLY.

It has a pioneering essence, but pioneers with insight. Negative indigo is the believer who has become a fanatic: blind devotion is an indigo failing. Addictions relate to negative indigo.

The flow of indigo energy creates an internal communication that manifests as profound thought processes, new insights, philosophy and intuition. The indigo vibration enhances and heightens awareness, while maintaining integrity. Stillness and contemplation can lead to a "super-cooled" state of indigo, in which intuition and sudden clarity of understanding can occur. The depths of indigo may seem mysterious, but its influence can yield pertinent information.

INDIGO AND THE BODY

The bone structure, especially the backbone, the pituitary gland, lower brain, eyes and sinuses are all represented by the colour indigo.

◀ THE INDIGO VIBRATION OPENS UP THE "THIRD EYE".

WHEN INDIGO CAN HELP

• Indigo is the strongest painkiller in the spectrum and is a great healer. It can be used to combat many illnesses, among them bacterial infections, and the results of air, water and food pollution.

• Indigo can help acute sinus problems (which psychologically are often uncried tears from childhood), chest complaints, bronchitis and asthma, lumbago, sciatica and migraine. Over-active thyroid, growths, tumours and lumps of any kind, diarrhoea and kidney complaints also respond to the use of indigo.

• The sedative influence of indigo can be helpful in lowering high blood pressure.

• Emotional and mental agitation can also be cooled and quietened by the calming effects of indigo. It is the perfect colour to induce a deep, healing peace.

The energy of purple

Purple can achieve great humility, even to the point of sacrificing itself for the benefit of others, without being a victim. It also has the ability to integrate psychic perception into everyday life.

THE CHARACTER OF PURPLE

The key to understanding the energy of purple is to see how its component colours, red and blue, work together: red is dynamic, while blue is quietening. Purple brings a new dynamism to blue's still qualities, and stability to the frenetic activity of red. Concepts and ideas are thus better able to find some real application. Purple is associated with imagination and psychic inspiration.

There is a danger that purple can become very arrogant. Where this happens inspiration becomes fanaticism and megalomania and imagination turns into fantasy and

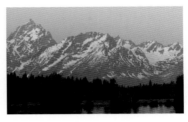

▲ PURPLE IS A GREAT PROTECTOR. IT IS RELIABLE AND SOLID, LIKE A HIGH AND MIGHTY MOUNTAIN RANGE.

delusion. The purple energy, because it seems to extend beyond current knowledge into unknown regions, can trap the spiritual dreamer in a world of unrealistic wishful thinking.

If fantasy about the unknown can be avoided, purple energy can bring enlightenment and healing. It integrates energies at all levels, and as healing requires the building up of new systems (red), according to accurate information (blue), so purple energy can accelerate healing, both physical and emotional.

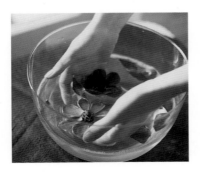

◄ PURPLE ENERGY COMBINES GENTLENESS WITH POWER.

◀ Purple is the colour of
the crown chakra, which
governs the brain.

The skill of integration is aided by purple. As the colour combines opposite energies, so it can help people who also need to work with an array of disparate things. It is often associated with the richness and diversity of ceremony, and with rulers and spiritual masters. Clergymen,

musicians and painters all work with the colour purple. Humility is a key aspect, but negative purple can be belligerent and treacherous.

Purple and the body

The top of the head – the crown, the brain and the scalp – is represented by purple, as is the pineal gland.

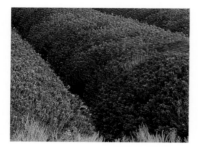

◀ Lavender is a gentle but very powerful healer.

When purple can help

• Purple can be used to treat any kind of internal inflammation, or heart palpitations or headaches. • The immune system and strained nerves can also benefit from the use of purple which enhances the natural healing energy of the body, strengthening the immune system.
• When there is a need to rebalance life, especially if it is lacking in a creative aspect, purple can increase the ability to use the imagination in practical ways and help to integrate new skills into everyday life.
• Purple can calm hyperactive states.

The energy of black

Black is connected to the secret mystery of darkness. It contains every colour within itself, absorbing all light that falls on it and giving out nothing except a promise. It is linked to unseen, hidden and fearful experiences.

THE CHARACTER OF BLACK

Black is the energy of gestation and of preparation. It has often been associated with winter and with the promise of seeds lying buried and dormant awaiting spring's growth and the new life to come.

Black is the colour of the person who keeps control by not giving information to others. Someone wearing black continuously may be saying that there is something absent from his or her life. Negative black believes that all is ended, there is nothing to look forward to. It is afraid of what is coming next.

When the energy of black is harnessed in a positive way, it can provide the discipline necessary to work through difficul-

◄ BLACK CLOTHES SUGGEST SELF-DISCIPLINE.

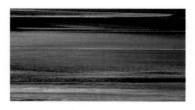

▲ THE COLOUR BLACK IS OFTEN SEEN AS NEGATIVE, BUT IT CAN BE THE PRECURSOR OF CHANGE FOR THE BETTER.

ties and achieve freedom. Working towards the light in any way will involve using the magic of black. Black can complete the incomplete. The mystic arts relate to black.

BLACK AND THE BODY

There are no parts of the body specifically connected to black except when seen on X-rays or in the aura as disease.

WHEN BLACK CAN HELP

- Use black in a positive way to encourage self-discipline.
- To break the stagnation of black, a small addition of colour will help the person trapped in black to reach out.

The energy of white

White is what is perceived as the entire visible light spectrum, the complete energy of light, and so it stands for wholeness and completion. White is next to the cosmic intelligence of brilliance – but has a denser brilliance.

THE CHARACTER OF WHITE

Many cultures associate white with purity and cleanliness, openness and truth. It is often used to denote holiness. It reflects all the light that falls on it, thus radiating all the colours of the rainbow.

White's fundamental characteristic is equality: all colours remain equal in white's domain. It is also a symbol of unity and faith. White has a sense of destiny. Everything is clear and explicit. It also has a cold quality. As a vibration of purification, white can help to clarify all

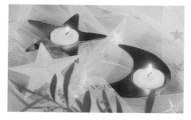

▲ BURNING PURE WHITE CANDLES WILL BRING A PURITY OF THOUGHT AND OPENNESS TO NEW EXPERIENCES IN YOUR LIFE.

aspects of life, giving the energy to sweep away all physical blocks and ingrained emotional patterns.

WHITE AND THE BODY

The eyeball is connected to the colour white: its differing shades of whiteness are used in the diagnosis of illness.

▼ "PURE AS THE DRIVEN SNOW", A PHRASE THAT LINKS THE TWO ASPECTS OF WHITE.

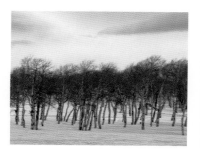

WHEN WHITE CAN HELP
• White has the ability to radiate out all colours, allowing development in any direction, so it is a good choice when you need some impetus.
• Wear white as a tonic to top up the colours in your body's system.

The energy of gold

 True gold has a belief in honour among men. It has the gift to release and forgive. Gold is related to the wise old sage. It is warm and sparkling, while its light-reflecting quality brings illumination to the mind and body.

THE CHARACTER OF GOLD

Gold is purity. It is the soul's experience of all that is past. It has access to knowledge and – most important – to knowledge of the self. Gold means "I am". It does not seek, it has already found. From its deep understanding it is able to forgive and let go of the past. It expands the power of love because it trusts completely and has no vice.

Negative gold's conceit is that of privilege and belief in itself as more worthy than others.

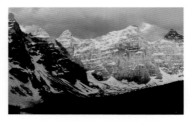

▲ THE GOLDEN LIGHT CAST BY THE SUN TURNS THE LANDSCAPE INTO A RICH AND UPLIFTING COLOUR.

It will blow its own trumpet, but true gold respects and appreciates the value of others.

GOLD AND THE BODY

No parts of the body connect with gold, an offshoot of yellow, but it can be seen in auras.

▼ GOLDEN BEACH HOLIDAYS CAN CAPTURE THE TRUE, NOBLE SPIRIT OF GOLD.

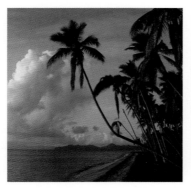

WHEN GOLD CAN HELP
• Physical and psychological depressions can be helped by gold as it is uplifting and dissipates negative energy.
• Any kind of digestive irregularity, rheumatism, arthritis, underactive thyroid can all be helped by gold. It will also reduce scars.

The energy of silver

Silver has a bright reflective quality which can create illusions and promote fluidity. It brings freedom from emotional restrictions. It is related to the moon and can light up our path.

THE CHARACTER OF SILVER

Silver is the thread of cosmic intelligence. An invisible silver cord is said to attach humanity to "the other side". It is able to still the emotions and is a great tranquillizer. Silver brings a clarity which helps resolve disputes. It takes an unbiased stand.

Negative silver shows up in relationships in which there is no substance, just delusion. People who fall in love with stars of the silver screen are under this negative influence. Professions that create make-believe also work under silver's influence.

▼ SILVER IS A COLOUR FOR THOSE WHOSE JOBS INVOLVE THE ART OF MAKE-BELIEVE.

◄ SILVER REPRESENTS ENDURANCE AND IS OFTEN USED TO MAKE TROPHIES.

SILVER AND THE BODY

The feminine dimension of the self is silver, whether it resides in a male or female body. Bathe in the moonlight to restore your equilibrium.

▼ SILVER CUTLERY CAN PROMOTE BALANCED AND FRIENDLY MEALTIME CONVERSATION.

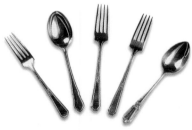

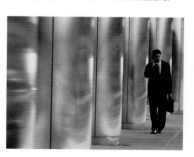

WHEN SILVER CAN HELP
- Silver brings freedom from emotional restriction: it is the great tranquilliser.
- Silver reflects mistakes without distortion. It harmonizes and brings about a fluid state of consciousness.

The energy of blends

Turquoise combines the calming, balancing qualities of green and the cool, quiet flow of blue with the warmth of yellow. Pink is also a blend, combining red and white. This mixture promotes consistency of affection.

THE CHARACTER OF TURQUOISE

In the body, turquoise is related to the throat and chest. The energy of turquoise allows self-expression, as the green quality of growth is added to the blue quality of communication, while the yellow explores information through feelings and emotions. A wonderful healing colour for the central nervous system, turquoise is a colour that allows you to stand still for a while and think only of yourself. The turquoise personality's basic motivation is to seek self-fulfilment in a personal relationship.

WHEN TURQUOISE CAN HELP
• When the throat and chest need soothing, there is low energy, or a failure to fit in, turquoise can help.

WHEN PINK CAN HELP
• In any turbulent or aggressive situation, pink can help to calm violent emotions and it will provide energy to move out of a negative situation.

THE CHARACTER OF PINK

The quality of pink energy depends on how much red is present. White stands for equality, red is the motivation to achieve a goal. Pink represents caring and tenderness and a limited exposure to pink can temper aggressive behaviour. The richer shades can help to improve self-confidence and assertiveness while the paler shades are more protective and supportive.

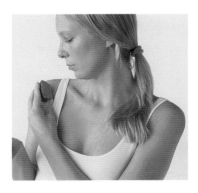

◂ PLACE THE COLOURED CRYSTAL OR STONE NEAR THE AREA THAT REQUIRES HEALING.

The energy of neutral colours

Brown is a colour of the earth and the natural world. It is the colour of solidity, preferring not to take risks. Grey is the true neutral colour, the bridge between white and black, where innocence and ignorance meet.

THE CHARACTER OF BROWN

Brown is a colour of practical energy. The brown personality is a deep thinker and can be very single-minded.

Like black, brown represents the seed waiting patiently to develop its full potential. It is the colour of hibernation. It suggests reliability and a state of solidity from which one can grow. Brown can suggest a quiet desire to remain in the background. However, it can also have a dulling effect as it lacks the ability to break out of established patterns. A touch of brown in a room can be warmly comforting.

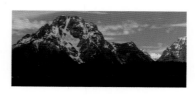

▲ ▼ THE DARK GREY OF THE MOUNTAIN, ABOVE, GIVES IT A FORBIDDING QUALITY, WHEREAS THE LIGHT GREY OF THE MOUNTAINS, BELOW, HAS AN ETHEREAL FEELING.

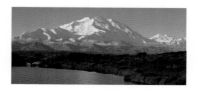

THE CHARACTER OF GREY

When grey contains a high proportion of white it tends to take on the qualities of silver's flow, but darker grey can be draining as the black in it can cause depression. However, grey can also help you to break free from the chains that bind. Negative grey is conventional to the point of narrow-mindedness. When the skin and nails have a grey tint, this can indicate congestion somewhere in the body.

WHEN BROWN CAN HELP
• Brown is a neutral and non-threatening colour which begets comfort and stability.

WHEN GREY CAN HELP
• Grey is not commonly used in healing, but light grey is extremely soothing. It can help to restore sanity.

Hidden colours

All colours, apart from the rainbow hues, are combinations of other colours. When using colour for healing, it is important to remember that these hidden colours will have a subtle effect that can be beneficial.

COLOUR COMPONENTS

When you are working with colour – particularly when you are using it for healing – it is important to be aware of what are known as hidden colours. For instance, orange is made up of the hidden colours of red and yellow. The eye will see orange but the body will also experience the red and yellow vibrations that are within the orange. Therefore, when working with orange for healing, you should take account of the psychological effects of red and yellow as well as those of orange.

The colour green has its own healing meaning, and also the meaning of the yellow and blue

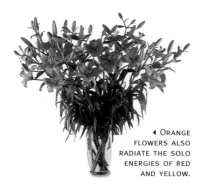

◀ ORANGE FLOWERS ALSO RADIATE THE SOLO ENERGIES OF RED AND YELLOW.

rays that make up green. Turquoise is a combination of all three of these rays. Similarly, purple has red and blue within it, so remember to evaluate these colour effects too. Grey, of course, consists of the hidden colours black and white. Brown is made up of various colours including yellow, red, and even black. Like all colours, brown has a wide range of shades or tints, each with a differing effect in healing. Every shade or tint has a unique combination of hidden colours.

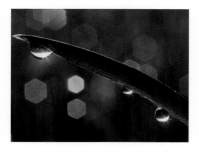

◀ GREEN'S HEALING QUALITY INCLUDES THE EFFECTS OF YELLOW AND BLUE

Complementary colours

Every colour of the spectrum has an opposite colour that complements it. Knowing these complementary colours will help you to identify which colours you need for healing, support and help.

OPPOSITES

The complementary colour of red is blue, that of orange is indigo and yellow's is purple. Green, the middle colour of the rainbow, has magenta, which is made up of red and blue.

A knowledge of complementary colours is often useful in everyday life. For example, if you feel extremely irritated by someone's behaviour, you will be reacting to an overload of red vibration within your system. To counteract this, just think of blue, put on some blue clothing or gaze at any blue object. Continue until you feel the anger pass. Or

▸ ALL COLOURS OF THE SPECTRUM HAVE A COMPLEMENTARY COLOUR. GREEN'S IS MAGENTA, AN EXTRA COLOUR MADE UP OF RED AND BLUE.

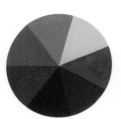

you may find yourself in a room with yellow decor that you find disturbing. Close your eyes and conjure up the colour purple – the complementary of yellow – to dispel the yellow vibration.

An understanding of complementary colours can be helpful when you are using a lamp with coloured slides for healing. Use a blue slide to relieve the red of irritability, for instance, or a red slide to pull you out of the blues. If you are ever in doubt about a colour, or have a feeling that too much colour has been used, just flood yourself with green light or visualize it. Green acts as a neutralizer, returning balance and order to any situation.

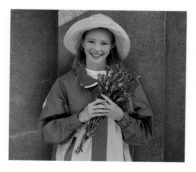

◂ WEARING THE COMPLEMENTARY COLOURS RED AND BLUE CAN HAVE A HAPPY EFFECT.

Hues, tints and shades

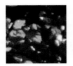

The description of a colour usually refers to the hue, that is one of the colours of the rainbow. Each colour can vary, it may be light or dark. These variations can be extremely beneficial when used for healing.

LIGHT AND DARK HUES

All variations of a hue share its underlying qualities, but their psychological meanings are modified according to whether they are a higher (tint) or lower (shade) tone. Tints are paler (higher) colours which have more white in them. This gives them a stronger healing quality. For example, the white added to red to create pink brings with it a compassionate and spiritual quality. The paler the pink, the greater the healing qualities it

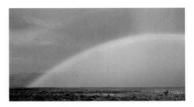

▲ THE RAINBOW CONTAINS THE SEVEN HUES USED IN COLOUR HEALING: RED, ORANGE, YELLOW, GREEN, BLUE, INDIGO AND PURPLE.

possesses. Shades of a colour are darker (lower) and are produced when the basic hue is mixed with black.

In general, the tints are considered positive and the shades negative. But this can be misleading as the darker shades can alert you to problems that you may need to address.

▼ WEARING A PALE TINT OF PINK CAN BRING A STRONG SENSE OF CALM.

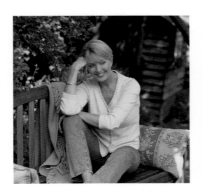

COLOUR DEFINITIONS

Hue: a basic colour in the visible spectrum, a ray

Tint: a hue plus white

Shade: a hue plus black

Colour categories

Colours can be grouped into practical categories, based upon the four elements (fire, earth, air and water) and the seasons. These colour groupings relate to personality types, and most people are drawn to one particular group.

COLOUR PREFERENCE

A colour grouping can help in your choice of colours for home decorations, clothes and belongings. You may be drawn to more than one category, which can be useful if you have to compromise with other people over room décor.

Occasionally, your second preference can be useful if you are choosing clothes to create a particular image for a specific purpose, but wearing colours to impress others may feel uncomfortable compared to wearing your natural, instinctive choice.

SPRING – WATER

Warm, light tints: turquoise, lilac, peach, coral, scarlet, violet, emerald, sunshine yellow, cream, sand.
Clear, almost delicate colours, that create a joyful and nurturing ambience.

SUMMER – AIR

Subtle tones, some dark, containing grey: maroon, rose, powder blue, sage green, pale yellow, lavender, plum, oyster, taupe.
Colours that are elegant, cool and contained, never heavy.

AUTUMN – FIRE

Warm shades (containing some black): mustard, olive green, flame, peacock, burnt orange, teal, burgundy.
Very rich, striking colours that suggest maturity and depth.

WINTER – EARTH

Sharp contrasts between hues, tints and shades: black, white, magenta, cyan, purple, lemon, silver, indigo, royal blue, jade.
Bold and powerful colours, with no subtlety.

Choosing colours

Your instinctive emotional response to colour can tell you a lot about yourself. It is possible to interpret your colour preferences through their known correspondences to your physical, emotional, mental and even your spiritual state.

SIMPLE CHOICE

Given a number of colours to choose from, the process of self-reflection and self-revelation can begin. The simplest approach is to make spontaneous choices. Which colour do you like most, and which colour the least?

The colour you like most will probably be evident in the way you have decorated your home or in your clothes. But it may also be a colour that you need now to help support you in your present situation. Look at the full range of characteristics of that colour for

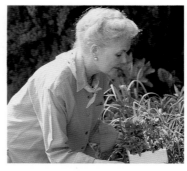

▲ YOUR CHOICE OF FLOWERS FOR THE GARDEN MAY REVEAL TENDENCIES TOWARDS CERTAIN COLOURS.

clues to other aspects that may help. If the colour you have chosen is an absolute favourite and you have no desire to make other choices, it could indicate that you have become stuck in a habitual pattern.

The colour you like least could suggest an area of your life that requires attention or healing. Bringing that colour energy into your life by adding it to your surroundings may be beneficial.

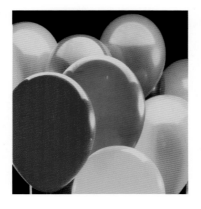

◀ A CHILD'S CHOICE OF BALLOON MAY GIVE YOU INSIGHT INTO THEIR MENTAL STATE.

Multiple choice

The process can be developed by making a series of choices. Decide beforehand what question each choice will represent. For example:

1 What are your physical needs now (activities, food, clothing)?

2 What are your emotional needs now (peace, fun, company)?

3 What are your mental needs now (time to study, assertiveness)?

How to do it

1 Use the chart overleaf, or collect together ribbons or buttons, at least one of each colour of the rainbow, plus a few other colours.

2 Lay them out at random on a plain background.

3 Close your eyes and have in your mind the first question.

4 Relax, open your eyes and pick up the colour you are immediately and instinctively drawn to.

5 Repeat the process for each question you ask.

Interpreting your choices

Look at your colour choice for each question and relate it to the meaning of that colour. You can then introduce the energy of the colour into your everyday life.

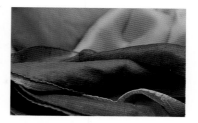

▲ A SIMPLE COLLECTION OF DIFFERENT COLOURED FABRICS CAN BE USEFUL FOR DIAGNOSING THE NECESSARY COLOURS.

Taking it further

You can invent any number of permutations for a series of questions. Here is just one possible list:

1 Where am I now?

2 What are my main difficulties?

3 What is at the root of those difficulties?

4 What are my priority needs?

5 What is the best way for me to move forwards?

▼ MAKE COLOUR CHOICES IN YOUR OWN MIND, SIMPLY IMAGINE THEM AND CHOOSE.

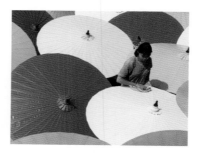

Using a colour-choice chart

You can use this colour chart to help you with your self-assessment or make your own chart using different paints or pieces of cloth. If you make your own you will be able to include as many colours as you like.

USING THE CHART

Before you begin to choose your colours, cover the meanings with a sheet of paper. This will help stop your eyes scanning the other page and will prevent the logical and judgemental part of your mind from interfering with your instinctive choice of colour.

Decide how many choices you will make and what each will represent, then close your eyes. For each choice, consider the question you are asking then open your eyes and see which colour you are immediately drawn to.

Record the colour you choose for each question. When you have made all your choices, remove the paper and study the key phrases and questions in the interpretation chart to help you focus your ideas. Where appropriate, introduce more of the colours you have chosen into your life, whether in terms of food, decor or clothing.

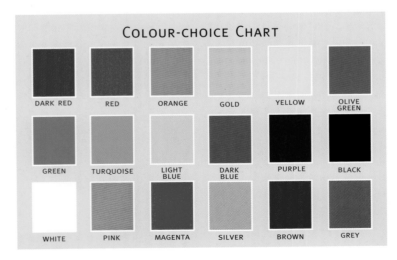

COLOUR-CHOICE CHART

DARK RED	RED	ORANGE	GOLD	YELLOW	OLIVE GREEN
GREEN	TURQUOISE	LIGHT BLUE	DARK BLUE	PURPLE	BLACK
WHITE	PINK	MAGENTA	SILVER	BROWN	GREY

Colour Chart Interpretations

Dark red
You need to keep your feet firmly on the ground. What is taking your attention away from where it needs to be?

Red
You need to take action, now. What is stopping you?

Orange
You need to let go of old emotions and ideas. What are you allowing to block your way?

Gold
You need to relax and enjoy life. What is it that is making you doubt yourself?

Yellow
You need to start thinking clearly. What are you afraid of?

Olive green
You need to reassess where you are going. What hidden factors are stopping your growth?

Green
You need space to gain a fresh perspective. What is it that is restricting you?

Turquoise
You need to express exactly what you feel. What are your strengths?

Light blue
You need to talk to people around you. What do you need to express to others?

Dark blue
You need time to think. What are you so close to that you cannot see clearly what is happening?

Purple
You need to heal yourself. What are you sacrificing to help others?

Black
You need to be quiet and listen. What do you want to hide from?

White
You need to make changes. What do you find painful in the real world?

Pink
You need to look after yourself more. Are you being too self-critical?

Magenta
You need to take time out to heal yourself. Are you risking your own health by overdoing things?

Silver
You need to restore your equilibrium. What are you deluding yourself about?

Brown
You need to focus on practicalities. What areas of your life have you been too dreamy about?

Grey
You need to disappear into the background. What do you want to hide and why?

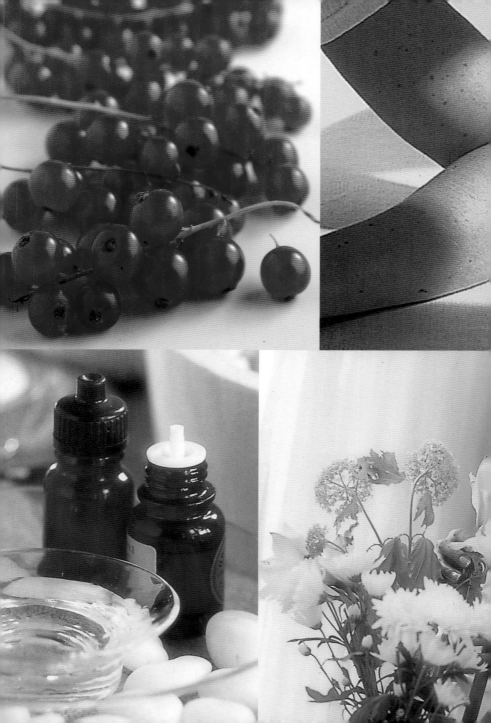

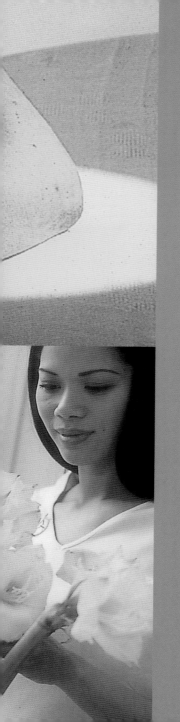

COLOUR
TREATMENTS

Now that you understand how the different colours of the spectrum can influence our moods and attitudes, you are ready to harness their therapeutic properties to rejuvenate the body, make decisions and enrich your life.

Choosing foods based on colour will help you to strike a healthy balance between your various dietary needs, and experimenting with coloured light will enable you to create an effective outlet for your ever-changing emotions. Colour essences and sprays are easy to make from flowers or gel, and are excellent tools for rapid healing. Plus, by incorporating colours into home decoration, dowsing and meditation, you will learn how to become totally at ease in your surroundings.

Colour and food

The colour of the foods we eat can have a powerful effect on our physical and emotional state. Eating the appropriate coloured foods can help to rejuvenate and balance the system, making you feel brighter and more alive.

FRESH FOODS

Wholesome, fresh food is full of colour energy. Seek out foods that are organically grown with no additives, as this will keep the colour vibration alive. Become aware of the colours of the different foods you choose, as your preferences can convey valuable information about yourself.

Your body will normally direct you to the foods that you need to rebalance your health, though habit or advertising may intrude on what should be an important guide for your health. Given a free choice, you will always tend to be drawn to those foods you need, and colour is an important factor.

If you have problems that correspond to certain colours you may wish to increase foods of that colour in your diet. Nutrients such as vitamins and minerals also resonate with particular colours, and these are included in the following lists, as are "non-foods" (foods with little nutritional value) which you may also crave at times when you need instant energy.

▸ RED FOODS PROMOTE TIRELESS ENERGY AND LIVELY ACTION.

FOOD COLOURS

Red: Gives extra energy, heals lethargy and tiredness
Orange: Creates optimism and change, heals grief and disappointment
Yellow: Encourages laughter, joy and fun, heals depression
Green: Improves physical stamina, heals panic
Blue: Brings peace and relaxation, helps concentration and heals anxiety
Indigo: Puts back structure into life, heals insecurity
Purple: Promotes leadership, heals and calms the emotionally erratic

Red foods and orange foods

RED FOODS

Foods that are red in colour are generally rich in minerals and are good sources of protein. They increase levels of vitality. Red deficiencies are shown through low energy, anaemia, light-headedness and lack of stamina. Red foods can also help heart problems of an emotional or physical nature. However, professional medical advice should also be sought.

FOOD FACTS

Fruits: strawberries, raspberries, cherries

Vegetables: red cabbage, beetroot, radishes, peppers (also green, orange and yellow), onions, tomatoes

Other foods: meat, pulses, nuts, fish

Vitamins: B12

Minerals: iron, magnesium, zinc (also orange)

Other nutrients: fatty acids

Non-foods: sugar (also yellow and purple)

ORANGE FOODS

The release of toxins and stress from the body is associated with orange. It also supports the reproductive system and encourages creativity on all levels: orange may help with writer's block. Vitamin C and zinc both resonate with orange and provide an excellent detoxifying combination to help the body rid itself of heavy metals and other pollutants. A lack of orange can cause problems in the area of the orange chakra such as constipation or fertility problems, and also stiffness in the joints.

FOOD FACTS

Fruits: oranges, peaches, apricots, physalis, kumquats, persimmon

Vegetables: pumpkin, peppers (also green, red and yellow), carrots

Other foods: brown rice, sesame, oats, shellfish

Vitamins: A, C

Minerals: calcium, copper, selenium, zinc (also red)

Yellow foods and green foods

Yellow foods

The sun is the main source of yellow during daylight hours, but most people work indoors and modern life uses up the yellow vibration dealing with pollution, chemicals, and high stress levels. Yellow foods can help. Lack of yellow leads to exhaustion, tension, restlessness, poor absorption of nutrients, digestive problems, lowered immunity, hot flushes, depression, poor memory and inability to make decisions.

Green foods

The foods that are of a green nature tend to be very rich in vitamins and minerals, though these can be lost in cooking or storage, so eat lots of fresh fruit and salad. Growing your own vegetables is a great way to ensure their freshness, as well as bringing you in touch with nature. Lack of green vibration creates an inability to relate, a feeling of being trapped, breathing difficulties and negative emotions.

Food facts

Fruits: lemon, bananas, grapefruit

Vegetables: grains, peppers, squash

Other foods: eggs, fish, oils, food rich in fatty acids

Vitamins and minerals: A, B complex, D, E, sodium potassium, selenium (also orange), phosphorus, iodine (also blue), chromium, molybdenite, manganese

Non-foods: food additives, alcohol, sugar (also red and purple)

Food facts

Fruits: apples, pears, avocado, green grapes, lime, kiwi fruits

Vegetables: cabbage, calabrese, broccoli, kale, sprouts, green beans, peas, leeks, other dark green leafy vegetables

Other: most culinary herbs – marjoram, basil, oregano, parsley

Vitamins and minerals: all vitamins, no minerals

▶ Eat plenty of fresh greens.

Blue foods and purple foods

BLUE AND PURPLE FOODS

Very few foods are naturally coloured blue or purple, but several work with a blue or purple vibration. Blue foods are useful when the voice and communication skills, glands or organs of the neck need a helping hand. Purple vibration foods can have a remarkable effect on the workings of the mind. Small amounts of basil, can help to relax the body while keeping the mind alert.

OTHER WORLDS, OTHER FOODS

Some foods with a purple resonance have long been used in healing. Used carefully, they can open the consciousness to other realms of experience and possibilities. In Central America the peyote cactus (*Lophophora williamsii*) is ritually harvested and used in religious and healing ceremonies, and ayahuasca (*Banesteriopsis caapi*) is collected throughout the Amazon basin for a similar purpose. Both are well known as purifiers of the body and can remove the causes of illness. The herb variety called holy basil is kept by many in the Indian subcontinent as a sacred herb of meditation.

FOOD FACTS

Fruits: plums, blueberries, black grapes, figs, passion fruit

Blue vibration vegetables: kelp and all seaweed products

Purple vegetables: purple sprouting broccoli, aubergines

Purple vibration plants: St John's wort

Vitamins: E

Blue minerals: iodine
Purple minerals: potassium

Non-foods: food additives and colourings, alcohol, sugar (also red)

◀ BLUE AND PURPLE FOODS OPEN THE MIND TO OTHER WORLDS.

Healing with coloured light

The human species has evolved to be reactive to sunlight, so living and working indoors, often under artificial lighting, may be an important factor in undermining health. Coloured light can counteract some of these harmful effects.

SEASONAL AFFECTIVE DISORDER

Studies of plants have demonstrated that full-spectrum natural sunlight, including ultraviolet (filltered out by most types of glass), plays an important part in maintaining the healthy functioning of plants and animals. The lack of sunlight in winter can be debilitating, and some people suffer from a condition called Seasonal Affective Disorder (SAD), with accompanying mood swings and low energy, when levels of the hormone-like melatonin are reduced in the body. The condition can be treated with several hours daily of bright full-spectrum light.

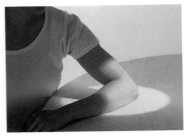

▲ YOU CAN USE CHROMOTHERAPY ON SPECIFIC AREAS.

CHROMOTHERAPY

On a basic level, chromotherapy, or light treatment, works by using different coloured gels or slides in front of high-powered lamps to bathe either the whole body or specific problem areas. The application of different coloured lights can bring about relief both for the body and spirit. The recipient of the treatment can either lie down or sit in a chair, with the lamp directed towards them. For any serious illness, however, you should always consult a medical practitioner.

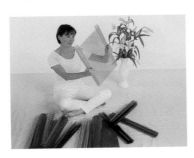

◄ USE COLOURED GELS IN FRONT OF A SPOTLIGHT TO CREATE HEALING COLOURED LIGHT.

Coloured lighting

By installing a lighting system that enables you to turn on any colour at will, you can flood the room with your chosen colour. This enables you to be bathed in a colour treatment for maximum health and well-being.

You can achieve the same effect very easily by acquiring a free-standing spotlight and selecting a coloured slide or gel appropriate to your needs. Place the gel over the spotlight, taking care to ensure it is not touching the hot bulb. Turn off any other lights in the room and turn on the spotlight. Sit with the spotlight shining on you and bathe in the coloured light for an instantly available, on-the-spot therapy.

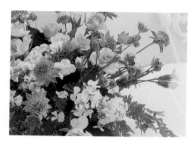

▲ PINK COUNTERACTS AN OVERLOAD OF WHITE, SO PINK FLOWERS ARE COMFORTING WHEN GIVEN TO SOMEONE IN HOSPITAL.

The all-white room

The perfect healing sanctuary for chromotherapy will be a white room. However, an all-white room in an everyday situation will cause an overload of white; if you are surrounded by it for too long it can cause agitation and frustration. Placing one red object in the room, or arranging flowers of the same hue, will dissipate the sterility that too much white can cause. You can help friends or relatives staying in all-white hospital rooms by taking in appropriately coloured flowers. Blue can help to calm fear and pre-operative nerves, while peach and pink introduce a little stimulation when the patient is recovering.

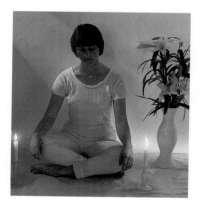

◀ SATURATE YOURSELF IN THE CALMING BLUE RAY FOR PEACE AND TRANQUILLITY.

Colour essences

Colour essences are vibrational remedies. They contain nothing other than water which has been energized by the action of natural sunlight passing through a coloured filter. They are easy to make and effective.

HOW COLOUR ESSENCES WORK

Some of the pioneers of colour therapy theorized that the atomic structure of the water was somehow altered and given particular life-enhancing properties. Current medical research is slowly coming to a very similar conclusion and is developing techniques to target specific light frequencies on diseased tissue to restore normal functioning to the cells. Vibrational remedies seem to work by helping the body to return to its natural state of balance after any kind of stress or shock has disturbed it.

▼ COLOUR ESSENCES CAN BE STORED FOR A FEW WEEKS IN BROWN GLASS BOTTLES.

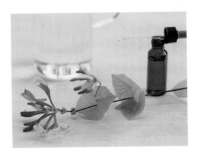

▶ SAVE SCRAPS OF COLOURED CLOTH TO MAKE COLOUR ESSENCES.

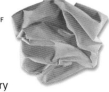

Although very simple to make, colour essences can be very effective tools for healing. Rapid release of stress can sometimes feel uncomfortable, and if this is experienced, simply reduce the amount, or stop using the essence for a day or two. Taking essences last thing at night, and then sleeping while they take effect, is a good way to comfortably restore a state of balance. They can also be taken first thing in the morning, which is a good way to make them part of your daily routine, but you may find that you need to take a bit more time getting up, if they affect you strongly.

Like all vibrational remedies, they have the advantage of being self-regulating: the body will only make use of the energy within the essence if it is appropriate.

USING ESSENCES

Colour essences can be used in many ways. A little can be drunk each day in water, or if you place an essence in a dropper bottle, it can be dropped directly on to the tongue. Because they are purely vibrational in nature, the colour essences only need to be within the energy field of the body to begin working, so other methods can also be used. You can spray it around your body for immediate effect; drop a little on to the pulse points at your wrists, on the side of your neck or your forehead; rub it on to the area needing help or the related chakra point; or add a drop or two to bathwater or massage oil.

HEALING COLOUR ESSENCE

YOU WILL NEED
Plain glass bottle or bowl
Spring water
Coloured gel or other thin coloured material
Brown glass storage bottle
Label
Preservative, such as alcohol, cider vinegar, honey or vegetable glycerine

1 Fill the bottle or bowl with spring water and cover completely with a coloured gel or cloth. You can also use a sheet of coloured glass laid over a bowl, but the essence will be most effective if only coloured light enters the water.

2 Leave the bowl or glass in bright natural sunlight for at least two hours.

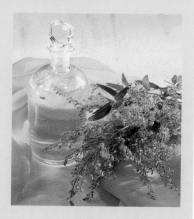

3 If you wish to keep the essence for future use, make a 50/50 mix of energized water and preservative, such as alcohol, cider vinegar or vegetable glycerine. It should be kept in a brown bottle away from light. It will keep in this way for many months.

Flowers and colour

For thousands of years plants have been used by different cultures to help to keep the body healthy and to fight disease. Many herbs indicate by their colour and shape how they can be used in healing.

FLOWER ESSENCES

Paracelsus, the 16th-century Swiss physician and occultist, is believed to have used the dew of flowers for healing and there is some evidence that flower waters were also an integral part of Tibetan medical practices. More recently, in the 20th century, Dr Bach rediscovered the healing properties of flower essences.

Colour flower essences are made by placing flowers in a bowl of water and energizing it with sunlight. As before, use flowers that you are instinctively drawn to.

Red flowers often boost energy levels. The flower essence of scarlet pimpernel (*Anagallis arvensis*), for example, can help to activate energy and clear deep-seated blocks. The elm (*Ulmus procera*) has deep red and purple flowers, and the flower essence helps to clear the mind when fatigue and confusion have set in. In this case, the red stimulates the energy reserves and the purple balances the mind.

Blue flowers will often bring a sense of peace and help with communication and expression. For example, the forget-me-not (*Myosotis arvensis*), as a flower essence, can aid memory and help those who feel cut off from deeper

▼ YOU CAN USE YOUR INTUITION TO CHOOSE PLANTS FOR FLOWER ESSENCES.

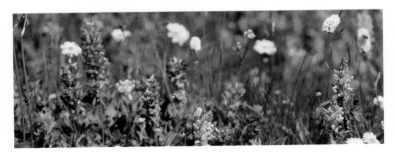

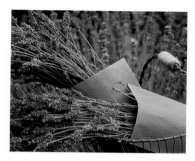

▲ THE COLOUR OF LAVENDER VARIES WITH THE SPECIES. USE THE DEEP PURPLE TYPES TO HELP CONNECT WITH YOUR INNER SELF.

levels of experience. Sage (*Salvia officinalis*) has violet-blue flowers that suggest it would be effective in the areas of the head and throat. The flower essence helps to give a broader outlook on life and a balance to the mind, encouraging the exploration of ideas.

Yellow flowers bring optimism and help to release tensions. The flower essence of dandelion (*Taraxacum officinale*) is a muscle relaxant which can also help to release rigid mental belief systems. The way in which the seeds disperse at the slightest breeze can be seen as a symbol of the quality of letting go.

Pink flowers are some of the most powerful healers, and there are many to choose from,

including the pink *(Dianthus)*, the rose (*Rosa damascena*), and the chive flower *(Allium schoenoprasum)*. Pink can help to counteract aggressive behaviour and it also encourages the qualities of generosity and affection.

Since white contains all the colours of the spectrum, white flower essences act generally, giving the body an overall boost. Common elder *(Sambucus nigra)* and chamomile *(Chamaemelum nobile)* are both useful flowers.

Although simple to make, colour flower essences can cause rapid release of stress, which can sometimes feel uncomfortable. If this is experienced, simply stop taking the remedy for a day or two or halve the dose from 6 to 3 drops a day.

▼ YELLOW FLOWERS HAVE ALWAYS BEEN ASSOCIATED WITH OPTIMISM AND CHEER.

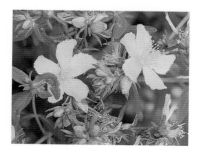

Meditation and visualization

Colour is a powerful tool in meditation because it has a profound effect on the nervous system, no matter what else may be happening in the mind. Meditating helps you to gather your scattered energies.

CELESTIAL HEALING RAYS

1 Close your eyes and visualize yourself sitting in a grassy, flower-sprinkled meadow with a cool and crystal clear stream running by you. The day is clear and bright, the sky is blue, with a scattering of soft white clouds and birds are singing in the trees.

2 Choose a colour that you need for your personal healing and well-being. Next, choose one of the clouds in the sky above you. Let this special cloud become filled with your chosen colour and start to shimmer with its coloured, sparkling light.

3 Allow the cloud to float over you; as it does, visualize the release of a shower of coloured stars cascading in all directions.

4 The mist settles on your skin and it gently becomes absorbed through your skin, saturating your system with its healing vibration.

5 Allow the colour to run through your body and bloodstream for a few minutes, giving your body a therapeutic tonic wash.

6 Allow the pores of your skin to open so that the coloured vapour can escape, taking any toxins with it. When the vapour runs clear, you can close your pores.

7 Stay quietly with your cleared, healed body and mind for a few minutes. Take in three slow and deep breaths, before slowly opening your eyes.

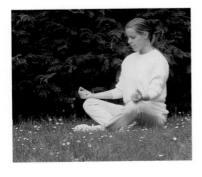

◄ MEDITATE OUT OF DOORS TO RECEIVE THE CALM OF GREEN.

Intuiting colour

You can use colour as a means of tapping into your intuition and developing your psychic ability. This is a sensitivity everyone has, and you can access it simply by making yourself available and clear of mind.

DOWSING WITH CRYSTALS

Use a crystal pendulum. Hold the chain between your first finger and thumb, with the crystal over the palm of your other hand. Direct a question to the stationary pendulum. If it swings round to the right the answer is "yes". Swinging to the left means "no". If it swings backwards and forwards the answer is inconclusive.

You can use crystals of different colours for different questions. For instance, if you are asking about relationships, use turquoise; for business and finance, use green.

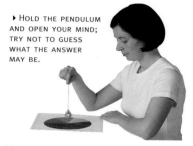

▸ HOLD THE PENDULUM AND OPEN YOUR MIND; TRY NOT TO GUESS WHAT THE ANSWER MAY BE.

USING A COLOUR WHEEL

Draw a circle on white paper and divide it into as many coloured sections as you wish. Hold a pendulum in the centre of the wheel and ask a question. Allow the pendulum to swing towards whichever colour it wants, to give you psychic colour clues. Refer to the profile of your chosen colour to analyse the information.

Remember that any intuitive process can give only indications as to the correct path you need to take. The art is in the interpretation. Monitor your findings – you will be surprised at how many of them materialize.

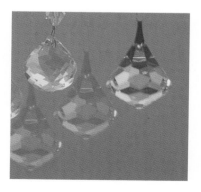

◂ DOWSING IS A MEANS OF TAPPING INTO YOUR PSYCHIC ABILITY.

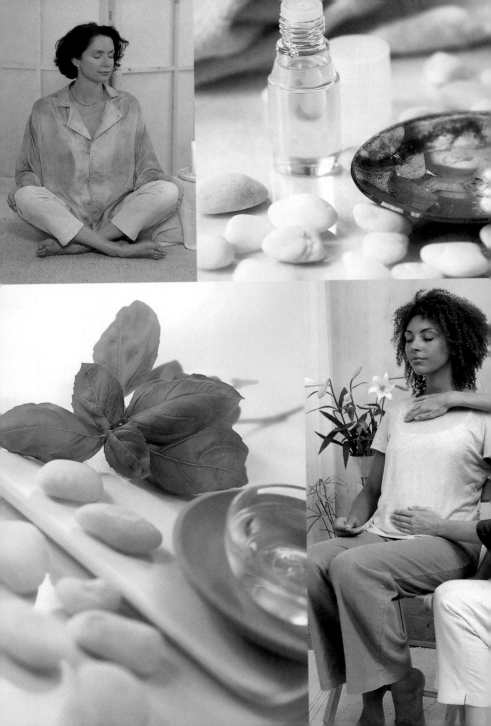

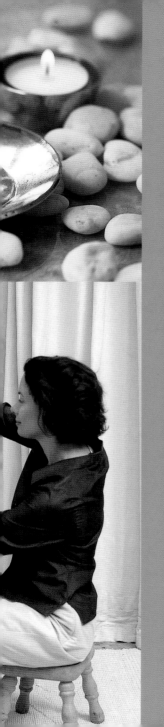

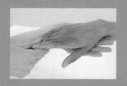

HEALING
HANDS

Since the earliest times, our hands have been a means of caring, comfort and giving. "Rubbing it better" is our natural response to a child's bumps and bruises and we respond to emotional pain with a hug or caress. Out of this basic instinct, healing traditions all over the world have developed their own unique methodologies, using the power of touch to relieve pain and stimulate the body's self-healing mechanisms.

The following chapter introduces four key hands-on therapies drawn from the East and West: massage, shiatsu, reflexology and reiki. With practice it is easy to include these disciplines in everyday life, using one-to-one contact to help us cope with the pressures of modern living, and to treat minor ailments the drug-free way.

The power of touch

We all need to be touched in some way. Touch is a basic human instinct with the power to comfort and reassure on many levels. It can relax the body, calm the mind and encourage healing and emotional well-being.

A NATURAL IMPULSE

The desire to touch and be touched is one of our most instinctive needs. The sense of touch is the first to develop in the embryo, and babies thrive on close physical contact with their mothers. The caring, loving touch of another is fundamental to the development of a healthy human being. This need to be touched does not stop with the end of childhood, yet as adults many of us have become afraid to reach out and touch one another. Mistrustful of our natural loving impulse, we have lost touch with

▼ YOUR BABY WILL ENJOY BEING MASSAGED AND STROKED BY YOU.

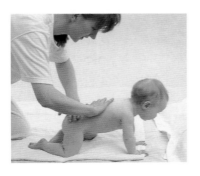

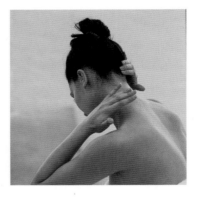

▲ WHEREVER WE FEEL PAIN OR TENSION, IT IS OUR INSTINCT TO TOUCH THE AREA.

ourselves and with the wisdom of the body. The beauty of practising therapeutic touch techniques is that we can begin to re-establish contact with ourselves – and others – in a way that is safe, caring and non-intrusive.

OUR SKIN

The skin is the body's largest sensory organ. By touching the skin, receptors in the dermis (the skin's second layer) react to the external stimulus and send messages through the nervous system to the

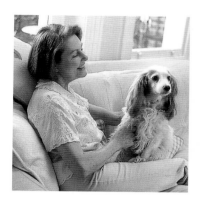

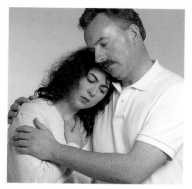

▲ PETS ENJOY A SOOTHING TOUCH JUST AS MUCH AS WE ENJOY GIVING IT.

▲ IF SOMEONE CLOSE TO US IS UPSET OUR NATURAL INSTINCT IS TO GIVE THEM A HUG.

brain. A gentle stroking technique can trigger the release of endorphins, the body's natural painkillers, and induce feelings of comfort and well-being. More vigorous touching techniques get to work on the underlying muscular structure of the body, stretching tense and uncomfortable muscles and easing stiffness in the joints.

BENEFITS OF TOUCH

Awareness of the therapeutic value of touch is growing and many touch-therapies are widely used in conventional healthcare to treat pain, ease discomfort and to improve the functional workings of the body. Given the pressures of modern-day living and the increased incidence of stress-related illness, touch therapies also have an important part to play in every-day life. Aching backs and shoulders after a tiring day at work hunched over a computer or stood on your feet, strained leg muscles after excessive exercise, or circulatory problems from a sedentary lifestyle are some of the occupational hazards of adult life. Through the healing power of touch we can learn to take care of ourselves better. Taking the time to channel healing energy or enjoy a soothing foot massage can ease some of the day-to-day tensions of life and put us back in touch with ourselves and our priorities, to feel relaxed and at home in our bodies.

Massage

Widely recognized as an effective method of holistic health care, massage is one of the oldest therapies in the world. It is based on manipulating the body's soft tissues with a few simple techniques.

HISTORY

For thousands of years some form of massage has been used to heal and soothe the sick. In ancient Greek and Roman times, massage was one of the principal methods of pain relief – Julius Caesar allegedly had daily treatments to ease his headaches and neuralgia. In the West, it seems to have

▼ REGULAR MASSAGE HELPS TO MAINTAIN THE COLLAGEN FIBRES, WHICH GIVE SKIN ITS ELASTICITY AND STRENGTH AND KEEP WRINKLES AT BAY.

played a vital role in health care until the Middle Ages, when it fell out of favour with the Catholic Church which regarded such contact as sinful. Its healing powers were rediscovered at the end of the 19th century by Professor Per Henrik Ling, a Swedish gymnast. Ling's methods formed the basis of modern massage – often referred to as Swedish massage. Support for this gentle, non-intrusive treatment has been growing ever since.

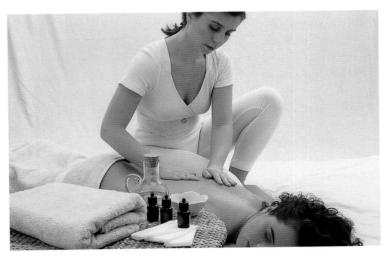

Healing powers

Massage is primarily about touch. When used with skill and care, it can evoke many beneficial changes within the body, mind and spirit. Massage can ease pain and tension from stiff and aching muscles, boost a sluggish circulation, improve the health and appearance of the skin, help the body to eliminate toxins, support the immune system, encourage cellular renewal and aid digestion. As tense muscles relax, stiff joints loosen and nerves are soothed, inducing an all-over feeling of relaxation and well-being. Receiving a massage is a nourishing and calming experience that can increase self-confidence and self-esteem.

Applications

As a therapy, massage can help strains and sprains to heal more rapidly after injury and is generally useful for treating muscle and joint disorders such as arthritis and back pain. However, massage is probably most widely used in the treatment of stress-related disorders. If you are constantly exposed to the adverse effects of stress, it can lead to problems such as anxiety, depression, lethargy, insomnia, frequent tension headaches, hypertension, breathing problems and digestive disorders, to name a few. While not a cure for specific complaints, the nurturing touch of another's hands helps soothe away mental stress and restores emotional equilibrium. There is also evidence to show that a massage treatment reduces the amount of stress hormones produced by the body, which can weaken the immune system. So, having a massage will help prevent as well as cure ill health.

▼ Everyone can benefit from the nurturing power of touch.

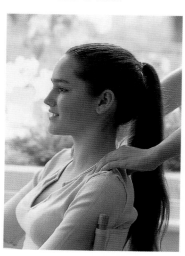

Choosing massage oils

It is usual to work with oils when giving massage. The oil helps the hands to flow and glide over the body and it also lubricates the skin. There are many different types of oil to choose from.

Vegetable oils

Probably the most popular and versatile massage oil is sweet almond. It is light, non-greasy and easily absorbed by the skin. Its neutral and non-allergenic properties make it suitable for all skin types – it may even be used on babies. Grapeseed oil seems to suit oily skins quite well, or soya oil is a useful alternative. Nut and seed oils are generally too rich and sticky to use on their own, but may be added to a lighter oil, such as almond, to create a mixture suitable for an individual skin type.

Essential oils

Fragrant essential oils have particular therapeutic properties, working on the mind and emotions as well as the physical body. They should never be used neat on the skin, but a few drops may be added to the

▼ Mix 5 drops of essential oil in 10ml/ 2 tsp carrier oil for a body massage.

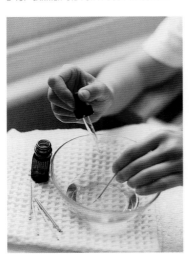

Nut & seed oils and their uses

- Walnut: balances the nervous system; helpful for menstrual problems.
- Sesame: for treating stretch marks.
- Apricot kernel/peachnut/ evening primrose: all promote cellular regeneration; useful for facial massage.
- Hazelnut: for oily skin.
- Jojoba: for oily and sensitive skin; helpful for acne.
- Wheatgerm or avocado: for very dry skin.

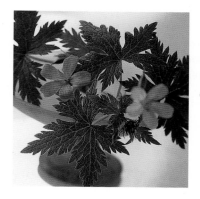

▲ A MASSAGE WITH GERANIUM OIL CAN HELP RELIEVE MOODINESS.

vegetable oil base mix (the "carrier"). You may blend up to three oils in any one treatment. Remember that essential oils are highly concentrated medicinal substances and should be handled with care. If in doubt, do not use them, and if any skin irritation occurs, wash the oil off with soap and warm water.

▼ ROSEMARY IS STIMULATING. IT CAN HELP RELIEVE DEPRESSION AND CLEAR THE MIND.

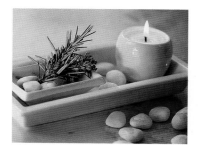

THE PROPERTIES AND USES OF ESSENTIAL PLANT OILS

- Basil: useful as a massage for regulating the nervous system. It is a good tonic and stimulant, and helpful for muscle cramp.
- Camomile: relaxing; useful for tension headaches, inflamed skin conditions, menstrual problems and insomnia.
- Geranium: refreshing, anti-depressant; useful in blends; good for nervous tension and exhaustion.
- Juniper: uplifting, warming; primary use as a detoxifier, useful for treating cellulite. Avoid in pregnancy and if you suffer from kidney disease.
- Lavender: balancing, refreshing; one of the safest and most versatile of all essential oils; useful for tension headaches, stress and insomnia.
- Orange: refreshing, sedative; a tonic for anxiety and depression; useful for digestive problems.
- Rose: sedating, calming, anti-inflammatory, aphrodisiac; useful for muscular and nervous tension, dry, mature and aging skins.
- Rosemary: stimulating; useful for mental fatigue and debility. Avoid in pregnancy and with epilepsy.

choosing massage oils **465**

Preparing for massage

Giving and receiving massage is a relaxing and enjoyable experience. It is important to work in a supportive environment – one that is warm, quiet and draught-free – and to choose a time when you won't be disturbed.

FIRST STEPS

Begin by gathering together all the necessary equipment and materials. This will include massage oils, a selection of clean, soft towels, tissues and perhaps some candles and soft music to set the mood. Make sure the massage area is firm but comfortable; the floor or a futon padded with a thick layer of towels is fine, but an ordinary mattress is generally too soft and springy. It is best to wear comfortable loose-fitting clothes, to take off any jewellery and to make sure your nails are short. Do a few

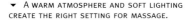

▲ A MASSAGE IS A RELAXING EXPERIENCE FOR THE RECIPIENT.

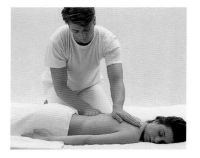

stretches and take some deep breaths to calm and centre yourself; giving a massage when you feel tense is counter-productive.

MAKING CONTACT

The initial contact is a key moment in massage. Gently place one hand on the top of the spine and the other near the base. When using oil, pour it on to your own hands first to warm it, never directly on to your partner's skin as cold oil can cause a shock and undo the relaxing effect. Using smooth, flowing strokes, spread the oil on to the skin then begin the massage.

▼ A WARM ATMOSPHERE AND SOFT LIGHTING CREATE THE RIGHT SETTING FOR MASSAGE.

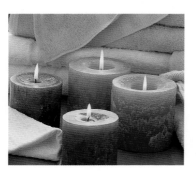

Massage strokes

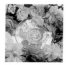

Massage techniques are relatively simple to learn. They range from a gentle, stroking action that relaxes the body to a more vigorous kneading, pummelling or hacking motion to stimulate and energize the system.

CIRCLING

This massage movement is useful for moving over large areas of muscle. The action releases areas of tension held in the muscles before deeper, stronger massage is used.

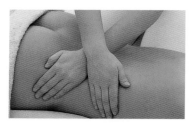

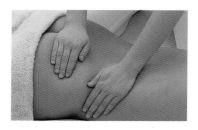

1 Lay both hands flat and parallel to each other about 10cm/4in apart. Circle both hands clockwise.

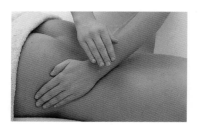

2 Lift up the right hand as it completes the first half-circle. Let the left hand pass underneath.

3 As the left hand continues to circle over the body, cross the right hand over it, dropping it lightly on the skin. Let the right hand form another half-circle before lifting off as the left hand completes its full circle. Repeat several times.

EFFLEURAGE

This technique describes long, soothing, stroking movements, using the flat of the hand (or fingers if you are working on small areas). These strokes are used at the beginning and end of the massage. They are also used in between other more stimulating strokes for continuity, and to establish contact with a new area of the body. They have a calming and reassuring effect and should be done slowly and gently.

PETRISSAGE

Kneading or petrissage movements stimulate the circulation and encourage the drainage of toxins. Generally, a single group of muscles or an individual muscle is worked on at a time. The basic kneading action is similar to kneading dough. Wringing movements also have a similar effect.

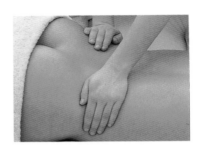

1 Place your right hand over the hip opposite to you and cup your left hand over the hip closest to you. Slide your hands towards each other with enough pressure to lift and roll the flesh on the sides of the body.

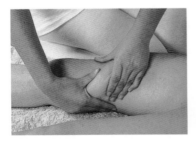

1 Grasp the flesh between fingers and thumb and push it towards the other hand. As you release the first hand, your second hand grasps the flesh and pushes it back towards the first hand. It is a continuous action, alternating the hands to squeeze and release.

WRINGING

Like petrissage, wringing relies on the action of one hand pushing against the other to create a powerful squeezing action.

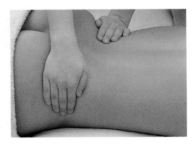

2 Decrease the pressure as you stroke across the back to your original position, hands passing each other to the opposite sides of the body. Without stopping, immediately begin to slide them back. Stroke your hands back and forth continuously while you wring up and down the lower back area.

FRICTION

Use friction techniques, such as pressure and knuckling, to work on specific areas of tightness and muscle spasm. Pressure techniques are less painful when performed along the direction of the muscle fibres.

1 To apply static pressure, press firmly into the muscle with the thumbs. Lean into the movement with the body, slowly deepening the pressure and then release.

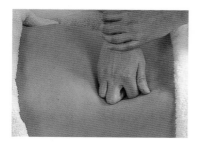

2 To release tension up the sides of the spine, use the knuckles in a loosely clenched fist on either side of the spine to produce rippling, circular movements.

CAUTION
Do not use tapotement on bony areas of the body. Never apply pressure on or below broken or varicose veins.

TAPOTEMENT

These movements are fast and stimulating, improving the circulation, and toning the skin and muscles. They are useful for working on fleshy areas of the body. Remember to keep your hands and wrists relaxed.

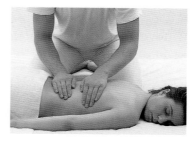

1 Cup the hands and make a brisk cupping action against a fleshy area, alternating the hands.

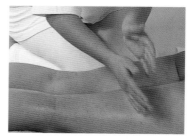

2 Use the outer edge of the palm and a chopping or hacking motion with alternate hands. Work rhythmically and rapidly.

Shiatsu

The word shiatsu means "finger pressure" in Japanese. It is a method of holistic healing that is based on applying pressure to key points on the body. Unlike most other forms of bodywork, you remain fully clothed during treatment.

HISTORY

Shiatsu was developed in Japan in the early 20th century and has its roots in Traditional Chinese Medicine (TCM). A basic idea in TCM is the concept of the life force, known as "chi" in Chinese and "ki" in Japanese. The life force is the fundamental essence or spirit of life. Invisible like the air that we breathe, it is the energy that animates and nourishes all living things. Ki flows through the human body, circulating through the cells, tissues, muscles and internal organs, and influencing health and well-being on a physical, mental and emotional level.

YIN AND YANG

This energetic life force or ki is recognized as having two polar, yet complementary, opposites called yin and yang.

◀ THE SYMBOL OF YIN YANG REPRESENTS BALANCING OPPOSITES.

Each of these represents different qualities: yin is feminine and passive, yang is masculine and active. The aim of shiatsu is to bring a harmony between the yin and yang energies of the body and its internal organs. This harmony can be disturbed through external trauma such as shock, or injury, or internal trauma such as depression or anxiety. This is when symptoms like aches and pains start to occur and

▼ BACKACHE IS JUST ONE OF MANY COMPLAINTS THAT CAN BE EASED WITH SHIATSU.

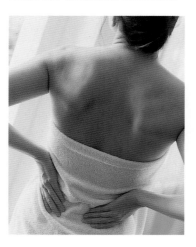

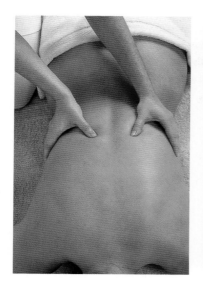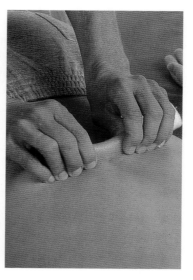

we start to experience a state of "dis-ease". In shiatsu, physical touch is used to assess the distribution of ki throughout the body and aims to correct any imbalances. This is done by applying pressure to specific points on the body where ki is concentrated, helping to release energy blocks and triggering the self-healing process.

BENEFITS

Shiatsu is particularly helpful for stress-related conditions, such as insomnia, tension headaches and digestive upsets, where the gentle, caring touch of another can help the

▲ ABOVE AND LEFT TOUCH IS THE ESSENCE OF SHIATSU. A SHIATSU TREATMENT CAN CALM THE NERVOUS SYSTEM, STIMULATE THE CIRCULATION AND BOOST THE IMMUNE SYSTEM.

body to relax and unwind. It is also useful for improving the circulation and easing out stiffness in the muscles and joints. This makes it useful for treating conditions such as back pain, arthritis or asthma for instance. However, you do not need to be ill to enjoy the benefits of shiatsu. It works very well as a preventive system of health care; it helps to keep the energy flowing freely in the body and has a balancing effect on the body, mind and spirit.

The meridians

Vital energy "ki" flows through the body along invisible energy pathways, or meridians. These meridians connect all the different parts of the body together and for good health it is essential that this energy can flow freely along them.

BALANCE AND HEALTH

Rather like the veins and arteries of the physical body, the meridians conduct ki, the invisible "blood" of life, to and from the body's cells and organs, bringing nourishment while taking away poisons. If a meridian is blocked, it means that one part of the body is getting too much ki and enters a state of excess, or "jitsu", while another part is getting too little and becomes deficient, or "kyo". The system or organ of the body connected to this meridian is then thrown out of balance and begins to produce symptoms of "dis-ease".

Shiatsu recognizes that any symptoms, however small and insignificant they may appear, are a sign that the energy within the meridian system is out of balance. It is therefore important to deal with minor symptoms, as they may be an early warning of a more serious health condition that could develop if they go unchecked, or may develop into a health problem.

TSUBO

Along the meridians are highly charged energy points, known as "tsubo" in Japanese, or pressure points in English. By using different shiatsu techniques on these

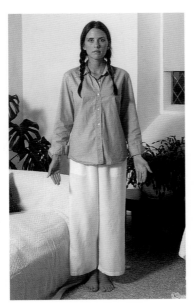

◀ THE MERIDIANS ARE ENERGY LINES RUNNING THROUGH THE BODY. THEY ARE NOT VISIBLE TO THE EYE AND WILL NOT SHOW UP ON AN X-RAY.

points, such as pressure or stretching for instance, you can help to release any blocked ki and encourage the meridian to "open". This will allow excess ki to disperse or provide a boost where it is stagnant or depleted.

THE HARA

Ki enters the body through the breath, circulates through the meridians and is stored in the abdomen or "hara", at a special point approximately three finger-widths below the navel. This is the body's centre of gravity and the seat of vital energy. The level of energy in the hara can be used to diagnose and treat problems in all of the meridian lines.

THE TWELVE ORGANS

There are 12 main meridians, each of which is linked to an "organ" of the body. All the meridians either start or end in the hands or the feet and connect internally to the organ whose condition they reflect.

In shiatsu the organs of the body are perceived in a broader and less literal sense than in conventional thought. In Traditional Chinese Medicine (TCM), the body is seen as a kingdom with each organ having a governing role, an "official" responsible for different functions. When the officials work together and co-operate there is peace and harmony in the land (body). If there is disagreement or disorganization between the different officials, imbalances start to occur.

LUNG

Official function: jurisdiction.

Responsible for: the intake of ki from the environment and the total

LUNG
HEART
HEART GOVERNOR
HEART

SMALL INTESTINE
TRIPLE HEATER
LARGE INTESTINE

KIDNEY
LIVER
SPLEEN

elimination of stagnant ki through exhalation.

Qualities: openness, positivity.

LARGE INTESTINE

Official function: elimination and exchange.

Responsible for: supporting the function of the lungs; the elimination of waste products from food, drink and stagnated ki.

Qualities: the ability to let go of clutter.

SPLEEN

Official function: storage.

Responsible for: general digestion of food and liquid; the flow of gastric juices and reproductive hormones; transformation and nourishment of the body.

Qualities: self-assurance and self-confidence.

STOMACH

Official function: in charge of the body's food store.

Responsible for: receiving and processing ingested food and drink; providing information for mental and physical nourishment.

Qualities: grounded, focused and reliable personality.

HEART

Official function: prime minister.

Responsible for: the blood and blood vessels; integrates external stimuli. The heart is the seat of the mind and emotions.

Qualities: joy, awareness and communication.

SMALL INTESTINE

Official function: treasurer.

Responsible for: converting food into energy; the quality of the blood and tissue reflects the condition of the small intestine.

Qualities: emotional stability, calm.

HEART GOVERNOR
HEART
LUNG

SMALL INTESTINE
TRIPLE HEATER
LARGE INTESTINE

LIVER
SPLEEN
KIDNEY

KIDNEY

Official function: energetic worker.
Responsible for: providing and storing ki for all other organs; governs reproduction, birth, growth and development; nourishes the spine, the bones and the brain.
Qualities: vitality, direction and willpower.

BLADDER

Official function: storage of overflow and fluid secretions.
Responsible for: purification and regulation.
Qualities: courage and the ability to move forward in life.

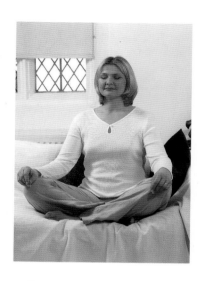

▲ TO EFFECTIVELY GIVE A HEALING TREATMENT YOU SHOULD FEEL CENTRED AND COMFORTABLE AND ATTUNED TO THE WORK IN HAND.

HEART GOVERNOR

Official function: joy and pleasure.
Responsible for: protecting the heart; is closely related to emotional responses.
Qualities: ability to influence relationships with others.

TRIPLE HEATER

Official function: plans construction.
Responsible for: transportation of energy, blood and heat to the peripheral parts of the body.
Qualities: helpful and emotionally interactive.

LIVER

Official function: planning.
Responsible for: storage of blood; ensures free flow of ki throughout the body.
Qualities: creative and full of ideas.

GALL BLADDER

Official function: decision making.
Responsible for: storing bile produced by the liver and distributing it to the small intestine.
Qualities: practical; ability to turn ideas into reality.

Basic shiatsu techniques

 Shiatsu uses the hands, elbows, knees and feet to apply pressure on specific meridian points. It can also incorporate passive stretching movements to help to loosen the body, manipulate the joints and ease tension.

FIRM PRESSURE

When giving a shiatsu treatment, focus on your breathing and posture. All movement should emanate from the hara (abdomen); this brings a calm, meditative quality to the mind and will be relayed through your healing touch. When applying pressure, lean on the appropriate point for up to 10 seconds before slowly releasing the pressure.

THUMB PRESSURE

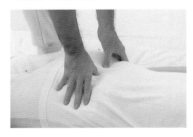

The bladder meridian is the largest and runs down each side of the spine to the sacrum (the triangular bone forming the back of the pelvis). A steady thumb pressure applied on the sacral points can relieve sciatica and lower-back pain.

PALM PRESSURE

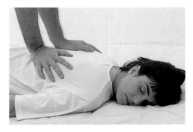

Relax and open out the hands. Shift your weight into the palms and heels of the hands to press firmly but gently along the bladder meridian points.

STRETCHING

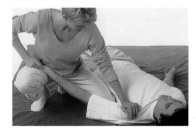

Gentle stretches along the meridians help the body. The practitioner opens the chest by gently stretching the lung meridian in the arm.

Do-in

This self-massage technique is designed to improve the circulation and flow of ki through the body. It will wake up your brain and aid concentration and mental clarity.

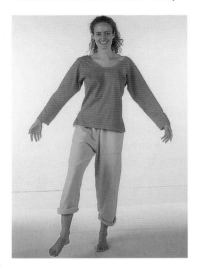

1 Shake your arms, hands, legs and feet, letting go of tension. Breathe deeply, keeping your back straight.

CAUTION
Seek the advice of a qualified practitioner if you suffer from high blood pressure, varicose veins, osteoporosis, thrombosis, epilepsy, if you are pregnant, or suffer from serious illnesses.

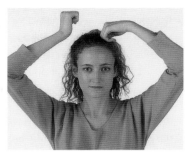

2 Make a loose fist with both hands. Keep your wrists relaxed and gently tap the top of your head with your fingers or knuckles. Adjust the pressure as needed and use your fingertips or palms for lighter stimulation. Work your way all around the head, covering the sides, front and back.

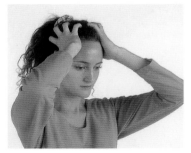

3 Finish by pulling your fingers through your hair a few times. This stimulates the bladder and gall bladder meridians that run across the top and side of your head.

Reflexology

The word "reflex" means to reflect. In reflexology, specific points on the hands or feet reflect another part of the body. By working on these points you can treat health problems elsewhere in the body-mind system.

HISTORY

Foot and hand treatments have been used in healing traditions across the world for thousands of years, but reflexology in its present form is a relatively recent discovery. In the early 20th century, an American doctor, William Fitzgerald, found that applying pressure to points on the hands or feet could help to relieve pain elsewhere in the body. Eunice Ingham, a physiotherapist, went on to map out these pressure points or reflex

▼ REFLEXOLOGY CAN BE PRACTISED ANYWHERE FOR RELAXATION AND HEALTH.

zones, matching up areas of the body with specific points on the feet and hands. Later, people discovered that these points also relate to certain emotional and psychological states.

BALANCING THE BODY

Reflexology is based on two important principles: that small parts of the body can be used to treat the whole, and that the body has the ability to heal itself. As a result of illness, stress or injury, the body's systems are thrown out of balance and its vital energy path-

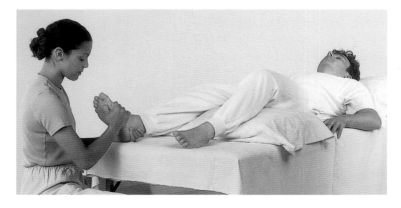

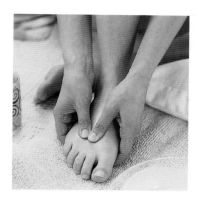

▲ You can practise the healing effects of reflexology on yourself.

ways are blocked. Messages between the brain and nervous system become distorted and the body begins to produce distress signals or symptoms in its call for help. These symptoms of "dis-ease" will show up in various ways (such as headaches or mood swings for instance) and toxic waste matter accumulates around the relevant reflex points. Places on the feet where there are toxic deposits will feel tender, sensitive or painful; or they may feel hard, tight or lumpy, or like little grains. Stimulating these points with massage helps the congestion to disperse and frees up energy blocks elsewhere in the system, encouraging the body to rebalance.

Treatment

Reflexology is becoming widely recognized as an effective treatment for many health problems. It works well for any condition involving congestion and/or inflammation, such as sinus problems, digestive disturbances, menstrual problems or eczema. It is also an effective method of pain relief and is useful for treating back pain, rheumatism, arthritis or headaches, for instance. A reflexology treatment is relaxing, making it popular for treating stress-related disorders, calming anxiety, alleviating tension and encouraging restful sleep. Many people enjoy reflexology because of its "feel good" factor.

▼ Reflexologists regard the feet as a map of the whole body.

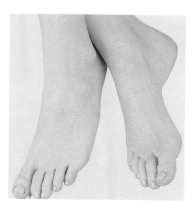

Reflex zones

In reflexology the fingers are used to apply pressure-point therapy to certain key points on the feet and/or hands. These points, known as reflex zones, are linked to the body's internal organs and systems and its external structure.

ENERGY CHANNELS

The body is divided into ten vertical energy zones that run from the head to reflex points on the hands and feet, five on the left, five on the right. These zones are similar to the meridians used in shiatsu. All parts of the body that fall into a particular zone are linked by nerve pathways and mirrored in a corresponding reflex point on the hands or feet.

If there is any imbalance within a zone, the body can produce a range of symptoms that relate to several different body parts that all fall within that zone. Problems with the eyes for instance may indicate an underlying problem with the kidneys. A reflexology treatment, therefore, would not only work on the reflex point related to the eyes, but would also treat the kidneys and any other relevant parts of the body in zone two.

CROSS REFLEXES

Reflexology also works with cross reflexes. Parts of the upper body correspond to parts of the lower body, so that the arms correspond to the legs (the elbows with the knees, the wrists with the ankles), the hips with the shoulders and the hands with the feet. This is useful when an area of the body is too painful to work on directly; for instance, to treat a dislocated right shoulder you can work on the reflex for the right hip.

ZONES ON THE FEET

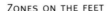

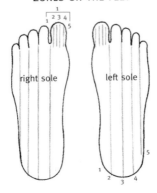

right sole   left sole

◀ LOOKING AT THE SOLES OF THE FEET, THE RIGHT SIDE OF YOUR BODY IS REPRESENTED BY YOUR RIGHT FOOT AND THE LEFT SIDE BY YOUR LEFT FOOT.

Zones on the body

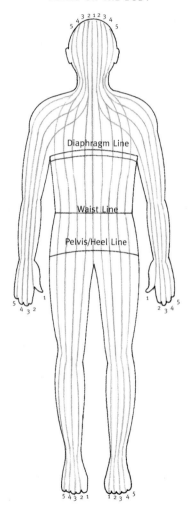

Diaphragm Line

Waist Line

Pelvis/Heel Line

▲ THE ZONES RUN VERTICALLY THROUGH THE BODY FROM HEAD TO FEET AND HANDS.

Parts of the body

Both feet together hold the reflexes to the whole body. It can be helpful to divide the body into different areas, tying these in with the relevant zones of the feet. Working from head to foot:

• The head and neck are represented by the toes: the right side of the head with the right big toe, and the left side with the left big toe. The eight little toes represent specific parts of the head, such as eyes, ears, mouth and so on. The kidneys and the eyes are both linked by the energy in zone two.

• The lungs, chest and shoulder areas are represented by the balls of the feet.

• The abdomen is represented by the area from the balls of the feet to the middle of the arch.

• The pelvic area is represented by the soles and sides of the heels and across the top of the ankle.

• The spine is represented by the line that runs along the inner edge of the feet.

• The limbs are represented on the outer edge of the feet, working from the toes to the heels are the arms, shoulders, hips, legs, knees and lower back.

A mirror of the body

The feet are believed to mirror the shape of the body, with the organs and body parts appearing in roughly the same position as they occur in the body. Each foot represents the left- and right-hand side of the body.

FOOT CHARTS

When you find a tender or congested part of the foot, you may look for that part on the charts and see approximately which reflex the tenderness lies on. However, picking out certain reflexes in isolation is only really effective in the context of working on the whole foot. Remember also that the charts are only guidelines for interpretation. Every pair of feet will be different and in reality your organs overlap each other, so everything will not "fit" neatly in exactly the same area as shown on the chart.

THE SPINE

Both feet together hold the reflexes to the whole body. The part that holds the spine therefore runs down the medial line along the inner edge of each foot. The spinal reflex is particularly important. It should always be massaged and the reflex worked thoroughly. The spinal column is not only our main bony support, but it also contains

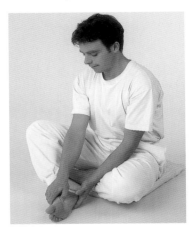

▲ YOU CAN TREAT YOUR OWN AILMENTS WITH REFLEXOLOGY.

the spinal cord, the central energy channel that transmits messages to and from the brain through the central nervous system.

PEDI-CURE

There are more than 70,000 nerve endings on the sole of each foot. By stimulating specific points on the feet, information is transmitted via the nervous system to the brain and a healing process is triggered.

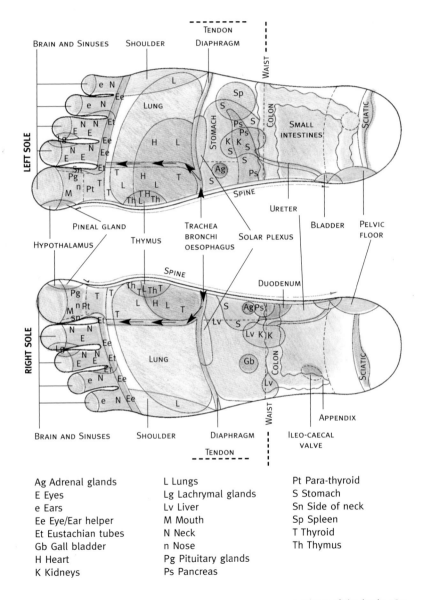

Ag Adrenal glands	L Lungs	Pt Para-thyroid
E Eyes	Lg Lachrymal glands	S Stomach
e Ears	Lv Liver	Sn Side of neck
Ee Eye/Ear helper	M Mouth	Sp Spleen
Et Eustachian tubes	N Neck	T Thyroid
Gb Gall bladder	n Nose	Th Thymus
H Heart	Pg Pituitary glands	
K Kidneys	Ps Pancreas	

Basic reflexology techniques

Applying thumb and/or finger pressure to the reflex points on the feet helps to release congestion and stimulates healing. There are several basic techniques which are simple to learn. The movements should be small and controlled.

HOLDING AND SUPPORT
When you practise any technique, always make sure that the hand or foot you are working on is secure. It will mean your partner will be more relaxed and you can work much more effectively.

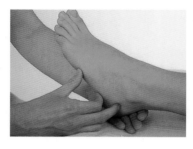

1 Use one hand to hold the foot and the other to work on it. Position your holding hand near the working hand, not at the other end of the foot as this can feel insecure.

THUMB WALKING
This is the most common method and a useful technique to use all over the foot. It is done with the pad of the thumb that "walks" forward in caterpillar-like movements.

Use one hand only, the other holds and supports the foot or hand you are working on.

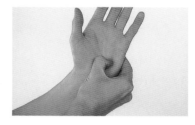

1 Press the thumb of one of your hands down on the skin of the other hand using a firm pressure.

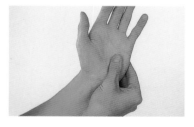

2 Ease off the pressure and slide or skate forward as you straighten your thumb in a caterpillar movement. Stop and press again. Keep your movements slow, continuous and rhythmic.

FINGER WALKING

This technique uses the fingers and is useful for bony areas.

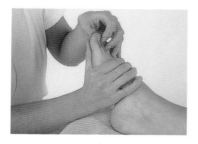

1 Hold the foot or hand with your right hand and fingerwalk from the tip of the big toe with your left index finger.

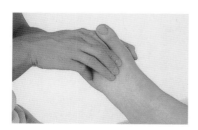

2 Firmly hold the foot or hand with one hand and fingerwalk down the top of the foot towards the toes, using the three middle fingers of the other hand together. This area can be very sensitive so take care not to press too hard with the fingers. Try to keep the pressure firm and even, but comfortable.

ROTATING

This technique is good for tender reflexes, or for when you want to work on a specific small point. Vary the pressure as is comfortable.

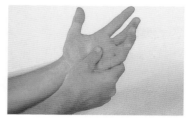

Using a firm pressure, press and rotate the thumb into the point.

PINPOINTING

Use this technique for deep or less accessible reflexes. Restrict it to the fleshy, padded parts of the feet as it can be quite painful.

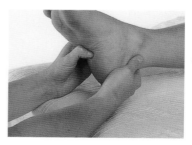

Supporting the heel, press deeply into the tissues with the inner corner of your thumb.

Top and sides of foot

It is not only the soles of the feet that relate to other areas of the body. These diagrams show the areas covered by the tops and sides of the feet. The whole body may be treated on the spinal reflex through the central nervous system.

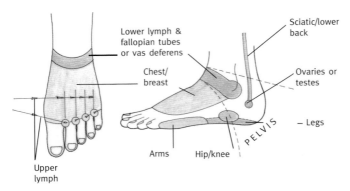

Lower lymph & fallopian tubes or vas deferens

Chest/breast

Sciatic/lower back

Ovaries or testes

— Legs

PELVIS

Arms   Hip/knee

Upper lymph

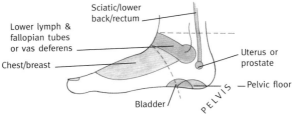

Sciatic/lower back/rectum

Lower lymph & fallopian tubes or vas deferens

Chest/breast

Uterus or prostate

— Pelvic floor

PELVIS

Bladder

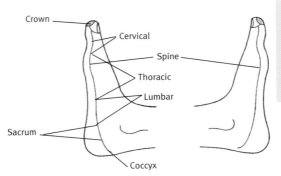

Crown

Cervical

Spine

Thoracic

Lumbar

Sacrum

Coccyx

THE SPINE

The spinal reflex should always be massaged, and worked thoroughly.

Hand charts

The hands reflect all the body, as do the feet. Once you have adjusted to the basic layout, the location of reflexes is quite straightforward. Use the hand reflexes when you cannot work the feet for any reason.

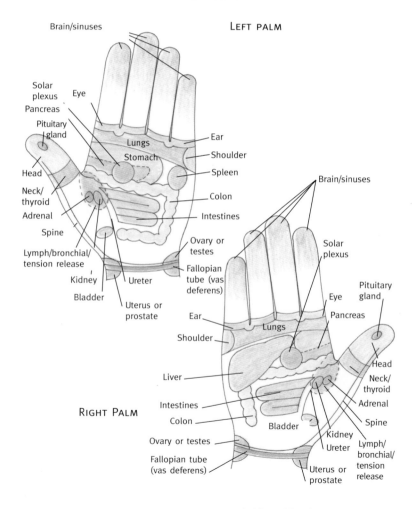

LEFT PALM

Brain/sinuses

Solar plexus
Eye
Pancreas
Pituitary gland
Lungs
Ear
Stomach
Shoulder
Head
Spleen
Neck/ thyroid
Brain/sinuses
Adrenal
Colon
Spine
Intestines
Lymph/bronchial/ tension release
Ovary or testes
Solar plexus
Kidney
Ureter
Fallopian tube (vas deferens)
Pituitary gland
Bladder
Uterus or prostate
Eye
Ear
Pancreas
Shoulder
Lungs
Liver
Head
Neck/ thyroid
RIGHT PALM
Intestines
Adrenal
Colon
Spine
Bladder
Ovary or testes
Kidney
Lymph/ bronchial/ tension release
Fallopian tube (vas deferens)
Ureter
Uterus or prostate

Reiki

Channelling divine or cosmic healing energy through the hands is one of the oldest and most profound methods of healing known. Reiki is a special technique that brings the ability to heal within the grasp of everyone.

History

Reiki (pronounced ray-key) means universal ("rei") life force ("ki") in Japanese. With its roots in Tibetan Buddhism, the ancient healing methods of reiki were rediscovered in the 19th century by Dr Mikao Usui, a Japanese mystic, during a vision. These methods were regarded as sacred knowledge, and the secrets were passed down from master to student in special initiation ceremonies. Today the tradition of master and student continues, and reiki practitioners have been through special "attunements" with a modern-day master to receive this ancient knowledge and open up a healing channel. It is relatively easy to find a reiki master and become a reiki initiate, but it is possible for anyone to channel healing reiki energy by understanding and applying a few basic principles.

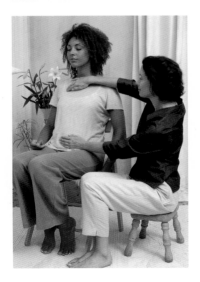

▼ A reiki practitioner channels healing energy through their hands.

Universal law

Reiki is about tuning in to the laws of the universe and working in harmony with them. The universe is a place of boundless energy that flows through space and time, and through everything here on Earth. We are not separate, isolated identities but connected to the universe and everything in it by this cosmic energy, the breath of life that nurtures and sustains us. This energy is sometimes known as the life force and its healing power is love. It is a force for good in the world that transcends time and place, colour and creed, and any negative, destructive impulses that threaten the health and well-being of life. Reiki invites us to open up and trust in this great love, allowing it to flow through us, bringing positive healing wherever it is needed. We can channel this healing energy for the benefit of ourselves and other people, as well as to treat plants, animals and even places.

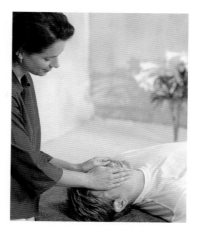

▲ WE CAN ALL BENEFIT FROM REIKI AND EACH OF US CAN CHANNEL REIKI ENERGY.

▼ REIKI CHANNELS THE ESSENTIAL ENERGY OF THE UNIVERSE TO CREATE WELL-BEING.

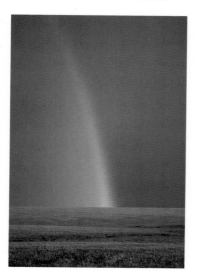

BENEFITS

Giving and receiving reiki is a relaxing experience. It is particularly effective for calming and soothing negative emotional states, for relieving pain and for treating stress-related conditions, such as insomnia, fatigue or tension headaches, for instance. A reiki treatment helps to rebalance the body's energy systems and generally promotes good health and well-being. Done regularly it can help to protect the body against illness and negative influences as it helps to realign the human energy system with the healing vibrations of love and light.

Reiki hand positions

In a reiki treatment, the hands are positioned at various places on the body. In order for the energy flow to be focused, the fingers and thumbs are held together, and the hands kept flat or very slightly cupped.

If you have not been officially attuned to reiki, prepare yourself at a quiet time, when your attention can be fully attuned to yourself. Visualize a stream of golden healing light entering your body through the crown chakra. See yourself as an open and receptive channel for this energy, allowing it to enter and pass through your body via the hands, on to the body of your partner.

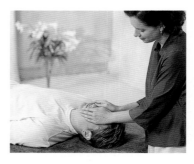

1 Place the hands over the eyes. This position aids clear vision and energizes the eyes.

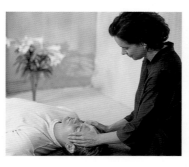

2 Slide the hands sideways on to the temples. This position helps to dispel tension in the face.

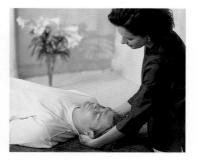

3 Bring your hands round to underneath your partner's head, just above the neck so that you are cradling it. This position balances the energy in both sides of the brain and releases mental tension.

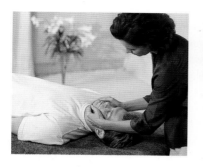

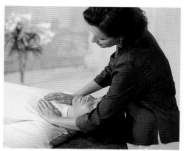

4 Remove your hands and place them with the heels of the palms on the side of the neck and with the palms and fingers lightly on the throat. This can help to release emotional trauma and upset.

5 Slide the hands on to the top of the chest. This position is relaxing and reassuring. Move to one side and continue down the trunk, placing your hands in a straight line across the chakra points.

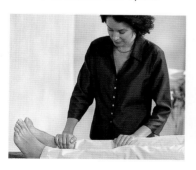

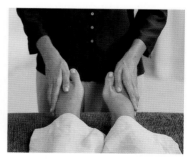

6 Continue working down, first one leg and then the other in as many stages as feels right. Working along the legs and channelling healing energy helps to balance and relax the recipient's lower body.

7 To finish, stand at the foot of your partner and finish by placing the hands on the feet, first the upper feet, then the soles. This helps to "ground" the energy so that your partner doesn't feel too floaty or light-headed at the end of the treatment.

Self-treatment with reiki

It is a good idea to practise reiki on yourself. This will increase your self-confidence when giving treatments to other people, as you will have experienced its healing powers first hand. It will also nourish and refresh you.

REIKI SELF-TREATMENT

You can give reiki to yourself at any time of the day. Some people like to start with it first thing in the morning in preparation for the day ahead. Others find it helpful to end the day with reiki, helping the body to relax and unwind in preparation for sleep. Ideally, it is best to set aside a full hour for a reiki self-treatment, but if this is not possible, 10–15 minutes set aside on a regular basis will bring good results and a healthier outlook.

Either sit in a comfortable upright position or lie down where you won't be disturbed. Set your alarm clock if you have appointments, and unplug the telephone. Close your eyes and centre yourself by breathing gently into the abdomen. Take in a deep breath, hold for a few moments and exhale. Repeat this a few times.

Imagine that golden, healing reiki energy is flowing into your body, circulating along the subtle energy pathways, nourishing every

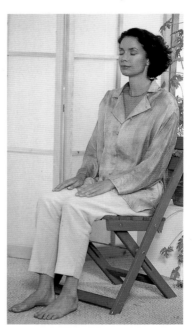

▲ A REIKI SELF-TREATMENT WILL LEAVE YOU FEELING REFRESHED AND READY FOR THE DAY.

cell and organ. Place your hands on any areas of your body that you feel need particular attention. Leave them there for as long as is comfortable. You may notice that the area of your body becomes warm as the energy circulates.

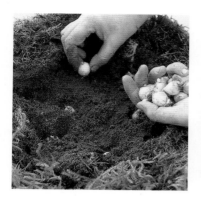

▲ THE FLOWERS, SHRUBS, EVEN BULBS IN YOUR GARDEN WILL BENEFIT FROM REIKI.

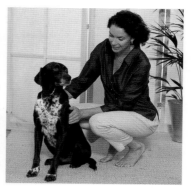

▲ PETS CAN BENEFIT FROM REIKI TOO — USE IT TO MAINTAIN GENERAL HEALTH.

Reiki Anywhere

Remember that there is nothing for your brain to "learn" with reiki. It is a question of being open to its healing powers and willing to let the energy flow through you. Cultivate the reiki habit and bring reiki treatments into other activities. Try relaxing back in a warm bath, and practise the hand positions on your face and torso. Reiki can be worked into a foot massage or a beauty treatment, or if you have a busy day, give yourself reiki as you go along. This can be done while watching television, queuing at the supermarket checkout or sitting in a traffic jam, for instance. Just put your palms anywhere on your body, imagine the healing energy entering you and say to yourself, "Reiki flow!" You will soon feel the benefits.

▼ GREETING THE DAY WITH A SALUTE TO THE SUN: ADDING AN ELEMENT OF RITUAL TO YOUR MORNING ROUTINE WILL CREATE A HAPPY DAY.

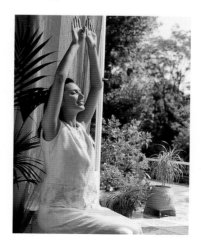

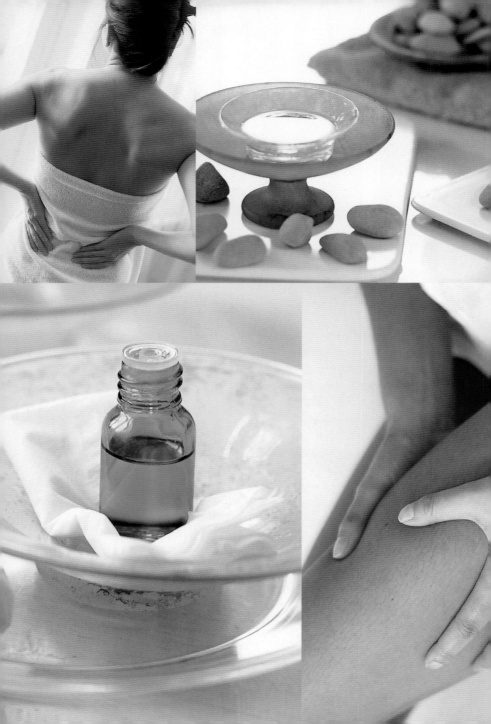

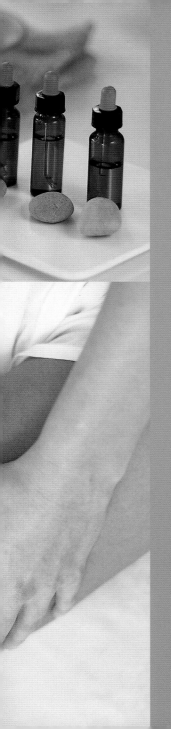

THE HEALING
TOUCH

Many common health problems are related to
stress and lifestyle. When we feel overwhelmed
and unable to cope, the body's fine-tuning is
knocked off balance and things start to go awry.
The body produces a range of annoying and
unpleasant symptoms. Many of these minor
ailments respond well to the healing touch of
massage, reflexology, reiki or shiatsu.

   The following section includes step-by-
step sequences and useful tips on treating a
range of minor complaints. Some of these
moves can be practised on yourself, while
others require a partner. Follow steps to
improve the circulation and digestion, to relieve
stress, tension, fluid retention, aches and pains,
and to enhance the quality of sleep.

Start the day sequence

To make the most of your potential, your bodily systems need to be functioning well as you start the day and to continue to do so throughout the day. The systems and senses can be stimulated with the following sequences.

INVIGORATING THE BODY

This sequence stimulates all your bodily systems, enabling you to make the most of your potential and start the day in the best way.

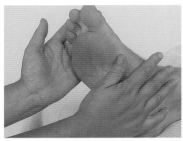

1 Massage the feet to establish good breathing and the instep to stimulate the nervous system.

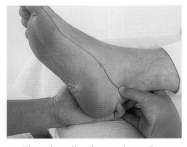

2 Thumbwalk the spine. Rotate the ankles and toes to stimulate circulation and free the nerves.

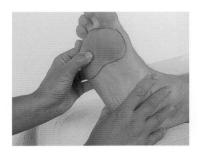

3 Work the diaphragm, and then across the chest to establish deep breathing to strengthen the body.

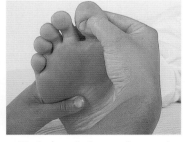

4 Work the pituitary reflex on the big toe in the centre of the toe-print: this is the master gland.

IMPROVING DECISIVENESS

By working the diaphragm, solar plexus and liver you are enhancing good breathing, which improves planning and decision-making.

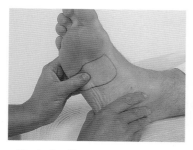

1 Work the liver.

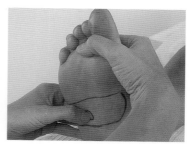

2 Work the gall bladder.

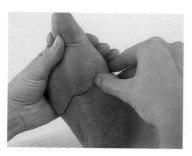

3 Work the diaphragm.

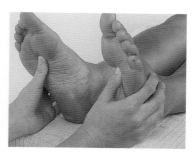

4 Work the solar plexus.

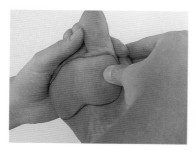

5 Work the lungs.

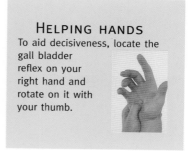

HELPING HANDS

To aid decisiveness, locate the gall bladder reflex on your right hand and rotate on it with your thumb.

Energy boosters

 If energy is flowing freely around your body you will feel well and find it easier to stay positive. Think positively: the power of thought influences physical health and, conversely, your moods are affected by hormonal balance.

ENHANCING ENERGY LEVELS

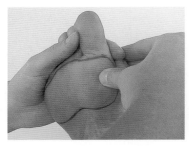

1 Work the lungs to improve your breathing patterns.

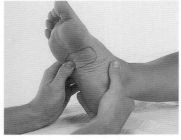

2 Work the liver, which is crucial to your general health.

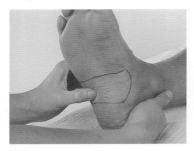

3 Work the small intestines to aid the uptake of nutrients.

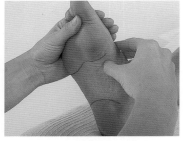

4 Work the whole digestive area. What you eat is turned into your energy during digestion.

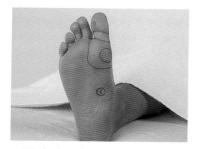

5 Work the glands on the big toe. Rotate the adrenals.

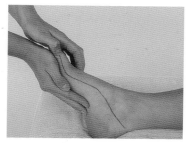

6 Work up and down the spine, your central column of energy flow.

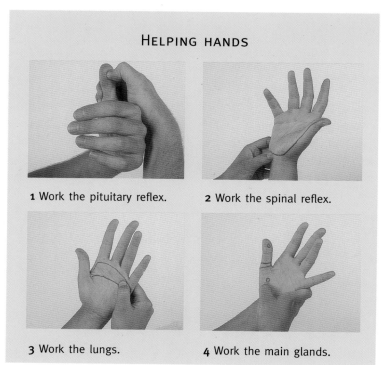

Improving skin, hair and nails

 To keep your skin, hair and nails in good condition you need hormone balance, good nutrition and effective removal of toxins through the excretory system. Stimulation of the circulation will aid the removal of toxins and the supply of nutrients through the bloodstream.

STIMULATING CIRCULATION

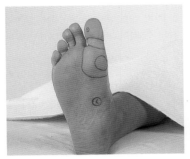

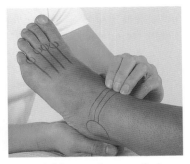

1 Work all the glands on both feet. Your skin, hair and nails are kept in good health by chemicals in your hormones, which are controlled by your glands.

2 In addition, make sure that you give attention to the lymph system on both feet to help remove toxins from the body.

HELPING HANDS

Work all the glands on both of your hands using the chart at the back of the book for easy reference.

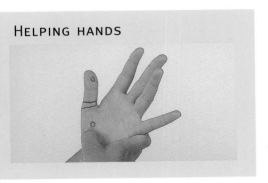

Invigorating the immune system

Where the immune system is strong, the body will deal naturally with threatening infections so that they cannot become established. Within the context of a full reflexology routine, pay particular attention to the liver, spleen and lymph systems.

IMMUNE BOOSTERS

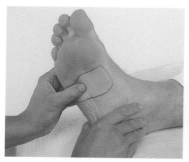

1 Work the liver to strengthen the whole body.

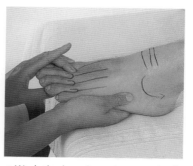

2 Work the lymph systems on both feet to aid the removal of toxins.

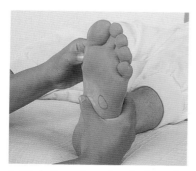

3 Work the spleen (marked on the left foot) and rotate the thymus gland (for both feet) positioned on the ball of the foot.

HELPING HANDS
Work the liver and spleen to strengthen your body, and the thymus gland and lymph system to fight off imminent infection. See the hand chart at the back of the book for the specific areas of the hand relating to these parts of the body.

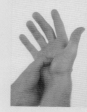

Easing colds, sore throats and sinuses

 Colds, sore throats and sinus problems all affect the respiratory system. To stimulate them to clear themselves of toxins and encourage uptake of nutrients, you need to work all the toes and chest area.

COLDS

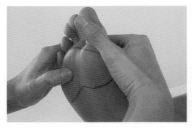

1 Work the entire chest area to encourage clear breathing.

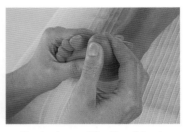

2 Beginning with the big toe, work the tops of all the toes to clear the sinuses. Then pinpoint the pituitary gland in the centre of the prints of both big toes to stimulate the endocrine system.

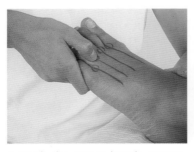

3 Work the upper lymph system to stimulate the immune system.

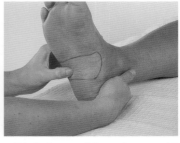

4 Work the small intestines to aid elimination of toxins and uptake of nutrients. Then work the colon to aid elimination. See the chart.

SORE THROATS

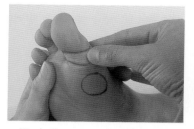

1 Work the upper lymph system, then the throat, and the thymus gland for the immune system.

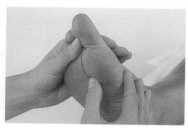

2 Work the trachea and the larynx so as to stimulate them both to clear and heal.

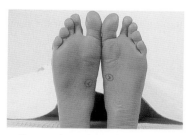

3 Rotate the adrenal reflex in the direction of the arrow.

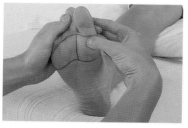

4 Work the thyroid helper in the chest section, then the whole chest area for the respiratory system.

SINUSES

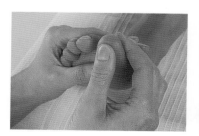

1 Work the sinus reflexes.

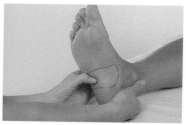

2 Work the ileo-caecal valve.

Backaches

More working days are lost through backache than from any other cause. Common causes of backache include poor posture, injury through straining and lifting, pregnancy, stress and muscular tension.

Back pain can vary from a dull, persistent, nagging ache to a sharp, searing pain. Tightness in the muscles around the spinal cord constricts the body's main energy pathway, affecting the central nervous system. The pain itself is also very draining. The soothing touch of another's hands can be very healing; reflexology and reiki are both helpful.

REFLEXOLOGY RELIEVER
A simple but effective reflexology treatment can help to release tension and relax the supporting muscles. The inside edge of the foot represents the spine.

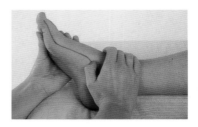

1 Thumbwalk along the spine, supporting the outer edge of the foot.

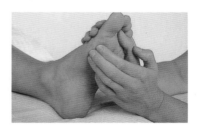

2 Fingerwalk across the spinal reflex, right down the instep, in stripes.

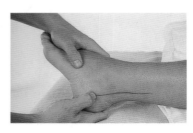

3 Thumbwalk up the helper reflexes.

TIPS FOR AVOIDING BACK PAIN
- Improve your posture; don't slump but sit straight, make sure your chair supports you.
- Take regular, gentle exercise, such as swimming or yoga.
- Invest in a firm mattress.
- Bend from the hips and knees when lifting heavy objects.

A gentle reiki treatment is another way of helping the body to relax. It can also address the underlying emotional and mental state that may be contributing to the problem. For instance, backache is often caused by worrying and feeling burdened. Lower back pain is linked to problems in the first chakra, indicating insecurity in material matters – such as worry about money.

Your partner should be sitting upright on a backless chair, or lying face down on the floor.

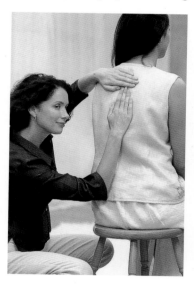

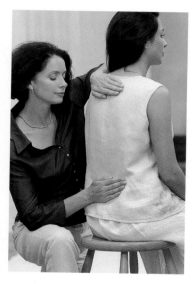

1 Place your hands in the shape of a T-cross between the shoulder blades and down the spine. This position treats the upper back and shoulder areas, stimulating the heart chakra and surrounding organs. Concentrate on the healing energy of your touch.

2 Allow your hands to be drawn to any other areas of the back where healing is needed. Finish by placing your hands at the top and bottom of the spine in the "spirit level" position, to balance the energy along the backbone and through the chakras.

Headaches

The majority of "everyday" headaches are caused by stress and tension. Other common triggers include eyestrain, hangovers, lack of sleep and exercise, caffeine overload, missed meals and hormonal swings.

REFLEXOLOGY FOR HEADACHES

A foot treatment can work wonders on a tension headache. Headaches generally mean there is too much energy in the head and eyes,

caused by excessive worry, mental work or eyestrain for instance. Reflexology can help to release the energy, encouraging it to disperse through the rest of the body.

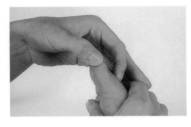

1 For pain relief, work the hypothalamus reflex. This controls the release of endorphins.

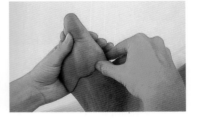

2 Work down the spine to take pressure away from the head. This will draw energy down the body.

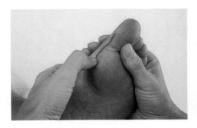

3 Work the cervical spine on the big toe. Work the neck of all the toes to relieve tension.

4 When we are tense our breathing is tight and shallow. Work the diaphragm area to encourage the breathing to become deeper.

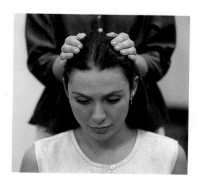

1 Place your hands on each side of the head at the back cupping the skull. This helps to dispel tension rising from the neck and balances energy in the brain.

REIKI HEADACHE SOOTHER
A reiki treatment can help to melt away tensions and restore peace and equilibrium. It is best if your partner sits upright for this treatment, although it can also be done with him or her lying down.

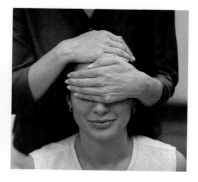

3 Finish by gently placing one hand across the brow, covering the eyes. Place the other hand on top of the head, touching the first hand. Hold the position firmly. This position helps relieve emotional stress and is soothing for the recipient.

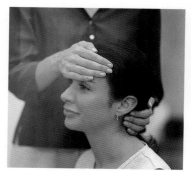

2 Place one hand on the forehead and the other at the base of the skull, cradling the head firmly in your hand.

Muscle pain and cramp

Muscles are the body's connecting tissue; their elasticity enables us to move. Pain in the muscles may result from injury or from overuse. Cramps are painful, involuntary muscle spasms.

MUSCLE RELAXING REFLEXOLOGY
Reflexology can help to reduce inflammation and pain in the muscles and nerve endings. It can also relax muscle spasm. Before concentrating on the specific area of pain, work the hypothalamus reflex first to help with pain relief.

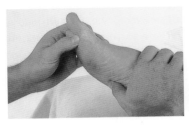

1 Work the adrenal gland reflexes on both feet thoroughly. These glands deal with inflammation and aid good muscle tone when working effectively.

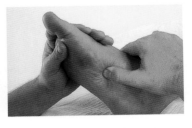

2 Thumbwalk along the spine to treat the central nervous system in the spinal cord.

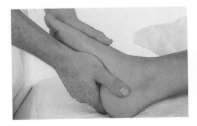

3 To ease cramp, hold the foot and massage the appropriate reflex using the foot chart as a guide.

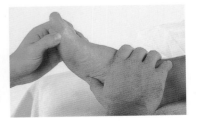

4 Work the parathyroid reflexes round the neck of the big toe.

Massage for calf cramp

Calf cramp can be triggered by exercise, repetitive action or sitting awkwardly. Cramp may indicate poor circulation or a deficiency of calcium or salt. Massage improves the circulation and alleviates pain. It also helps eliminate lactic acid, a waste product stored in the muscle tissue after exercise.

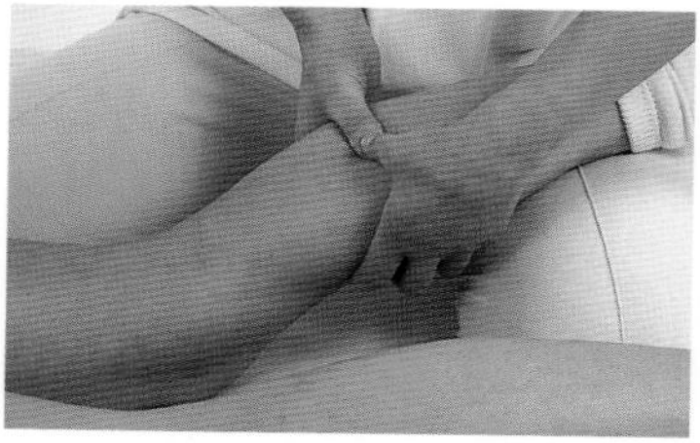

1 Apply thumb pressure into the cramped muscle for 8–10 seconds.

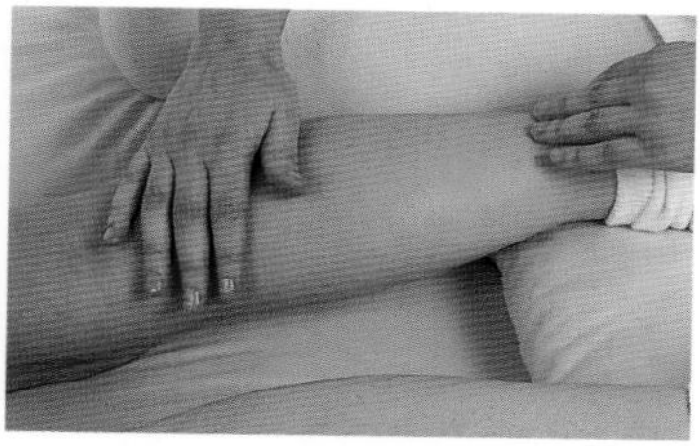

2 Work from the ankle to the thigh using long effleurage strokes.

Hamstring cramp massage

It is usually underused or ill-prepared muscles that go into cramp during exercise.

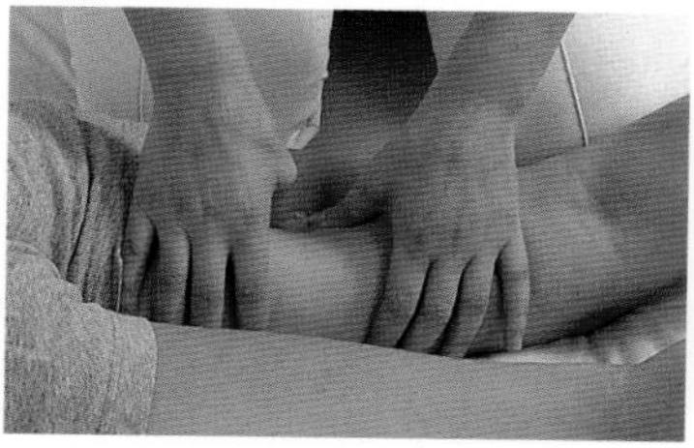

1 Raise the ankle on a small pillow and begin by massaging the back of the thigh using alternate hands in slow, rhythmical stroking movements. Then apply static pressure to the middle of the thigh with the thumbs, holding for 8–10 seconds.

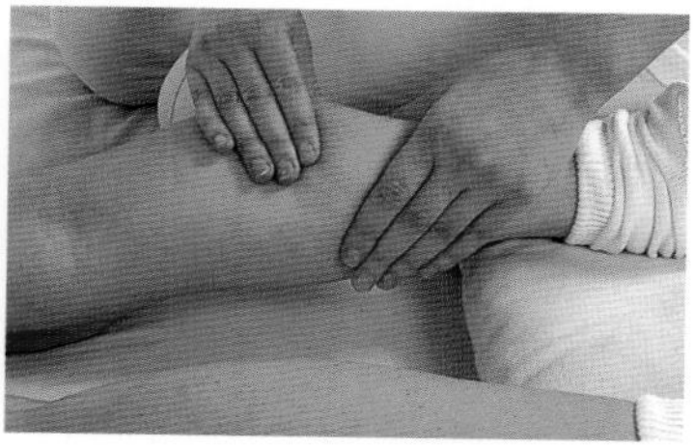

2 Firmly knead the calf muscle. Squeeze, press and release the muscle using one hand after the other. Finish the massage by doing some soothing effleurage strokes up from ankle to thigh and back down again.

Tennis elbow and repetitive strain

 Overuse of any part of the body puts a strain on the muscles and tendons and can result in painful conditions, such as tennis elbow or repetitive strain injury (RSI). Both of these conditions can be helped with touch therapies.

TENNIS ELBOW MASSAGE
Inflammation of the tendon running along the forearm to the elbow creates pain. Sportspeople and gardeners are particularly at risk. Massage can help to ease the pain.

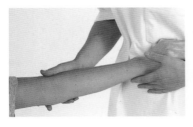

1 Support your partner's wrist in one hand and use soothing strokes along both sides of the arm from the wrist to the elbow and back again. Repeat several times.

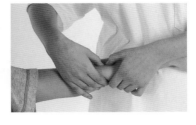

2 Rest the hand against your side. Work up the arm, from wrist to elbow and back, making small circular movements.

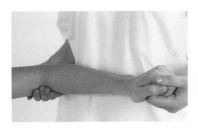

3 Stand to one side of your partner, secure their hand in yours and support their elbow with your other hand. Flex the elbow forward.

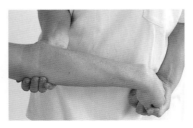

4 Bring the hand back to give the tendons that are attached to the bones a good stretch.

REFLEXOLOGY FOR REPETITIVE STRAIN
Repetitive strain can affect any part of the body that is overused. It is an occupational hazard for keyboard operators, where a stiff neck and shoulders, aching wrists and pain and weakness in the forearm are increasingly common problems. Reflexology can help to ease some of the discomfort.

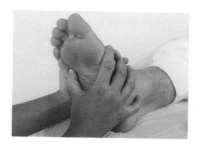

1 Work the shoulder reflexes thoroughly by using the thumbwalking technique. Gently fingerwalk across the same area on the top of the foot, with the three middle fingers held together.

2 Rotate the ankles to ease aching wrists and stimulate healing within the joints. Work down the outside of the foot to relax the shoulders and arms.

TIPS FOR KEYBOARD WORKERS
• Make sure your wrist is well supported. Mouse mats are available with inbuilt wrist supports.
• Take regular breaks away from the keyboard.
• Flex and rotate the fingers and wrists, to keep them supple and stop them from aching.
• Massage hands and forearms on a regular basis.

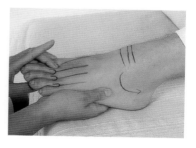

3 Work the lymph system on both feet to encourage toxins to drain away. Fingerwalk down the lines from the toes towards the ankle, then work around the ankle.

Fluid retention

A heavy feeling in the legs and puffy, swollen ankles are typical signs of fluid retention. The problem is often aggravated by hot weather, prolonged periods of standing, premenstrual tension, long haul flights and pregnancy.

MASSAGE TO IMPROVE CIRCULATION
Excess fluid indicates that the kidneys and/or circulation are not working properly. Massaging the legs and the thighs will improve the local circulation and so bring more blood and oxygen to the muscles. Firm effleurage movements are particularly helpful. They should always be done in one direction, towards the heart.

TIPS TO AVOID FLUID RETENTION
- Drink plenty of water to help the kidneys flush out (at least six glasses a day).
- Remember to increase your water intake in hot weather.
- Include raw food in your diet.
- Regular massage will improve the circulation and drainage of toxins.
- Avoid prolonged sitting or standing in one spot.

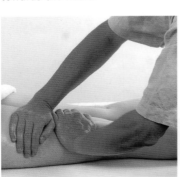

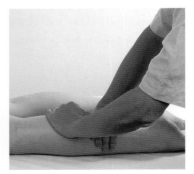

1 Place your hands on your partner's thigh and stroke upwards to the buttock several times using smooth effleurage strokes. Keep the pressure light but steady, letting one hand follow the other.

2 Move your hands down to the calf and stroke up to the back of the knee a few times. Repeat these two steps, always starting the massage on the upper leg and always stroking towards the heart.

Shiatsu menstrual treatment

Used on the feet, shiatsu can help to stimulate the body's energy system, improving circulation and the drainage of toxins. There are also specific points that can help with menstrual problems.

1 With a loose fist, tap the sole of the foot. Then gently massage the whole foot thoroughly with both hands.

2 Massage the web between each toe and then massage the toe joints. The point between the big toe and the second toe is good for period pains (do not use this massage during pregnancy).

3 Come to the sole of your foot and apply pressure to it with your thumb. This will have a revitalizing effect upon your body and stimulate energy flow.

4 Use your thumbs to massage the area under the ankle bone. This is a good point to use for any menstrual disorders. Use your thumb and press firmly.

▶ Instead of suffering from period pains, try a shiatsu self-treatment.

Useful aromatic oils

- Pine: reducing puffiness in the legs, particularly after prolonged standing and in late pregnancy.
- Geranium, juniper, rosemary: premenstrual fluid retention.
- Fennel, juniper, lemon: detoxifying oils.
- Cypress, geranium, pine: after long-haul flights.

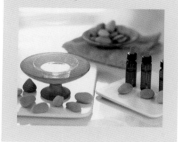

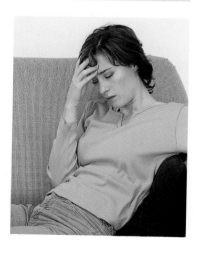

Improving circulation

The circulatory system connects all the systems of the body. Its tone and vitality is fundamental to life and to the integration of the whole body. There are many steps we can take to help it function effectively.

HAND AND FOOT MASSAGE

Cold feet and hands are a sign of poor circulation. When we breathe in, oxygen from the air is absorbed into the blood and carried to the heart. It travels around the body, carrying vital nutrients to every cell and returning waste products for disposal. Poor circulation means that the body's tissues and organs are inadequately nourished and that toxins are not removed properly, leading to many other health problems. A massage will help to warm hands and feet, and improve the circulation.

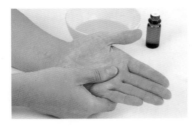

1 Using a little oil, massage the palm of the hand with a steady, circular movement of the thumb.

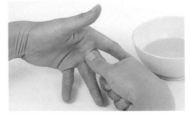

2 Squeeze down each finger to stretch and loosen the joints, pushing towards the palm. Repeat.

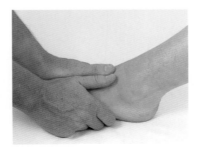

◀ **3** To stretch the foot, use both hands with the thumbs on top and fingers underneath the foot. Keep a loose but firm grip. Move the thumbs outward, as if breaking a piece of bread. Repeat several times, keeping the fingers still while moving your thumbs.

Shiatsu techniques

Working a shiatsu treatment on each side of the spine is invigorating and relaxing. Rubbing and rolling techniques are useful for improving the circulation – of both blood and energy – throughout the whole body.

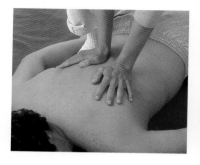

1 Use the palms to apply gentle but firm pressure down each side of the spine.

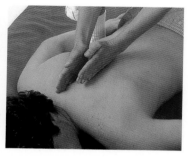

2 Using the side of your hands, vigorously rub down each side of the spine a few times.

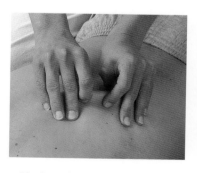

3 Pinch and take hold of the skin on the lower part of the spine. Lift the tissue and gradually roll it up the spine. Roll the skin from the spine, out towards the sides to cover the entire back.

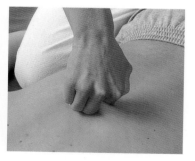

4 Use your index and middle fingers to pinch and take hold of the tissue. Twist and lift the skin at the same time. Work within your partner's pain threshold. Cover the whole back using this technique.

Improving digestion

If we are what we eat, then the healthy functioning of the digestive system is essential. Stress and tension are responsible for many digestive disturbances, including bloating, constipation, abdominal cramps, diarrohea and indigestion.

SHIATSU TREATMENTS

In shiatsu, the Stomach meridian is vital for the production of "ki" in the body. These movements help to relax the body and ease any digestive disturbances.

▸ **1** Sit at your partner's side and place your right hand on the stomach. Note the breathing rate: fast and shallow indicates tension. When you are attuned to your partner's breathing, continue.

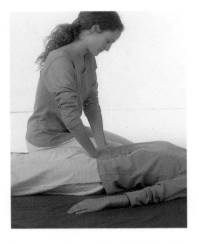

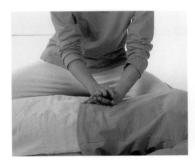

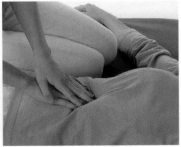

2 Using one hand on top of the other, apply pressure in a clockwise movement around the stomach. If you find tension, increase the pressure until it dissolves.

3 With one hand on the other, rock and push from one side of the belly to the other, pulling back with the heel of the hand until you feel the stomach relax.

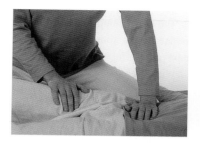

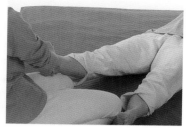

4 Stretch your partner's leg out and place your knee or a pillow underneath your partner's knee for support. Apply palm pressure along the outside frontal edge of the leg following the Stomach meridian. Start from the top of the thigh and work down to the foot.

5 Move down to your partner's feet and take a firm hold of the right ankle. Lean back and stretch the leg out. Repeat with the other leg. To finish the treatment, come back to the "hara" (abdomen) and tune in again, checking for any tension and relaxation of the muscles.

REIKI INDIGESTION TREATMENT

These hand positions aid the digestion of food and can also help to free any blockages that are caused by emotional problems – often a cause of bad digestion.

Kneel beside your partner and place one hand on the sternum and the other on the solar plexus at the centre or bottom of the rib-cage. If there is a stomach upset, constipation or diarrhoea, place the second hand lower down on the second chakra. Focus your attention and channel healing energy to the area.

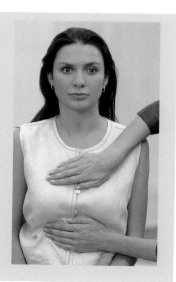

Relieving stress

When we are under stress, the body pumps extra adrenalin in its "fight or flight" response. If this goes on for extended periods of time it has a damaging effect on our health and results in many common complaints.

REFLEXOLOGY EASY BREATHING

When we are stressed, our breathing becomes quick and shallow and our digestion is upset. By breathing more deeply and slowly, we can help ourselves to cope with stress: it is not possible to panic while you are breathing well. This reflexology treatment works to open up the chest and lungs. It will calm you down, settle your nerves and increase the supply of life-giving oxygen to the body.

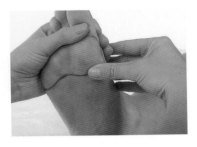

1 Thumbwalk along the diaphragm line to release tension, pain and tightness. When it is contracting and relaxing freely, the abdominal organs are also stimulated.

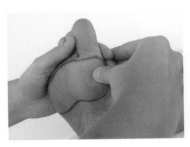

2 Work the lung reflexes on the chest area so that once the diaphragm is relaxed, the breathing can open up, increasing the supply of oxygen to the body.

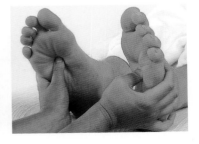

3 Take both feet together and position your thumbs in the centre of the diaphragm line. As your partner breathes in, press in with your thumbs. Release as they breathe out. Repeat this several times.

SHIATSU SHOULDER MASSAGE
Stress causes the neck and shoulders to tighten, creating pain and stiffness. This treatment gives relief.

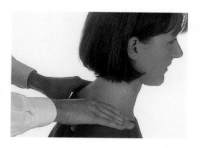

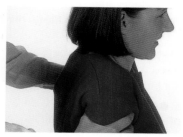

1 Place your hands on your partner's shoulders and take a moment to tune in. Grip and hold the shoulder muscles on each side of the neck. Squeeze them a few times in a rhythmic kneading action.

2 Take a firm grip of the upper arms. Ask your partner to breathe in as you lift the shoulders up and breathe out as you allow the shoulders to drop back down again. Repeat the shoulder lift three times.

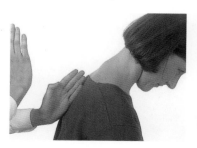

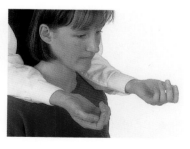

3 Use a gentle hacking action with the sides of your hands. Move rhythmically across the shoulders and base of the neck. Keep the movement consistent, then increase the intensity as you feel the muscles relax.

4 Place your forearms on your partner's shoulders. As you breathe out, press down with your arms on to the shoulders, applying gentle but firm, perpendicular, downward pressure. Repeat several times.

Relieving tension

Tension held in the body is usually the result of stress, pain or shock. The muscles tense or tighten up in an attempt to ward off the unpleasant stimuli. The healing touch of another's hands can help us to relax.

HEAD AND NECK MASSAGE

When we feel tension, we usually hold it in our shoulders and neck, keeping ourselves taut. This unnatural posture can result in a thumping headache and aching around the eye area.

A good head massage helps the facial muscles relax and worry lines disappear. You may be able to make your partner look almost 10 years younger with this tension-relieving treatment.

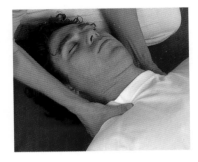

1 Place your hands on the shoulders, fingers underneath and thumbs on top. Firmly massage the shoulders using a kneading action.

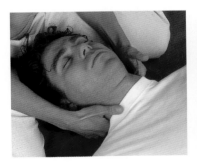

2 Move your hands to the neck. With your thumbs on the side and fingers underneath, stretch out the neck by gently pulling away. Repeat several times.

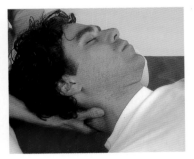

3 Lift your partner's head off the floor and firmly squeeze the muscles of the neck.

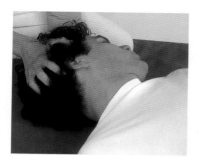

4 Rub the scalp using your finger-tips and then run your fingers through the hair.

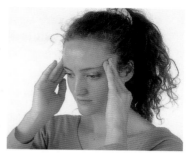

5 Using the fingers of both hands, work on the delicate facial tissue, moving symmetrically across the face to cover all the facial muscles.

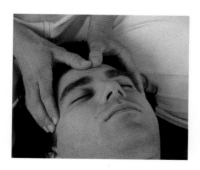

6 Place the thumbs side by side on the centre of the forehead and stroke out to the temples, working in strips. Smooth any worry lines.

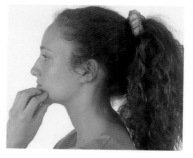

7 Take the chin between thumb and fingers and gently pinch your way out along the jaw, relaxing and releasing any tension.

TIPS FOR RELIEVING TENSION

• Take regular exercise to help diffuse tension and change the focus of your attention from any worries.

• Set aside some quiet time for yourself each day.
• Unwind in an aromatherapy bath before you go to sleep.

Improving sleep

A good night's sleep is essential for health. During sleep the body's cells renew and repair themselves and we relax. To prepare yourself for sleep, help the body to unwind before going to bed.

RESTFUL SLEEP ENHANCER
A foot massage and reflexology treatment will help the body to relax. It will also improve the circulation and accelerate the removal of toxins. Try this treatment to make the most of the healing properties of sleep.

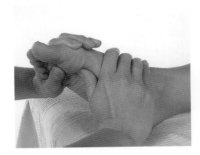

1 Holding the foot with one hand, bring the foot down on to the thumb of your other hand and lift it off again. Move your thumb one step to the side and repeat, working your thumb methodically across the foot to the outer side, following the boundary line of the ball of the foot.

▸ **3** Thumbwalk along the spinal reflex from the heel to the big toe. Support the outside of the foot with your other hand.

2 Firmly thumbwalk along the diaphragm line. It is important to relax the diaphragm, because this area helps to calm the whole body and to steady the breathing.

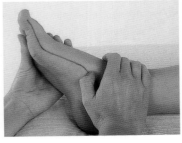

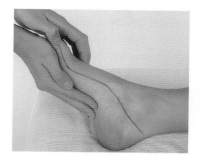
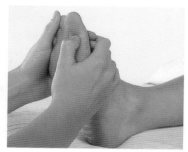

4 Repeat, going down the spinal reflex several times. Rotate gently around any tight or sensitive areas.

5 Gently thumbwalk up the back of the toes: do this with care as there is likely to be tenderness there.

AROMATIC HAND AND FOOT MASSAGE

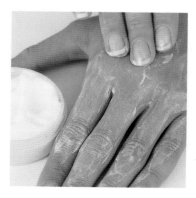

Massaging the hands and feet will help to relax the whole body. Use small, circling strokes on the soles and palms, repeating the movements on the other foot and hand. Use firm pressure to avoid tickling and irritating movements.

SLEEPY-TIME AROMAS

Try adding a few drops of essential oil to your massage oil or lotion.
• Lavender: for relaxing and balancing.
• Camomile: for soothing and calming.
• Neroli: for calming stress and anxiety.
• Clary sage or marjoram: for a strong sedative action.

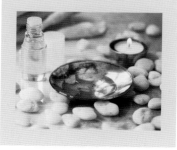

Looking after your hands

We rely on our hands to perform countless everyday tasks. Our hands are one of the most overworked parts of the body, yet it is easy to take them for granted, forgetting to give them the care they deserve.

SIMPLE HANDCARE

Everyday of our lives our environment has an impact on our hands. Freezing winter temperatures, biting winds, central heating, water, detergents and strong sunlight all have a damaging effect on the delicate skin of our hands. As we get older, our skin loses its elasticity and becomes increasingly dry.

There are a few simple things that we can do to look after our hands. Exposure to the sun is believed to be the main cause of skin aging, so it's essential to protect your hands from the damaging effect of the sun's harmful

▼ USE A MOISTURIZER CONTAINING A SUN-SCREEN TO PROTECT YOUR HANDS FROM ULTRAVIOLET LIGHT AND TO KEEP THE AGING EFFECTS OF THE SUN AT BAY.

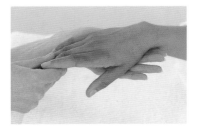

NAIL & HANDCARE TIPS

• To remove dead skin cells: add a teaspoon of salt to warm olive oil and massage into the hands.
• To strengthen the nails: rub a little neat lavender oil into the cuticles every night.
• For dry, brittle or weak nails, or nails with white flecks: make sure you have enough calcium, zinc and B vitamins.

ultraviolet rays: use a good-quality moisturizer containing ultraviolet filters. Get into the habit of wearing rubber gloves for washing up and always use a moisturizer after exposing them to water.

Age spots on the back of the hands are made worse by cold weather and sunlight. Protect your hands from wintry winds by investing in warm gloves, and use a richer moisturizer at this time of the year. Saffron oil or a few drops of lemon juice mixed into yogurt and rubbed into the hands can help to reduce age spots.

AROMATHERAPY PAMPERING TREATS
As well as looking after our hands on a day-to-day basis, a weekly manicure will keep the nails in good shape. Use essential oils to strengthen your nails.

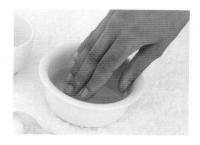

1 Soak your fingertips in either warm water, warm olive oil or use cider vinegar if the nails are weak. Gently clean the surplus cuticle from the nail area.

▼ HANDS THAT ARE NEGLECTED AND WORN-LOOKING ARE SAID TO AGE A WOMAN.

2 Gently push the cuticles back with an orange stick wrapped in cotton wool. Use a cotton bud (Q-tip) to apply neat lavender oil to each cuticle.

▼ FOR CRACKED, DRY SKIN MIX PATCHOULI OIL IN A CARRIER OIL AND APPLY TO HANDS.

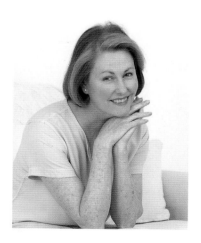

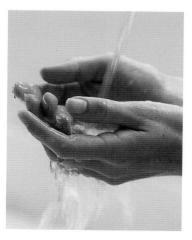

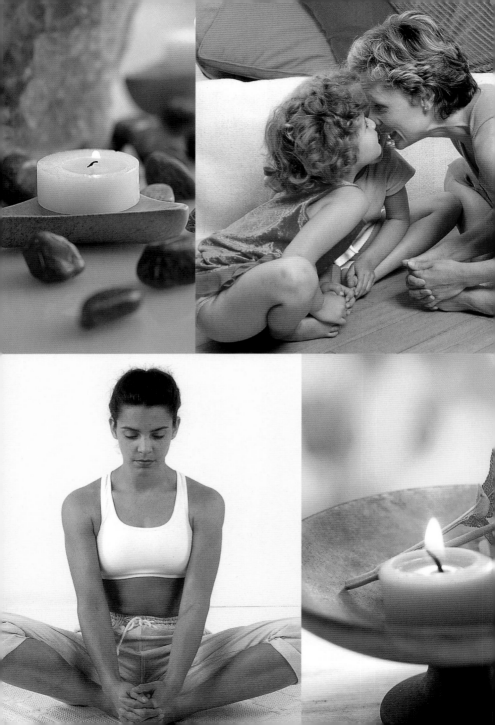

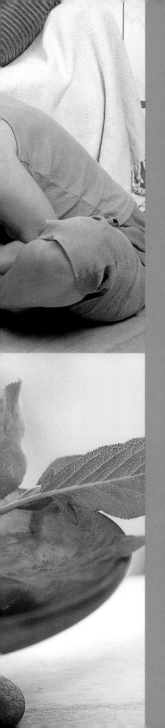

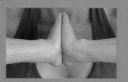

HEALING WITH
YOGA

In the Sanskrit language, the word "yoga" refers to union, harmony and balance. Many forms of this ancient discipline have been practised throughout the East since antiquity, and in more recent times it has taken hold in the West.

Beginning with a look at the koshas – our "five states of being" – this chapter shows how yoga can be used to heal, both by rebalancing the nervous system and by promoting the flow of energy through the body. Yoga has been described as a state of relaxed alertness, and you will see how, through techniques that include postures (asanas), breathing (pranayama), and resolve (sankalpa), the negative attitudes and habits we have learned make way for a new, positive relationship with our environment.

Healing and self-healing

We all need healing, which simply means changing for the better at one or more levels of our being – the physical, energetic, nervous, thinking and attitudinal aspects. These five levels, called the koshas in yoga, are interactive.

THE KOSHAS

These levels can be pictured as invisible layers, emanating outwards from the solid physical body (the first level). We feel the energy body as we approach someone or when they invade our space. The nervous system picks up signals from outside via our five senses. Our thoughts travel across space and even time. Our attitudes shape our destinies through eternity.

When we meditate we can become aware that these five levels of our being also flow inwards, contacting the vibrations of the spirit. These levels make up "who we are".

Successful healing brings us – the whole person – into our optimum state of harmony and well-being by treating not only our physical symptoms but also any energy disruptions, nervous imbalances, mental overload or deep

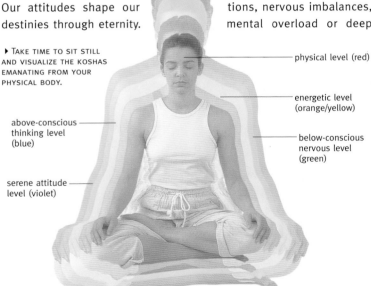

▶ TAKE TIME TO SIT STILL AND VISUALIZE THE KOSHAS EMANATING FROM YOUR PHYSICAL BODY.

physical level (red)

energetic level (orange/yellow)

above-conscious thinking level (blue)

below-conscious nervous level (green)

serene attitude level (violet)

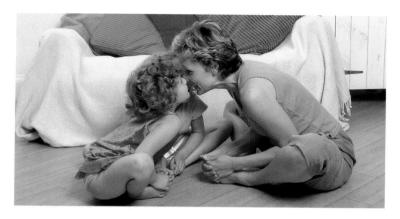

"soul sickness" that may be affecting us. This alters our whole outlook on life, even allowing us to live peacefully with symptoms or circumstances that previously caused us great distress.

SELF-HEALING WITH YOGA

In yoga we take responsibility for our own well-being through the practice of self-discipline, self-awareness and self-surrender. Self-discipline simply means "sticking at it", practising yoga regularly, with enthusiasm and commitment. A few breaths and stretches here and there during quiet moments, plus a regular daily session of half-an-hour or so, is ideal – but any yoga is better than none at all and will still bring great results over time. Joining a weekly yoga class is a good idea and can inspire us to develop our practice further.

Self-awareness is essential for safety in practice. If anything feels wrong, stop doing it. Yoga is non-competitive, so we learn to know and accept how we feel today and to practise accordingly. Yoga is a state of relaxed alertness at all times. Self-surrender means letting go of our comfortable habits and familiar mindsets to make room for healthier ones. Our body lets go of its worn-out cells as new ones are formed. In the same way, we must let go of our worn-out opinions, prejudices, habits, self-image and other burdens.

The nervous system

The nervous system is related to the middle kosha that links our physical and energetic states (or "body" koshas), with the thinking and attitudinal levels (or "mind" koshas). The system has several branches; yoga works on them all.

The middle kosha contains all the unconscious aspects of the mind, such as the memory, instinct, and programmed responses, as well as the nervous system that allows the conscious mind to communicate with the body and to turn thoughts into physical actions. The brain and spinal cord provide the main "motorway" for nervous impulses to travel along the nerve cells to and from all parts of the body. It is vital to keep this "traffic" flowing freely.

Yoga makes us more aware through the sensory nervous system: our sight, hearing, touch, taste and smell become more alert and responsive. It makes us more skilful in movement through the motor nervous system, which tells each muscle when to contract and by how much. It even allows us to access the autonomic nervous system, so that we can choose consciously when to be keyed up or relaxed while maintaining our inner serenity.

▼ YOGA TEACHES US THAT WE CAN CONSCIOUSLY CHOOSE WHEN TO RELAX.

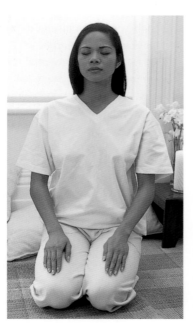

THE AUTONOMIC NERVOUS SYSTEM
This system maintains homeostasis (internal harmony) by controlling the respiratory, cardiovascular, digestive, hormonal, immune and other involuntary body systems.

Its two complementary branches work together like the accelerator and brakes in a car. One branch "revs up" certain systems to help us deal with imminent physical danger. This is known as the "fright-fight-flight" response and it is needed for surviving external threats. The other branch deals with nourishment, long-term maintenance, rest and repair. It is responsible for ensuring our longer-term health and survival. Most of us fail to appreciate that we do not have the resources to attend to both these aspects at the same time. If we spend too much time in fight-or-flight mode, we are neglecting to digest our food or repair our damaged cells, and tiredness and poor health will inevitably follow.

Our nervous systems have not yet evolved to cope with the profound changes in lifestyle wrought by our technological society, which is only about 200 years old. Today, our lives are highly stressful, competitive and go-getting, making us feel angry, frustrated, confused and anxious a lot of the time, and it is not surprising that many of us get

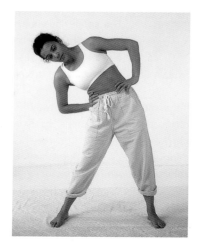

▲ KEEP YOUR SPINE LOOSE AND SUPPLE TO HELP YOUR NERVOUS SYSTEM DO ITS WORK.

stuck in the fright-fight-flight syndrome. Since there is no physical enemy for us to kill or escape from, the stress hormones in our bodies remain unused. These can build up to dangerous levels and eventually lead to serious diseases. Our nervous systems may become totally out of balance, with the accelerator on full throttle nearly all the time.

The autonomic nervous system may seem to be beyond our conscious control, but fortunately we can influence it through yoga, helping us to regain internal harmony and balance.

The spine's energy motorway

The spine houses a subtle "motorway" that carries the life force in our energy body. As it enters or leaves at the "roundabouts" or chakras, this life force is a blend of all our energies: physical, vital, nervous, mental and attitudinal.

If the spine's energy "motorway" is obstructed the "side roads" become blocked and their territory is deprived of essential nourishment, communications, and the ability to remove toxic wastes. The resulting distress is called "illness". You can keep the traffic flowing smoothly in the spine through the use of posture, movements with breath awareness, visualization, relaxation and meditation.

THE CHAKRAS

Energy enters and leaves our spine through the chakras. These are also associated with the three important cavities in our bodies. The abdominal cavity protects our vital organs and houses three major chakras dealing with the energies of Life: survival, social interaction and self-confidence. The legs and feet are extensions of our survival chakra. Great emphasis is placed in yoga upon strengthening the lower body so that we can cope with the challenges of living.

The skull cavity lies at the top of the spine and protects the brain. It houses two major chakras concerned with the energies of

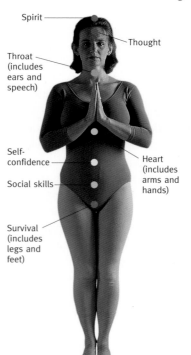

Spirit

Thought

Throat (includes ears and speech)

Self-confidence

Social skills

Heart (includes arms and hands)

Survival (includes legs and feet)

◀ THE CHAKRAS REPRESENT THE THREE ENERGIES OF LIFE, LIGHT AND LOVE.

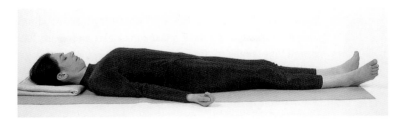

awareness and wisdom or Light. Breathing and balancing exercises switch on the Light in our heads, giving us greater understanding in both yoga and daily life.

Lying between the skull and abdominal cavities is the thoracic cavity. This protects our hearts and lungs and houses the two chakras concerned with relationship or Love energies. The arms and hands are extensions of the heart chakra (for reaching out to others) and the ears and mouth are extensions of the throat chakra (for communicating). Simply thinking about someone engages relationship (Love) energies, even if we don't actually like them. Yoga gradually increases our capacity for unconditional love and cancels out

negative thoughts and feelings. Backbends and chest expanding exercises help to open and lift the upper body, allowing Love energy to flow more freely. It also improves our breathing and circulation.

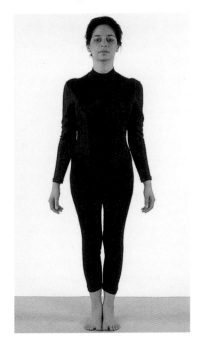

▶ IN *TADASANA*, YOU ARE ALIGNING YOUR SPINE WHILE FIGHTING THE FORCES OF GRAVITY. IT IS A SIMPLE YET STRONG POSE.

the spine's energy motorway **533**

Breathing patterns

Yoga helps us to change our breathing. Slow, deep breathing through the nose relaxes the heart and sends "all is well" messages to the brain. Once we have learned yoga breathing habits we can lessen our stress and anxiety.

A fast, shallow breathing pattern, with panting or gasping through the mouth to "snatch" more air, is usually the result of stress. This type of breathing strains the heart and makes the stress worse. It also sends panic messages to the brain, which then revs up the fright-fight-flight response and a vicious circle is created: "Quick! Fight harder! Run away faster!" Since we cannot physically fight the boss nor flee from a traffic jam, we end up feeling even more anxious and stressed.

The diaphragm is the chief "breathing muscle". It lies across the base of the chest, separating it from the abdomen above the waist (and stomach). When we breathe in, it flattens downwards, massaging the abdominal organs. When we breathe out it relaxes upwards into the chest. "Deep" yoga breathing is diaphragmatic breathing. In yoga postures the breath is co-ordinated with both stretching and moving energy.

KNEELING POSE, *VAJRASANA*

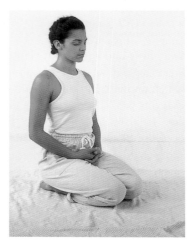

▲ Sit on your heels, with big toes touching underneath you. Tuck your tailbone under and tilt your pelvis backwards, to avoid hollowing your lumbar spine. Clasp your hands in your lap and stretch the spine up, lifting and opening your chest. Keep your chin and shoulders down. Breathe slowly and deeply a few times in this position and focus on feeling the breathing movements within.

ARM AND CHEST STRETCH WITH BREATH

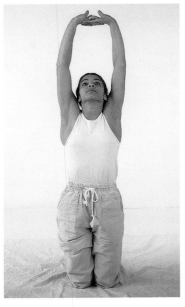

BODY-MIND BREATHING CYCLE

Now add the feeling of moving energy up and down the spine, which calms, balances and heals the nervous system. The general rule is to move energy upwards through the spine on the breath IN and to stretch and energize the limbs on the breath OUT. You may need several breaths to perfect a posture. End by breathing OUT to bring energy down and relax.

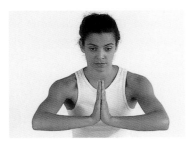

▲ Sit in *vajrasana* (see opposite). Now, as you breathe IN, kneel up and stretch your clasped hands directly overhead, with your palms up. Breathe OUT and stretch up even more. Breathe IN to sit on heels and OUT to lower hands to lap. Repeat the sequence a few times, co-ordinating breath and movements. The arm stretch, with the breath, can also be done when standing or sitting on a chair.

▲ Put palms together with your elbows out to the side. Stand in a comfortable upright position. Pull the spine up and breathe IN, squeezing the inner thighs and pelvic floor muscles. Breathe OUT, squeezing corset muscles at waist. Breathe IN, pressing palms together and squeezing spinal muscles behind the heart to lift and open the chest. Breathe OUT to relax. Repeat three times.

Spinal alignment

Good spinal posture is vital to the health and well-being of all five koshas. It allows free passage of nervous impulses between the body cells and the brain, and of vital energy within and between the chakras.

DANGERS OF POOR POSTURE

Many common health problems are linked to poor posture. Besides causing compression in certain nerve pathways and disharmony in the chakras, poor posture also causes physical problems around the areas where the spine is out of alignment. Blockages in the structural, nervous or energy systems will reveal themselves in time through congestion, distress, pain and eventually disease around the area involved.

COMMON PROBLEMS

Rigidity in the pelvic and sacral area puts pressure on the hip, knee, ankle and foot joints, and the ligaments. This pressure eventually makes movement, and walking, difficult and painful.

▼ DO YOU RECOGNIZE ANY OF THESE COMMON POSTURAL PROBLEMS IN YOURSELF?

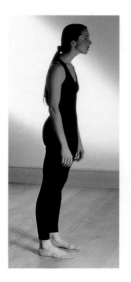
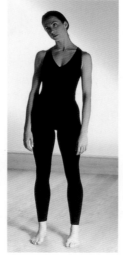
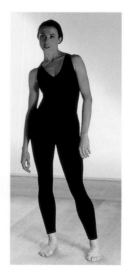

Compression of the digestive organs results in insufficient oxygenated blood causing them to malfunction. This can lead to infection as the stale blood is not removed.

Compression of the cervical spine (causing a jutting chin) is a frequent cause of headaches and mouth breathing, which can itself cause nasal and sinus congestion.

A weakness in the thoracic spine (which causes a concave chest) can

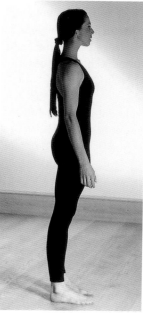

▲ WHEN STANDING CORRECTLY, THE BODY IS BALANCED AND THE SPINE STRETCHED UP.

result in the compression of the diaphragm and intercostal muscles. This can lead to poor breathing, chest infections, lung congestion and heart and circulation problems.

Compression in the lumbar spine (caused largely by weak abdominal muscles) results in all kinds of lower back and leg pain (including trapped nerves and sciatica) and failure to hold the lower organs in place. This can lead to problems such as prolapse and incontinence.

Some problems are caused by structural abnormalities, and yoga can often help. Most of the above problems, however, are due to poor posture, which is apt to deteriorate further with age or excessive weight gain. Fortunately, they can be halted and even reversed through gentle and persistent yoga practice, especially those practices that improve spinal alignment through movement and isometric "muscle squeezing" done standing, kneeling, sitting or lying.

The chakras, or vitality centres, can also be energized and balanced when breathing and visualization practices are combined with an awareness of spinal alignment. A strong lower body allows the upper body to lift and open.

Improving posture

This isometric "muscle-squeezing" exercise will improve your posture. Do it lying on your back, sitting, kneeling or standing. Practise it anywhere and often, to replace poor postural habits with good ones.

ISOMETRIC EXERCISE

1 Stretch up through your spine. Press the palms together at heart level before lifting your elbows to shoulder height.

2 Begin by tightening the muscles of the inner thighs (at the top near the groin). Involve the backs of the thighs as well, but keep the buttocks relaxed. Squeeze an actual or imaginary jar between the thighs. These muscles help to support the trunk when standing.

3 Next tighten the pelvic floor muscles. These muscles also help to support the weight of the trunk. Squeeze as though pulling the base of the body up inside. Weakness in the pelvic floor muscles causes lower back pain, sexual problems and also incontinence (especially after childbirth).

▼ ISOMETRIC EXERCISE INVOLVES ALMOST IMPERCEPTIBLE BUT POWERFUL MOVEMENTS.

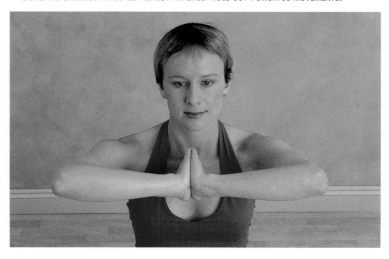

4 Now tilt the pelvis slightly by tucking the tailbone under. Lift the pubic bone by tightening the lower abdominal and groin muscles. These muscles help to hold the sacral spine in alignment, correcting excess lumbar curvature and pressure on the sacroiliac joints.

5 Tighten the corset muscles (the transverse abdominals), pulling the waist and navel back towards the spine. This holds the lumbar spine in place and prevents abdominal sagging. Your energy will sweep spontaneously up through your chest, neck, head and crown, as you realign them by opening the chest, lifting the ears away from the shoulders and bringing the head in line with the spine.

6 The sacrospinalis muscles on each side of the thoracic spine

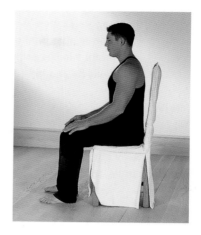

▲ TIGHTENING THE CORSET MUSCLES KEEPS THE TORSO ERECT AND ENERGY FLOWING.

hold it upright and keep the chest open. Pressing the palms hard together activates these muscles and lifts the chest. Breathe IN strongly, drawing your energy down from the crown, bringing Light into your body and mind, and opening yourself to the Love energies radiating from your "divine core".

7 To release this posture, breathe OUT slowly and deeply. Take your energy down to your feet then relax, releasing all physical, mental and emotional "waste products". Let them become neutralized by the Earth. Do three rounds only. Repeat this exercise frequently.

WATCHPOINT
Do not squeeze the pelvic floor or abdominal muscles if you are pregnant, after recent abdominal surgery or have serious digestive problems. Instead, focus on lifting up through the lower, middle and upper spine.

Letting go

Deep relaxation is an essential part of yoga practice, whether it is a short rest between exercises or fifteen blissful minutes ending with your resolve, or *sankalpa*. The shoulders and hips hold tension and should be eased first.

MAKING A RESOLVE

We feel happy and at peace when we relax. We can retain this feeling afterwards by changing some of our unhelpful attitudes towards life while we are in the relaxed state. If life is a journey we can choose either to "climb mountains" (difficulty and struggle) or to "go with the flow" (relaxing and letting go). It is up to us, but making room for change means letting go of negative or outdated beliefs and trusting the Cosmos (or God, the Universal Life Force or Spirit) to guide us into the future.

SANKALPA

Meaning "resolve", *sankalpa* is a yoga practice for changing our attitudes. We can change the energies in any of our chakras, building up more vitality (Life), awareness (Light) or positive attitudes in our relationships (Love) by practising *sankalpa* in deep relaxation.

Before entering into relaxation, we choose how we want to be and

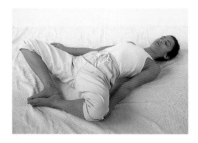

▲ THE BUTTERFLY STRETCH IS A RELAXING POSE FOR DEEP BREATHING AND LOOSENING THE HIP JOINTS.

form a statement in simple words, starting with phrases such as "From this moment on I am becoming more and more ..." or "I am feeling more and more ..." or simply "I am ...". Use only positive words that make you feel good about yourself. Be positive. Avoid words that suggest the possibility of failure, such as "try", or words that reinforce your present condition, such as "less tired/negative/depressed" and so on. Avoid projecting into the future with statements saying "I will be/feel/ become ...", remembering that change can only happen in the here and now.

Choose only one quality at a time for your *sankalpa*, and stick with it until it is no longer needed. Repeat the same *sankalpa* every time you relax, also upon waking and before going to sleep. Meanwhile live your life as if you already have the quality you are developing. When your *sankalpa* is established, make a new one.

SAVASANA, CORPSE POSE

This is a great relaxation position and is called the corpse pose because all the muscles relax. Your body temperature will drop, so you may need a light blanket.

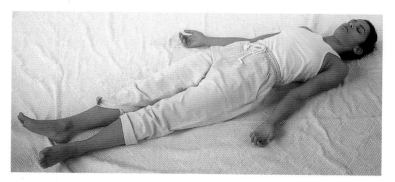

1 Roll the feet and hips in and out to find the best position, then roll the hands and shoulders in and out. If your chin juts up, place a small cushion under your head.

2 If your waist arches away from the ground, place a cushion under your knees. It takes time and awareness to find and settle into your most relaxed position.

How to practise yoga

We practise yoga techniques – posture, breathing, movements with breath and energy flow, classical poses, relaxation, resolve and meditation – in order to become "yogic" and to live daily life in the state or attitude of "yoga".

YOGA MEANS UNION

Both yoga and true healing involve creating harmony between the five koshas – the physical, energetic, nervous, thinking and attitudinal levels of our being. The result is more abundant Life (energy), Light (awareness) and Love (receiving and giving).

WHAT YOU NEED FOR PRACTICE

Choose a quiet warm space, with enough room to lie down and stretch. Wear loose clothing. Have a rug or shawl handy for relaxation

▼ GATHER TOGETHER EQUIPMENT TO SUPPORT YOU IN YOUR POSTURES.

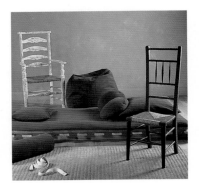

and meditation. It is best to work on a non-slip mat or piece of carpet, roughly 180cm x 60cm (6ft x 2ft) and use a firm cushion or upright chair to sit on for breathing and meditation. Some extra small cushions are also useful.

Set aside a regular time and place each day, to establish your "yoga habit". Practise yoga before eating, with an empty bladder and bowels. Wait about two hours after a large meal.

WHICH TECHNIQUES TO PRACTISE

Always involve all five koshas, however short your practice. Begin with a breathing exercise and careful spinal alignment to harmonize the nervous system. Continue with some stretches to release physical tension and get your energy flowing. End with relaxation and/or meditation to relax your mind and release negativity. Repeat your *sankalpa* (see earlier in this chapter) for healing, and to create beneficial changes in attitude.

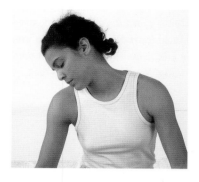

▲ SIMPLE MOVEMENTS RELEASE TENSION AND ENCOURAGE ENERGY TO FLOW.

Several sequences are shown for you to "mix and match" to suit your energy levels. Choose to lie, sit or kneel if you feel weak or tired. When you feel energetic practise vigorously while standing, in order to develop strength and stamina. Rest briefly between sequences and for longer at the end. Practice should be regular rather than long: 15–30 minutes once or twice a day is ideal, plus a weekly yoga class if possible.

Every day is different and yoga brings improvements very quickly. Your own body is your best guide. Practise at what is a comfortable pace for you today, and for only as long as the exertion is enjoyable. If you feel breathless or shaky, take a rest and slow down your breathing. Resume your practice later when you feel better, perhaps choosing an easier sequence.

MAKE YOGA PART OF YOUR LIFE
Stay focused in your yogic attitude, whatever you are doing. Use odd moments for stretching, alignment, breathing or repeating your resolve – waiting for the kettle to boil, after long sitting or telephoning. There are many such moments in a day.

▼ YOGA CAN BE PRACTISED WHENEVER YOU HAVE A MOMENT TO SPARE.

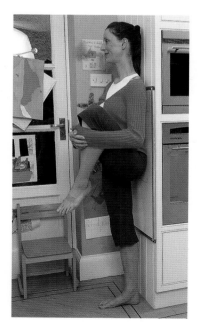

Getting started

Start your yoga practice lying down if you feel stiff, tired or unwell. Allow gravity to help and support you as you breathe slowly and deeply and limber up gently to get your circulation and energy flowing. You will soon feel great.

BE GENTLE WITH YOURSELF

Before you start, make sure that you are comfortable. Use pillows or cushions if you need support. If you are feeling unwell or are recovering from illness, take things very easy. If in doubt, consult your health practitioner before starting – but remember that yoga can work wonders at many levels, even if "exercise" is contra-indicated.

BREATHING

Lie comfortably, with knees bent and head supported if necessary. Feel your energy moving as you breathe, travelling up through your body as you breathe IN, and down again as you breathe OUT. Let your

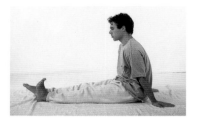

▲ USE YOGA TO DISPEL SLUGGISHNESS AND GET YOUR CIRCULATION MOVING.

breath soften and lengthen as you connect with the "tide of life" and float upon it for a few moments.

MOVING THE EXTREMITIES

Before you begin the postures, flex and stretch your fingers and toes, then your ankles and wrists. Move your feet and hands in circles in every yoga session and at odd moments during the day. Moving the extremities is the easiest and quickest technique to get the circulation and energy moving through the whole body. Practised regularly, this helps to remove congestion, stagnation, sluggishness and fluid retention, and wakes up the nervous system.

▼ *SAVASANA* IS A TRADITIONAL YOGA POSE – IDEAL FOR GENTLE EXERCISE WHEN UNWELL.

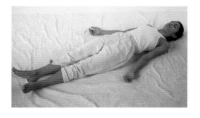

Pelvic lift

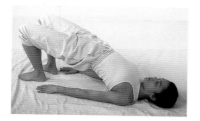

▲ Lie on your back with knees bent. Breathe IN to tighten pelvic floor and lower abdominal muscles. Breathe OUT to tilt pelvis and tuck tailbone under. Breathe IN to lift pelvis. Breathe OUT to lower. Repeat.

Knees to chest

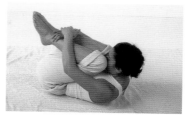

▲ Lie on your back and clutch your knees to your chest. Hug with your arms and lift your head gently to your knees. Roll gently from side to side, then vigorously forward and back to sit up.

Lying twist

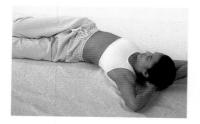

▲ Lie on your back with knees bent. Keep ankles, knees and inner thighs pressed together through-out. These muscles support the groin, pelvic floor and lower spine. Breathe OUT to lower the knees to the floor. Breathe IN to raise them (still pressed together). Repeat.

Seated forward bend

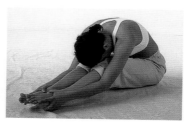

▲ Place your head over bent knees and gradually stretch out your legs. Keep your spine long and relaxed. Breathe deeply into the back of your chest a few times. Breathe IN to move energy up the spine and OUT to move it down. Unfold and return to *savasana* to relax.

Energy (Life) and balance (Light)

These sequences charge you with energy (Life) and wake up your mind (Light). Use them to start the day, or after too much mental work or enforced sitting. Always practise yoga in bare feet – unless stretching in public places!

DYNAMIC STANDING WARM-UP

Simply walking about on tiptoe is one of the best energizers there is. Standing on your toes strengthens your feet and ankles and relieves congestion, stagnation and fluid retention in the legs (Life). To stand on tiptoe and look up calls for balancing skills that sharpen the brain (Light). If your sight or hearing is impaired you will find balancing a challenge, so hold on to something, or practise with your back against a wall for support.

▼ STANDING ON TIPTOE STRENGTHENS MUSCLES AND SHARPENS THE MIND.

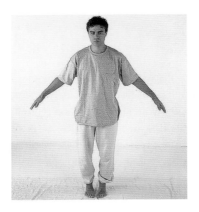

SQUATTING

To begin squatting, try leaning against a wall for support. Keep your heels a little way away from the wall to help you balance.

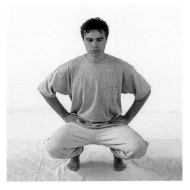

▲ Stand with your feet apart and hands on hips. Align the spine and tighten the muscles of the lower trunk. Breathe OUT as you bend your knees to the sides and lower into a squat, keeping your spine upright. Breathe IN as you rise to standing again. Avoid bending forward as you lower yourself down – hold on to the edge of a table if needed.

STANDING STRETCH

Stretching your arms overhead strengthens the chest muscles and opens the chest to allow better breathing. Keep your spine aligned and your arms well back, in line with your shoulders, to stretch the pectoral muscles and lift the sternum. Poor posture, fatigue and depression shorten these muscles and reduce the lung area. This worsens the poor breathing that created these problems in the first place. If, when you stretch your arms overhead, you feel breathless (through weakness or chest or heart problems), practise this exercise with your hands in *namaste* (prayer position) at heart level.

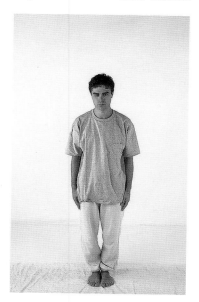

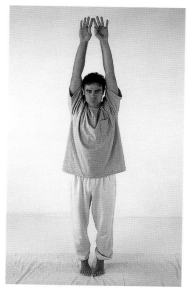

1 Stand tall, aligning your spine and distributing the weight evenly on both feet. Tighten the muscles of the lower trunk (Life) for strength to stretch up and open chest (Love).

2 Breathe IN, raising arms to sides and overhead, and coming on to your toes. Breathe OUT to lower arms and heels. Repeat vigorously until glowing with energy.

energy (Life) and balance (Light) **547**

Positive feelings

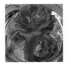

These arm-circling, side-bending and twisting movements should all be done while keeping the lower body strong and unmoving and the spine in alignment. The movement is all from the waist upwards, in the thoracic area (Love).

OPENING THE CHEST FROM A STRONG BASE

These movements should be able to cheer up the gloomiest and most lethargic person, since they cleanse the lungs, improve the circulation and open the heart centre. Stand firmly with feet about hip-width apart, arches and inner knees lifted, back and inner thighs strong, pelvic floor drawn up, abdominal muscles holding the pelvis and spine in good alignment.

As you practise the movements, take your attention and your energy right into your fingertips. They are extensions of your loving heart, reaching out to embrace the world and everyone in it, including yourself. Feel that streamers of light are flowing out from your fingers in big circles up, down and around you, brightening up the atmosphere as you stretch and move through your whole body. For a less energetic version, the movements can also be done while kneeling or sitting cross-legged.

ARM CIRCLING

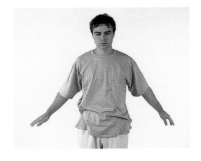

1 Stand with feet about hip-width apart and arms out to sides.

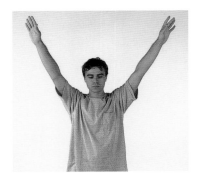

2 Breathe IN to raise arms forward and up. Breathe OUT to lower them back and down. Repeat several times, making big circles.

CHEST OPENING

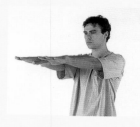

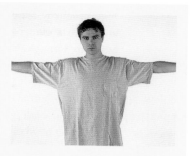

1 Stand tall with feet apart and arms in front at shoulder level. Keep your shoulders down and neck long throughout.

2 Breathe IN to take straight arms to sides at shoulder level. Breathe OUT to return them to the front. Repeat vigorously.

SIDE BENDING

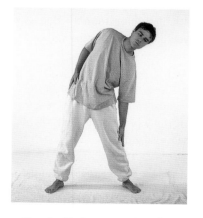

▲ Stand with feet apart. Breathe IN, stretching your spine up. Breathe OUT to bend to the right, keeping the left shoulder back and in line. Repeat to left. Repeat both sides.

ROTATING TRUNK

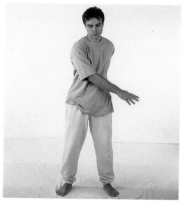

▲ Standing with feet apart, swing the arms and rotate the upper trunk from side to side, keeping the spine upright, the arms loose and breathing naturally and vigorously.

Breathing exercises

Yogic breathing removes stress. With practice, we can learn to de-stress ourselves in almost any situation, simply by breathing through the nose and engaging the diaphragm in slow, deep breathing movements for a few moments.

Shallow, stress-related breathing emphasizes the top and middle parts of the chest, similar to when we are panting from unexpected exertion such as running for a bus. Peaceful, rhythmical breathing engages the lower part of the chest and especially the diaphragm.

Yogic three-part breathing uses all the breathing muscles around the bottom, middle and top of the lungs. Stand, sit or lie and settle your breathing before you start. Just three deep yogic breaths may be enough to trigger the "all is well" response when we are feeling

THE YOGIC THREE-PART BREATH

1 Place your hands on your waist to feel the movement of the diaphragm and lower ribs as you breathe deeply IN and OUT.

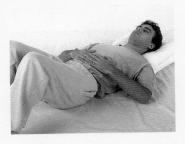

2 Now place your hands around the sides and front of the chest and feel the ribs opening and the

sternum (breastbone) rising as you breathe IN. Breathe OUT and feel them retracting.

3 Then move your hands to your collarbones. As you breathe IN fully you may feel them move slightly.

4 Breathe IN from the base of the lungs to feel as though your chest cavity is filling with air up to the collarbones. Breathe OUT as fully and slowly as possible (residual air always remains in the lungs) to release tension.

stressed. This is the quickest and easiest way to control our nervous system and to calm it down when our mind and emotions have revved it up.

All yoga techniques exercise and relax mind and body. *Alternate nostril breathing* also restores the balance between them. Being too introverted makes us depressed or mentally exhausted and being too extroverted makes us physically exhausted. Mind and body are designed to work in harmony. People who spend too much time "in their heads" as well as those undergoing physical exhaustion, trauma or a life crisis, can benefit greatly from this simple exercise, followed by deep relaxation. You need to practise it on a day-to-day basis though, before turning to it in a crisis. Build up the number of rounds very gradually.

ALTERNATE NOSTRIL BREATHING

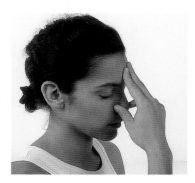 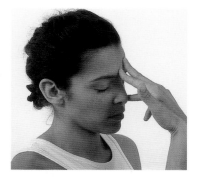

1 Sit erect on a chair. Place index and middle finger of right hand on forehead with left hand in lap. Close right nostril with thumb and breathe IN through open left nostril. Close left nostril with ring finger and open right nostril. Breathe OUT through open right nostril.

2 Breathe IN through open right nostril. Close it with your thumb and open left nostril. Breathe OUT through left nostril. This is one round. Do several rounds then rest a moment with natural breathing, and observe how you feel. Repeat several times.

Balancing stretches

The focus here is on keeping the spine stretched and aligned all along its length while holding your balance – whether standing on one leg or both – and performing the different movements with deep concentration.

These stretches all require balance, focus and concentration, so they are good for Light energies (the mind). They also require a strong lower body (Life) and with regular practise, help you gain an open chest with relaxed arms, shoulders and neck (Love).

ISOMETRIC BALANCING

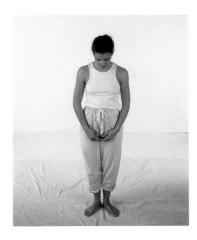

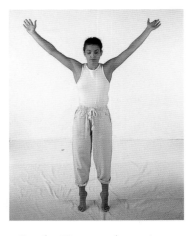

1 Stand with hands clasped and head bowed. Breathe IN to focus on tightening inner thigh and pelvic floor muscles. Breathe OUT as you raise arms to the sides a little and focus on squeezing "corset" muscles around the navel, pulling the navel back towards the spine.

2 Breathe IN as you rise on to your toes, raising your arms high to the sides and opening the chest by focusing on and squeezing the muscles along the upper spine. Breathe OUT to relax arms, feet, head and squeezed muscles. Do three rounds.

CHEST AND THIGH STRETCH

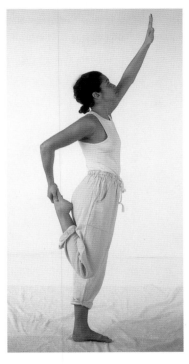

⏶ Stand on one leg and bend the other knee, holding the foot against your buttock with the bent elbow pointing back. Raise your other hand high in front, as though pressing it against a wall. It is helpful to practise this pose while standing about 15cm (6in) away from a wall, so that you have to stretch up and really open the chest.

LOOSENING ROLLING TWIST

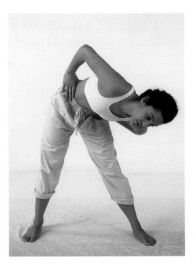

⏶ Rolling twists are energetic, so do them slowly and with awareness and stop if your breathing speeds up. Stand with feet about 75cm (2½ft) apart and hands on hips. Stretch up through the spine and push the pelvis forward with knees loose as you breathe IN. Breathe OUT to lean back from the upper trunk. Twist forward and clockwise in a fluid motion. Breathe naturally, focusing on maintaining strength and stillness in the lower body, with all the movement from the waist and upper spine. After a few rounds, repeat anticlockwise.

The tree pose

This sequence is excellent for spinal alignment and energy flow, as well as working the abdominal muscles. It works the legs strongly, opens the chest, raises the arms and engages the optical and balancing mechanisms in the brain.

STANDING IN THE TREE POSE
Nearly all the classical *asanas* (yoga poses) work on all the energy centres along the spine, and the tree pose is a good example.

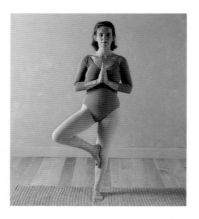

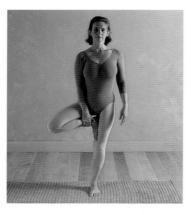

1 Stand with your feet hip-width apart and parallel, toes evenly spread. Feeling rooted to the floor, allow your right leg to float up, bent at the knee. Take hold of your right foot and position the sole firmly against the inner thigh of your strong, standing leg, with the bent knee out to the side, feeling the opening in the hip joint.

2 If you cannot achieve this position, place the sole wherever comfortable on the inside of the straight leg – what is important is to keep the knee back so as to open up the hip area. Realign your pelvis, tucking your tailbone under, and softly fix your gaze on a point in front of you to help you balance. When you feel steady, join your palms in *namaste*, breathing freely. Hold the position for several breaths, then breathe OUT to bring the leg and arms neatly down. Repeat the movement with the opposite leg.

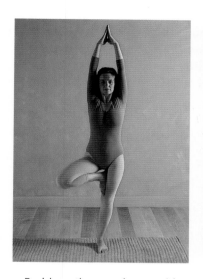

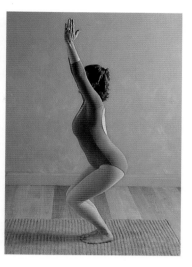

3 Feel how the muscles on either side of your leg and trunk are working together, co-operating in the job of holding you upright and steady. Come out of the pose if you start to wobble. Once you feel rooted and secure in this pose, raise your arms slowly overhead, palms together, breathing in. Breathe deeply and hold the pose. Repeat on the other side.

4 When you have worked equally on both sides, stand calmly to settle your body and breath. When you are ready, breathe IN to raise your arms over your head, being careful not to arch the lower back. Stretch right through from your heels to your fingertips and take a few breaths. Then breathe OUT to bend your knees as though you are sitting down. Keeping your spine as vertical as possible, lower yourself until you are almost squatting. Keep your heels on the floor. Take a few deep breaths in this position, then breathe IN to stand again. Repeat this "standing seat" several times.

Forward and backward bending

Many people bend forward by stretching their lumbar spine, with rigid hips and knees. This puts great strain on a very vulnerable area. Practising correct forward and backward bends gives you greater flexibility and a fully stretched back.

PREPARATION

This sequence is strong and dynamic. It requires some limbering movements first, especially in the upper spine, such as *opening the chest*. Movements such as *dynamic standing warm-ups* or *squatting*, strengthen the legs and feet and make the hips, knees and ankles more flexible. *Squatting* also trains the spine to remain upright when you are bending down.

PROTECTING THE LOWER BACK

Bending incorrectly – usually from the lumbar spine – is the most frequent cause of lower backache, especially when lifting. When you practise any kind of standing forward bend in your yoga sessions, first tighten your spine-supporting muscles and always bend forward with knees well bent and spine as straight as possible.

Your upper trunk and head are very heavy, especially if you let them sag like dead weights – so stretch the spine out and forward

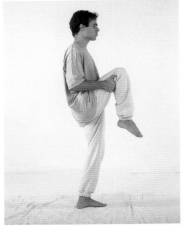

▲ LIMBER UP FOR THE BENDS BY LIFTING YOUR KNEES TO STRENGTHEN LEGS AND HIPS.

as you bend from the hips and take your body weight into your strong thighs. Your spine is precious and you can protect it by developing both awareness and lower body strength. Bend forward only as far as you can. Place your hands on your shins, ankles or the floor to support your upper body weight before attempting to straighten your knees. It is more important to stretch your spine than your legs.

Forward bending

Experiment with picking up a light but bulky box from a squatting position and then rise by straightening your legs – there should be no stretching in your lumbar spine (below and behind the waist) because your legs are strong enough to lift the weight of both your own body and the box. The muscles that hold your spine in place, which you have been strengthening through sessions of *body-mind breathing,* are protecting your lower back at all times. While in a forward bending position, with knees well bent and your head hanging down, you can release tension in your neck and shoulders by gently rotating your head.

Standing forward bend

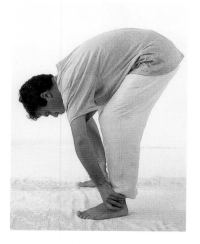

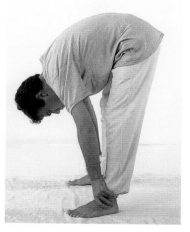

1 Stand with feet about 75cm (2½ft) apart and knees well bent. Breathe OUT to bend forward and clasp your ankles or shins. Breathe IN. Breathe OUT to relax and let the spine lengthen, keeping legs bent.

2 On each breath OUT let gravity stretch your spine more, to get your best stretch for today. Finally straighten your legs if you can. Roll up very gently and stretch your arms up.

Backward bending

The aim is to increase flexibility in the thoracic spine (chest) without overarching the lumbar spine or the neck (cervical spine). Chest expansion exercises are a good way to do this. Practise this movement frequently as it's very good at relieving feelings of tightness and for improving breathing capacity. It is also a good way to warm up your spine before the back bends.

The neck carries all the nerves from the brain to the body. Congestion here is often caused by hunched shoulders, as we unconsciously attempt to "carry the world on our shoulders". Dropping the

Chest expansion

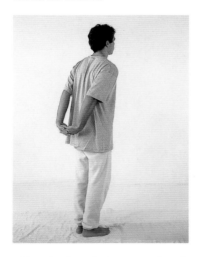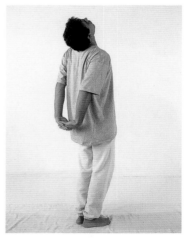

1 Stand tall and clasp your hands behind your back. Breathe OUT as you straighten your arms and lift them up behind you, keeping your lower body firm. Breathe IN to return your arms and stretch up through your spine.

2 Breathe OUT to bend the upper spine backwards, keeping your knees bent and lifting your straight arms up behind you. Take a few breaths in this position. Breathe IN to straighten up. Drop your head back only if it feels comfortable.

shoulders and opening the chest, as in back-bending poses, relieves this congestion, which is a common cause of headaches and feelings of acute tension. People who look and feel uptight are apt to have stiff shoulders, necks and thoracic spines because they are habitually "holding themselves together".

STANDING BACK BEND

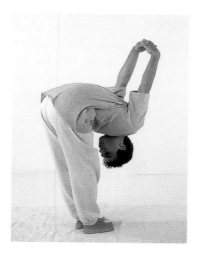

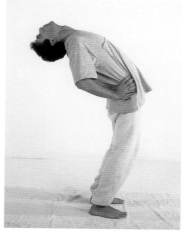

3 Breathe OUT to bend forwards with knees bent, lifting your straight arms up behind you. Take a few breaths in this position. Breathe IN to straighten up. Repeat this sequence frequently to open the chest and improve posture.

1 Stand with hands on waist or lower back. Breathe IN and stand tall. Breathe OUT, pushing pelvis forward, bending knees and arching upper spine backwards. Remember to take a few breaths. Breathe IN to come up slowly.

Twisting the spine

Spinal twists stimulate and strengthen the muscles on either side of the spine. These hold it in alignment by working equally on both sides. They also increase flexibility by contracting on one side and releasing on the other.

PREPARATION

Before twisting the spine extend it fully and avoid leaning forward or back. This allows the spine to twist from the waist upwards through the thoracic and cervical areas, opening the chest and stimulating the nerves that radiate outwards from the upper spine. A spine that is not fully stretched will twist too much in the lumbar area, rather than evenly along its whole length.

This imbalance is a common cause of backache. Practise twisting movements after warming up well.

HELPING THE HEART AND CIRCULATION

All movement helps the heart and circulation (especially the diaphragm's movement when breathing slowly and deeply). Twisting movements also help to flush out the "used up" blood and toxic waste products that result

SIMPLE SEATED TWIST

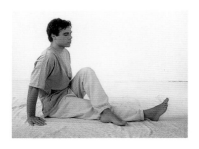

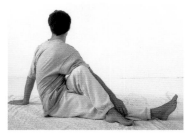

1 Sit tall, with your legs in front and your hands beside you. Place the sole of the left foot on the floor on the far side of the right leg. Breathe IN and stretch your spine up.

2 Breathe OUT to bring your right arm over the left knee and take hold of your right leg for leverage. Breathe IN to stretch up. Breathe OUT to twist. Repeat other side.

from energy production in the cells, and to get freshly oxygenated blood to every cell – especially in parts of the body that can be hard to reach in other ways.

STRETCHING THE SPINE

First practise three rounds of *body-mind breathing* to tighten the muscles that support the spine.

Keeping your mind on these muscles and the spine stretched up, breathe OUT and twist. This squeezes stale blood out of areas that can get congested – the abdominal organs, spinal muscles, lungs and neck. As you breathe in again and untwist, freshly oxygenated blood rushes into the areas that you have just squeezed.

FORWARD TWISTING

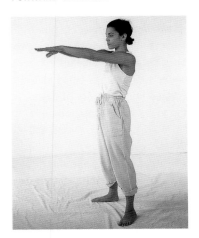

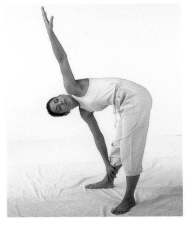

1 Stand with feet about 75 cm (2½ft) apart and arms stretched out in front of you at shoulder height. Breathe IN. Breathe OUT and bring the right hand down your right leg and your left hand up above you in a straight line.

2 Turn your head (if comfortable) to look at your left hand. Breathe IN to straighten up into starting position. Breathe OUT to bring left hand to left leg. Repeat vigorously. For more twist, slide your hand down your opposite leg instead.

Kneeling sequence

Kneeling or sitting is less tiring than standing, because gravity is with you rather than against you. These yoga poses work to loosen your upper back and shoulders, as well as your knees and ankles.

PREPARATION

Sit on your heels, with big toes turned in to touch each other. If your knees are stiff, place a cushion between your shins and your ankles. If your ankles are stiff, place a cushion beneath them until you are more flexible.

CHILD POSE

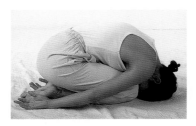

▲ Sit on your heels and breathe IN. Breathe OUT to bend forward. Place your forehead on the floor, bringing your arms close to your feet. If your chest or bust feels compressed, you may prefer to rest your forehead on your fists or on a cushion. Breathe into your ribs at the back to expand your breathing for a few moments.

FLEXIBILITY IN THE LOWER BODY

Stiffness indicates poor circulation, usually due to lack of movement. Our skeletal and muscular systems are designed for movement – animals move from place to place and human "animals" have learnt to move on two legs, freeing the upper limbs. However, this puts great strain on the pelvis and lower back because they bear the body's whole weight. Yoga helps alleviate congestion, pressure and pain in the lower half of the body.

STRENGTH IN THE UPPER BODY

The upper spine, shoulders and arms are also often out of balance because they do not carry enough weight to keep them strong. Again, yoga brings our awareness to this tendency. Bearing the body weight more equally in the all-fours position allows us to regain flexibility and relieve strain and congestion in the lower back, and develop greater strength in the muscles of the upper trunk.

CAT STRETCH

BACK ARCH

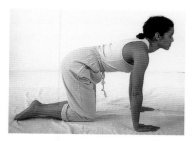

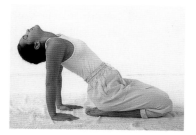

1 Sitting on your heels, stretch your hands forward along the floor, then raise your buttocks so that your shoulders are over your wrists and your hips are over your knees. Stretch out your fingers to make a broad base to take your weight. Breathe IN with your back flat and your neck relaxed.

▲ Sit on your heels with your big toes turned in and touching. Place your hands on the floor behind you with fingers pointing towards your buttocks. Spread your fingers and lean back with your wrists under your shoulders. Breathe IN, lifting the chest high. Breathe OUT to lower the chest. Repeat.

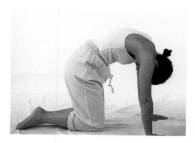

2 Breathe OUT as you arch your upper back. Drop your head and look at your navel, tucking your tailbone under. Feel the stretch in the upper back. Repeat.

WATCHPOINT
When practising the *cat stretch*, ensure that your hips are directly over your knees. Keep the arms straight, with wrists directly below the shoulders and the fingers spread. It is the upper body that is being worked here, not the weight-bearing joints of the lower body, so focus on moving the upper spine, neck and head and keep your hips fixed.

Classical inspiration

 Here we show an expert performing two modern classical poses taught in most yoga classes: swan stretch and dog stretch. This level of grace and flexibility is inspiring but all of us will benefit from our own practice of these positions.

INVERTED POSES

Wonderfully energizing, inverted poses are popular with yoga practitioners. The two best known poses – the headstand and the shoulderstand – are difficult to get into and dangerous to topple out of. A good alternative is the inverted *dog stretch*, where your head is held lower than your heart for a few minutes, but you are in a stable position. Begin with the swan stretch to elongate your spine and neck in preparation.

BENEFICIAL CHANGE IS HEALING

Even if we cannot yet achieve the perfect *dog stretch*, we can nevertheless work on those three basic activities that bring about the beneficial changes in us that we call "healing": self-discipline, self-awareness and self-surrender. More than two thousand years ago, the great yoga master, Patanjali, called them the "practical steps on the path of yoga". They underlie all healing and achievement – not only in yoga but also in other

SWAN STRETCH

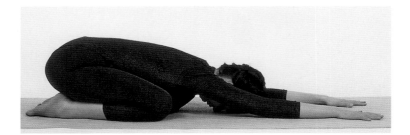

▲ Sit on your heels with toes touching and spine straight. Bring your head to the floor (with your buttocks still touching your heels). Stretch your spine, taking your arms forward into the swan stretch.

aspects of our lives. Everything worthwhile requires enthusiastic practice, commitment and understanding of the principles involved. We need to let go of our negative conditioning, bad habits and poor self-image to move forward.

DOG STRETCH

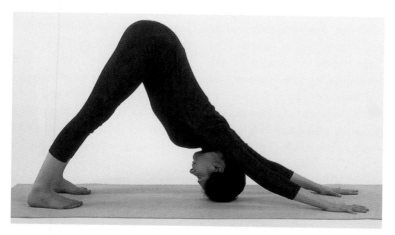

1 Begin in the *swan stretch*. Shift your weight forward on to hands and knees in the *cat stretch*. Tuck your toes under. Lift your buttocks into the air, keeping your knees bent. Stand on your toes, taking your weight forward into shoulders, arms and hands. In this position, work to open your chest and bring your shoulders closer to the floor.

2 Finally, straighten your legs and bring your heels to the floor (if you can). Breathe deeply throughout, holding the position for as long as you can without strain. To come out of it, lower your knees to the floor and rest your heart in the *swan stretch* for a few moments before raising your head and trunk into an upright position, sitting on heels.

Final relaxation

Every yoga session should end with winding down, final relaxation and a "grounding" ritual. These practices may be the most important part of your yoga session, as they promote an attitude that brings healing at many levels.

WINDING DOWN

End your yoga session with some final stretching and some deep breathing. These are very relaxing activities, highly recommended at any time, and especially before going to sleep at night. They "switch on" the branch of the autonomic nervous system that activates the body's essential maintenance and repairs necessary for healing. Feel that "all is well" – as it nearly always is in the Now. This is a deeply peaceful and healing attitude in itself. We can always feel that way, even when stuck in a traffic jam. Why get fearful and uptight about something that is not a physical threat? Usually it is because we are reacting according to our outdated mental patterns of thinking.

These patterns, these basic attitudes, can soon be changed by practising our "all is well" yoga techniques at every opportunity, many times each day – especially when feeling stressed.

▼ *SAVASANA* IS AN IDEAL POSITION FOR MENTAL AND PHYSICAL RELAXATION.

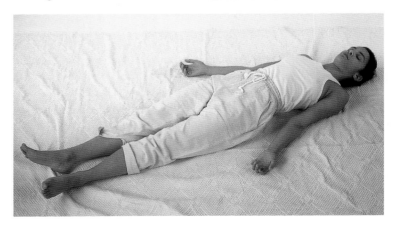

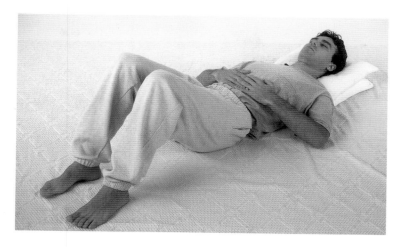

Final relaxation

This is "winding down" practised in a position (such as *savasana*) where the body is totally supported so that all muscles can relax completely. This, in turn, reinforces the attitude that "all is well" – otherwise the large "fighting and fleeing" muscle groups in the arms and legs would be clenched, and probably the jaw too.

As you relax, take your mind on a journey around your body to discover whether any muscles have tightened up again. If so, breathe OUT slowly while sending a message of letting go into those places that are holding on to tension. Final relaxation is not

▲ IF THE SMALL OF YOUR BACK ARCHES AWAY FROM THE FLOOR, SUPPORT YOUR HEAD AND BEND YOUR LEGS.

a time to fall asleep. Rather, keep an attentive mind in an inert body, watching out for the slightest tension in order to dissolve it.

Grounding

After 5–15 minutes' deep relaxation, come out very slowly, maintaining the inner attitude of peace and trust (Love), while being ready for and aware of (Light) the challenges of Life. Become conscious of your body and surroundings before sitting up. Once sitting, you can touch the ground with your head (Light) and hands (Love) as you celebrate your Life.

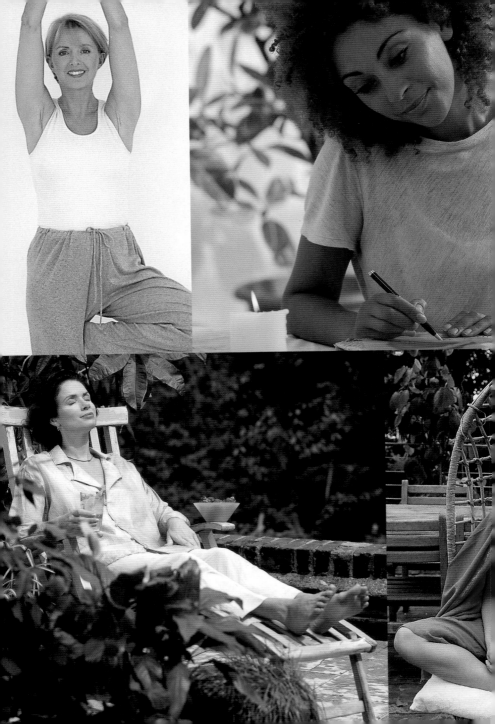

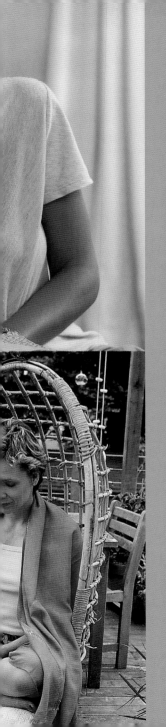

YOGA
TREATMENTS

The pace of life is fast and demanding and it is easy to get lost in the outer world. More and more people are suffering from stress-related illnesses ranging from everyday tension headaches to depression and serious nervous disorders. Many of these health problems can be related to imbalances in the chakras (energy centres).

Beginning with more about chakra healing – and its relationship to life and love – this section encourages us to "come back" and explore our inner world using deep relaxation and meditation techniques. These have the power to heal old wounds, bringing clarity of vision and purpose. There are also specific exercises to boost immunity, aid circulatory, digestive and respiratory problems, and ease aches and tension.

More about the chakras

The chakras correspond to points along the physical spine and seem to co-ordinate the emotional qualities and basic attitudes that create our "inner" world and reflect out into our lives. Balancing the chakras balances our lives.

We can change the state of our autonomic nervous system from the fright-fight-flight syndrome to "all is well" by working with the chakras. Use awareness, movement and stillness in those areas of the body that feel closed or weak and are in need of energy, healing and rebalancing.

▼ STRONG, EARTHBOUND POSTURES DRAW ENERGY TO THE LIFE CHAKRAS.

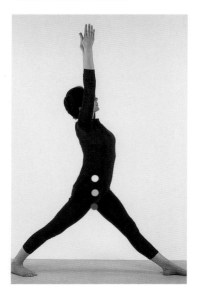

THE THREE LIFE CHAKRAS
These correspond to points on the spine in the abdominal cavity:
1 At the base (including the legs and feet). This chakra is concerned with physical safety/survival. Here we trust (positive) or fear (negative) the world. Yoga helps us to stand firm with strength and courage.
2 At the sacrum. This chakra is concerned with sexual/social inter-action. Here we enjoy (positive) or shrink from (negative) the company of others. Yoga helps us to have more fun and friendship in our lives.
3 Behind the navel. This chakra is concerned with self-confidence. Here we work to succeed (positive) or are obsessed with self-image (negative). Yoga helps us to live our lives with enthusiasm and commitment.

THE TWO LOVE CHAKRAS
These correspond to points on the spine in the thoracic cavity:
4 Situated behind the heart (and including the arms and hands). This chakra is concerned with personal

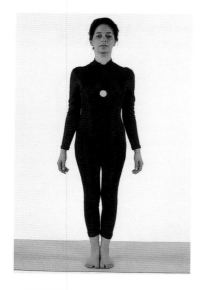

▲ STRAIGHTEN YOUR SPINE AND OPEN YOUR CHEST TO BALANCE THE LOVE CHAKRAS.

relationships. Here we share with others (positive) or "keep ourselves to ourselves" (negative). Yoga helps us to accept both the joy and the vulnerability of relating.

5 Situated behind the throat (and including speech and hearing). This chakra is concerned with creative communication. We express our thoughts and feelings while listening to those of others (positive) or we choose to "hide behind words" without hearing (negative). Yoga helps us to share our truth more honestly.

THE TWO LIGHT CHAKRAS

These lie in the skull cavity:

6 Situated behind the brow. This chakra is concerned with mental activity. We focus our thoughts clearly (positive) or live in a mental fog (negative). Yoga helps us to relax and be more aware that "all is well" beneath the noise of our mental chatter.

7 Situated on the crown. This chakra is concerned with our attitudes and spiritual purpose. We grow in wisdom (positive) or stagnate in self-centredness (negative). Yoga helps us to relax and embrace ourselves and others.

▼ PRACTISE FORWARD BENDS TO SEND BLOOD TO THE LIGHT CHAKRAS.

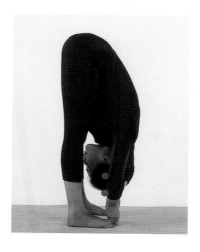

Relaxing body and mind

After relaxing body and mind we can unwind at those deeper levels where old fears, hurts and resentments lurk, sapping energy and joy. Once accessed, these "sore places" in our psyches can be healed.

YOGA RELAXATION

Follow the instructions, moving systematically "inwards" and then "outwards" again. With practice you will know what you can do in ten minutes or in twenty. Allow time to "return" to the everyday world and to ground yourself thoroughly. Practise daily and this technique will bring deep and healing changes. You could tape the instructions to play while you relax.

1 Remember your *sankalpa*.
2 Settle your body in *savasana* – you can cover yourself with a blanket if needed. Have your spine and head totally supported and your shoulders and hips loose. Once settled, do not move.
3 Settle your breathing.

4 Take your mind to each part of the body in turn and connect with that part. Always use the same order: right thumb, each finger in turn, palm, wrist, forearm, elbow, upper arm, shoulder, right side of chest, of waist, right hip, front of thigh, back of thigh, front of knee, back of knee, calf, shin, ankle, heel, ball of foot, top of foot, big toe, each toe in turn. Repeat on left side. Go around twice if you have time. This practice connects our minds with our bodies and heals the body-mind split that can cause many problems.
5 Move energy from the feet and up the spine – through the chakras – as you breathe IN and down as

▼ PLACING BLANKETS UNDER YOUR BACK HELPS TO OPEN UP YOUR CHEST.

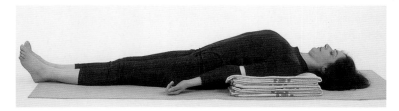

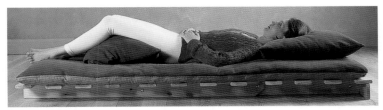

▲ YOU MAY FIND *SAVASANA* EASIER IF YOU SUPPORT YOUR KNEES AND HEAD.

you breathe OUT, healing and restoring balance at all levels. Wash away all burdens on the tide of energy moving back down to the Earth through your feet.

6 Visualize a place that means "spiritual home" to you – inside a sacred building, in a garden or by the sea, or in your own heart space where the Eternal Flame burns brightly. Settle yourself quietly and reverently in this space and feel its vibrations healing you.

7 Silently repeat your *sankalpa* three times, with deep commitment and intent.

COMING OUT OF RELAXATION

When you are ready, start to come out of relaxation. Look at the place you are in and say goodbye to it, remembering that it is always there for you to return to. Begin to breathe consciously and deeply, revving up the "engines" of your body, ready for movement. Move your fingers and toes, your wrists and ankles. Stretch your limbs with a long, contented sigh, then a yawn, then a sigh again. Curl up, roll on to your side and sit up slowly when you are fully awake. Ground yourself thoroughly before getting up.

▼ FIND YOUR MOST COMFORTABLE POSITION. SETTLE INTO IT AND RELAX.

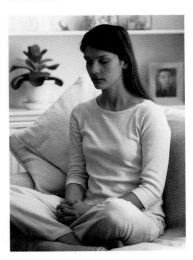

Yoga and common health problems

Prolonged stress contributes to many health problems by overworking some systems and causing congestion or stagnation in others. Yoga rebalances the nervous system, removes toxic build-up from the body and is holistic.

POLLUTION IN THE BODY

The immune system is programmed to remove (through activities such as pain, inflammation, fever, etc.) all foreign bodies that enter the body. These can be bacteria, viruses, food additives, poisons in food, water and air, recreational and medicinal drugs (the side-effects). We ingest so much that is unnatural nowadays that the body gets stressed and confused as to what is friend and what is foe and starts attacking itself.

▼ A HEALTHY DIET PLAYS AN IMPORTANT PART IN BOOSTING YOUR IMMUNE SYSTEM.

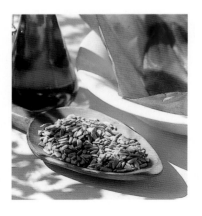

Many common conditions such as addiction, allergies, asthma, auto-immune diseases or chronic fatigue, are largely due to environmental stress.

The yogic answer to stress from pollution is two-fold. First, it works to reduce overall stress by rebalancing the autonomic nervous system so that the fright-fight-flight response is less easily triggered and the "all is well" response becomes the norm. Secondly, it tries to avoid ingesting pollutants through lifestyle and diet. This includes our diet of mental and emotional negativity as well as physical poisons. In the end, if we attend to the warning signals of distress, we create a happier and more fulfilling lifestyle.

ADDICTION

All yoga is very helpful. Relaxation with *sankalpa* and meditation brings release, healing and recovery when practised persistently with other (especially group) therapies.

Allergies

Regular yoga practice can reduce the need for medication. Consider your diet, as this is often how substances that are poisonous (to you) enter the system. Practise relaxation and meditation to reduce stress, as this can trigger allergic reactions.

Arthritis

Gentle exercise brings relief. If only some joints are affected, practise in the evening, having loosened up during the day. If inflammation is general the morning may be better. Avoid all exercise during a period of "flare up". Take great care with replacement joints and try to avoid positions that put pressure on weight-bearing joints. Choose sitting or lying positions for initial limbering and breathing and then do standing sequences slowly, with deep breathing and rests.

Asthma

Do what feels comfortable, slowly and without strain. Use your breath as a monitor, breathing deeply through your nose. Stop to rest at the first signs of breathing

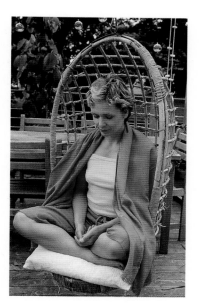

▲ Do you have a favourite spot? Relax and spend time "just being".

discomfort. Relax propped up. Watch your diet to avoid constipation. Relaxation and meditation reduce the levels of stress that can trigger asthma attacks.

Auto-immune diseases and chronic fatigue

Keep active and cheerful through regular yoga practice, but avoid stress and fatigue by relaxing mind and body and working with *sankalpa* for serenity and a positive attitude.

Back, neck and head pain

Pain and discomfort in these areas may be caused by poor posture, which can result from prolonged stress (feeling overwhelmed or defeated), lack of exercise and too much sitting.

Improving posture

Realigning the spine, gently and persistently through regular yoga practice, can change both posture and attitudes. Practise relaxation and chakra meditation (propped up to be upright and comfortable) to strengthen the positive aspects of the chakras – especially those in the region of the pain. Reduce stress by practising *alternate nostril breathing* and deep relaxation in any comfortable position. Work on the muscles that hold the spine in place with *body-mind breathing* and gentle isometric "muscle squeezing" to improve spinal posture and to reduce injury and the body's need to protect itself by going into spasm.

Lower back pain

Lie on the floor with knees bent to take all pressure off the spine. Move the spine gently to ease discomfort. The upturned beetle is also helpful: move the knees gently in all directions to ease the lower back. Move the head from side to side and loosen the shoulders for the upper back and neck. Keep the chin tucked in.

Headache

Pressure in the cervical or thoracic spine through habitually jutting the chin forward and/or slouching creates "traffic congestion" and is

▾ BACK PAIN CAN BE RELIEVED BY GENTLY MASSAGING YOUR SPINE AGAINST THE FLOOR.

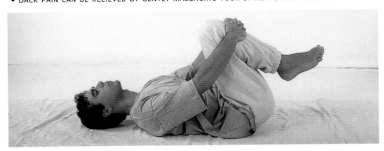

a common cause of headaches. Loosen the neck muscles with the head upside down in a forward bend, standing, sitting on a chair or lying prone over the edge of a bed. Take short yogic breaks between daily activities, especially those involving the eyes.

CARDIOVASCULAR/RESPIRATORY PROBLEMS

These conditions can result from prolonged stress, when the nervous system's fright-fight-flight response is switched on more or less permanently, ready for "action" and "excitement". Eventually the overused systems falter, while the underused systems are unable

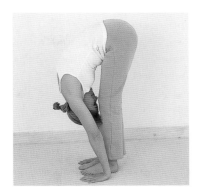

▲ INVERTED POSTURES CAN HELP A HEADACHE, BUT BE WARY IF YOU HAVE CARDIOVASCULAR OR RESPIRATORY PROBLEMS.

to provide essential nourishment, repair and recuperation. When the "all is well" response is blocked through prolonged stress we probably feel angry and exhausted. The yogic answer is to change our whole outlook upon life, to slow down yet keep as active as possible, and to learn to enjoy simple pleasures and a peaceful life.

Yoga exercise is helpful. Use your breath as a monitor, stopping if the breathing speeds up. Deep slow breathing, focusing on the OUT breath, induces a slow pulse rate and reduces stress. Avoid head-below-heart and arms-above-head positions if they make you feel breathless or dizzy. Relax and meditate regularly.

▼ TO CALM THE MIND, TRY THIS SIMPLE MEDITATION. LOOK AT A CANDLE FLAME, THEN CLOSE YOUR EYES, KEEPING THE IMAGE IN YOUR "MIND'S EYE" AS LONG AS YOU CAN.

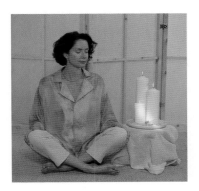

Depression

The term depression is often loosely used to describe anything from "feeling the blues" for a day or two to a prolonged and severe condition that requires medical treatment and supervision.

Yoga can alleviate this painful mental and emotional stress by rebalancing the Life, Light and Love energies. Focus on activating the Life chakras to increase vitality. Go for brisk walks and practise strong, invigorating standing postures to get the energy flowing. Depression can create deep fatigue, so exercise in short bursts with rests between each sequence – but do keep at it. Start and end your sessions with *alternate nostril breathing*. Avoid meditation and do not practise deep relaxation for longer than ten minutes, focusing on a positive *sankalpa*. Keep a spiritual diary to record and release distress. Re-read it periodically and notice how much yoga is lifting your spirits.

Digestive and other problems

The fright-fight-flight response, while revving up (and eventually exhausting) some systems, denies

▾ BE POSITIVE AND VALUE YOURSELF – YOU ARE ALWAYS YOUR OWN BEST FRIEND.

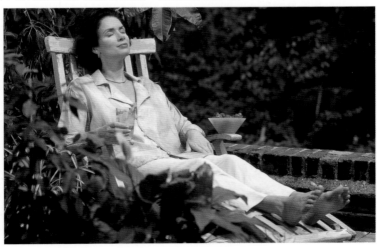

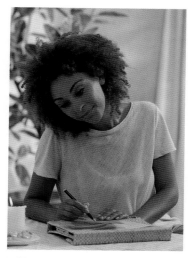

▲ WRITING THINGS DOWN EASES THE BURDEN ON THE MIND AND REDUCES ANXIETY.

Breathe deeply and relax often to reduce stress. Use *sankalpa* and meditate on the chakras and how both their positive and negative qualities promote or block the "all is well" response that creates healing and a balanced lifestyle.

▼ STANDING POSTURES CAN INVIGORATE AND LIFT YOUR SPIRITS.

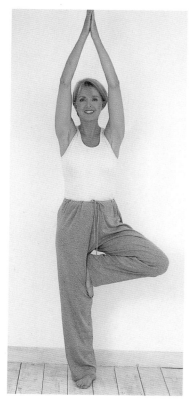

energy to all non-essential functions at the same time. If this response becomes your habitual pattern, many of the body's systems (such as the digestive, eliminatory and hormonal systems) become depleted and will then malfunction or become diseased.

Yoga helps to rebalance the nervous system and reduce anxiety (and therefore the production of adrenalin). Avoid lying prone, or putting pressure on the abdomen in postures. Improve spinal alignment with deep breathing. Practise yoga before eating.

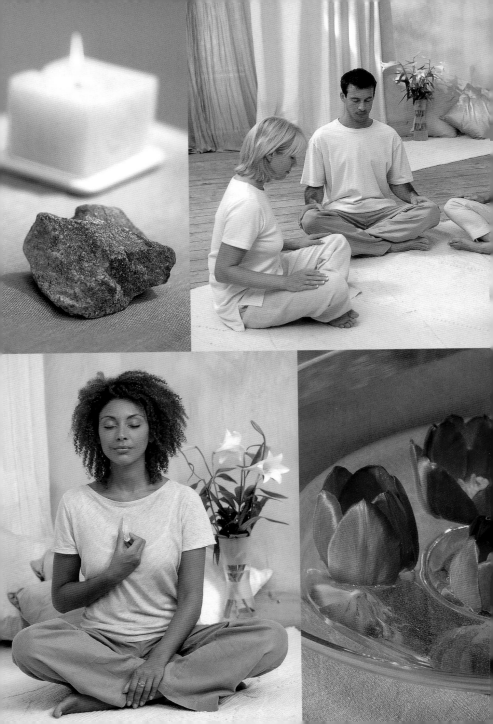

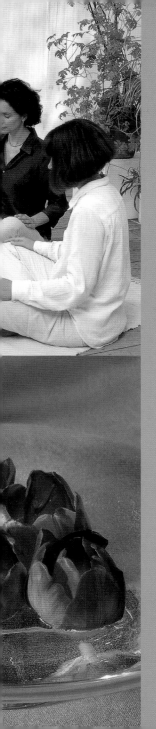

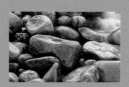

HEALING WITH
MEDITATION

Meditation can help to bring the body and mind into a state of harmony, so that relationships with people are more fruitful, work flows more efficiently and problems are more easily solved. It is a means by which to balance an active life with calming periods of inner reflection.

This chapter introduces you to a number of simple meditation techniques and offers you suggested ways in which to practise them. It provides guided meditations for specific purposes, such as those to help improve confidence and make important decisions. Whether at home, on a crowded train or in a busy office, you can let go of the stress in your life and bring yourself to a greater state of awareness and tranquillity,

What is meditation?

People have always had the need to seek inner peace and relaxation, for spiritual and health reasons and self-realization. By practising just 20 minutes a day, you can achieve and enjoy the wonderful benefits of meditation.

Just what is meditation? Most simply put, it is sitting and relaxing. Many people find that their lives are so full of the demands of work, family, friends and organized leisure pursuits that they have no time to "stand and stare". Some are so caught up in planning and working towards the future that they take little pleasure from the here and now. In their bustle to "get on", they miss out on the simple pleasures of life: the changing seasons, birds singing or children discovering the beauty of life.

Beauty and joy, however, can be experienced in the most industrial of landscapes or the most difficult living situations. Meditation is a good way of taking time out and allowing yourself to tune into and appreciate the moment, whether you happen to be walking along the seashore, sitting by a stream, or just noticing and enjoying the intensity of silence in a still room.

▼ MEDITATION CAN HELP YOU TO REACH YOUR INNER RESPONSES TO THE WORLD AROUND YOU.

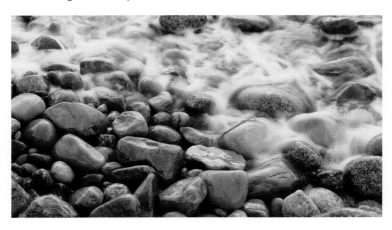

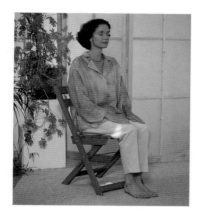

▲ SIT WITH YOUR FEET FLAT ON THE GROUND AND YOUR HANDS RESTING IN YOUR LAP.

GETTING COMFORTABLE

Rather than push yourself to adopt some strained physical position for meditation, just relax – sit in a chair or stroll through your favourite landscape at a steady pace. It is better not to slump or lie down when you are learning to meditate, as this could lull you into sleep: a state of relaxed attentiveness is what is desired. If you sit on a chair, do so with your feet flat on the floor, hands resting in your lap or on the arms of the chair, and your head comfortably balanced. If you are walking, take slow, careful steps – be aware of the movement of each foot, and its contact with the ground beneath.

BEING HERE AND NOW

Above all, meditation is about staying with the moment, about being in touch with your surroundings and your inner world. To experience this spirituality, you need not be a part of any organized religion. Although most religions do use some form of focused contemplation to promote spiritual awareness, meditation is also a technique that can be used for stress management or simply as a method to gain self-awareness.

Meditation is a pleasant way to gain deep relaxation, one in which you allow precious time for yourself. Simply meditating on a regular basis can be beneficial, but using words and images while practising can promote a marked improvement in your general well-being or in a specific area of life. It can even help you gain confidence when planning for upcoming events.

The benefits of meditation come from regular use. If under stress, you may find that meditating twice daily will restore composure and reduce irritability. It is best to allow at least ten, and ideally 20, minutes in meditation at each session.

A brief history of meditation

Meditation has been used throughout the world in all cultures. From informal reflection to the formal prayers held at retreats and on pilgrimages, meditation can lead us to a greater understanding and acceptance of ourselves and others.

In many people's minds, meditation is perhaps most closely linked with Buddhism – indeed, it was the main practice through which Buddhism's founder, Gautama, finally realized the state of enlightenment. Buddhism has defined many stages of meditation that are commonly practised for the purpose of achieving the ultimate level of purifying the mind and clearing away all thoughts and

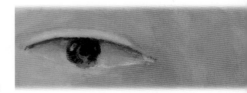

mental images. Meditation is a kind of "emptying" of the mind of distracting thoughts and ideas.

THE PRACTICE OF YOGA

From the Hindu tradition, one of the best-known practices of meditation is yoga, the yoking or harnessing of mental and physical powers. Most of us think in terms of "hatha" or royal yoga, which is a series of physical exercises and postures performed to gain physical, and therefore mental, control. Less well known is "bhakti" yoga – a focusing of the mind, a style that is akin to the meditation outlined in this book; this is practised in Christian religions, as well. According to this

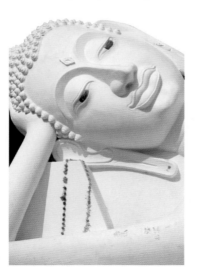

◀ A REPRESENTATION OF THE BUDDHA, WHICH FOLLOWERS USE AS A FOCUS FOR MEDITATION.

discipline, the practitioner sits and focuses his or her attention upon an aspect of their god. In doing so, they gain insights into their own responses to the

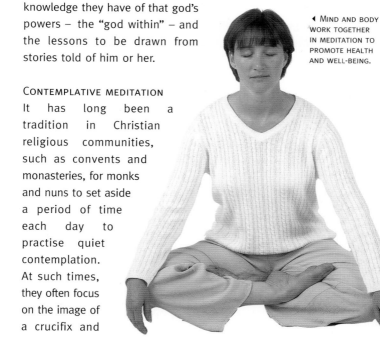

▲ MEDITATION IS A PART OF ALL THE WORLD'S RELIGIONS.

knowledge they have of that god's powers – the "god within" – and the lessons to be drawn from stories told of him or her.

CONTEMPLATIVE MEDITATION

It has long been a tradition in Christian religious communities, such as convents and monasteries, for monks and nuns to set aside a period of time each day to practise quiet contemplation. At such times, they often focus on the image of a crucifix and

contemplate the passion of Christ, and all that it symbolizes for the believer. This is, of course, meditation, and it has all the benefits of helping the individual come to an understanding of his or her inner beliefs and response to their faith. In recent years, the practice has also become increasingly popular among many lay Christians.

◀ MIND AND BODY WORK TOGETHER IN MEDITATION TO PROMOTE HEALTH AND WELL-BEING.

a brief history of meditation **585**

Mental and physical benefits

A potent physical and psychological therapy, meditation can be as strong as a commercial drug in helping the body and mind to keep illness and depression at bay. Practised regularly, it can promote a continued state of good health.

An individual emerging from a period of meditation, however brief, will notice a change in their emotional state from when they began the exercise. This can present itself in many ways, often as the sensation of being refreshed, with a more positive attitude and a general feeling of well-being. Situations and people that had been irritating and worrisome before may now be seen in a new and more positive way. The meditator may feel more in control, and less anxious.

These reactions have been known for years, but it is only in recent times that a physiological explanation has been available. Knowledge gained from brain scans and the measurement of brainwave patterns has given medical experts new information about the "alpha state" that results from meditation.

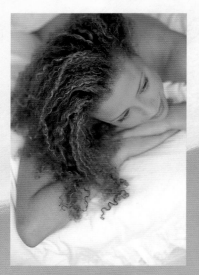

THE ALPHA STATE
When we are truly relaxed there are stages of change in the brainwave pattern, until it predominantly falls into the alpha state. Within this state, the brain triggers chemicals called endorphins – it is these substances that produce the feelings of well-being. Endorphins have even been called "nature's own opiates", and the good feelings that they induce can

◄ THE CHANGE IN BRAINWAVE PATTERNS CAUSED BY REGULAR MEDITATION CAN GIVE YOU A FEELING OF ALERT CALMNESS AND INCREASED MENTAL COMPOSURE.

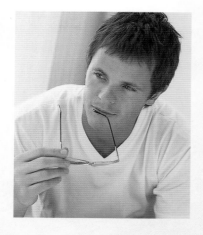

continue for some time after the meditation has ended. The length of time will vary from one individual to another.

There is also a very real physical benefit: since these same endorphins also boost the immune system, they help the body to fight infection and disease, promoting a state of enduring good health.

Meditation for a busy work life

The pressures of modern life often mean that people are so busy, they maintain a level of constant activity throughout the day. Not only are they stifling their emotional responses, they are also pushing their health to the limit.

Many experts on stress management emphasize the need for a period of mental and physical relaxation at different stages during the day. They point out that by taking this time out, one actually gains rather than loses when it comes to productivity, as the brain simply cannot maintain intense activity for long periods and remain efficient.

THE 20-MINUTE RULE

Writer Ernest Rossi has formulated the "20-minute rule", which is based on the theory of ultradian rhythms. Ultradian rhythms are biorhythms that the body works through during each day – a little like hyperbolic curves of energy that repeat every 90 to 120 minutes or so. Naturally, it would be best to work only at peak performance times, but in lieu of this, timing your work breaks to coincide with the mind/body slow-down pattern every 90 minutes ensures maximum productivity and inhibits the build-up of stress.

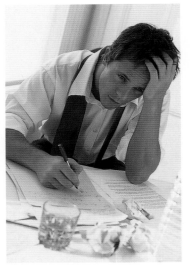

▲ STRESS CAN BECOME DAMAGING WHEN WE ARE NO LONGER ABLE TO CONTROL OUR RESPONSES TO IT.

Rossi suggested a pattern of working for 90 minutes and then taking a 20-minute break, so as to completely change the mind/body state. Ideally, you should stop all work activity and experience a change of physical status (stand rather than sit, look into the distance rather than close up, for example) and mental focus. A 20-minute meditation is ideal, and you should be able to feel the benefits instantly.

TAKE A BREAK

Is it coincidence that workers throughout the world have evolved breaks at approximately 90-minute intervals (coffee, lunch, tea)? This has grown up through experience, and has occurred in all types of work environment. On returning to work after the break, you will view tasks and challenges afresh and be able to deal with

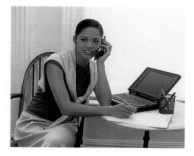

▲ MEDITATION HELPS YOU TO REMAIN CALM WHEN UNDER STRESS.

them more quickly and efficiently, as the mind and body are alert and ready to climb up to peak performance again on the biorhythmic curve. The feeling of well-being will continue well into the next 90-minute period.

Unfortunately, the intense demands of modern work practices, instant communication, and rising numbers of self-employed workers have meant that more people take their breaks at the desk, or ignore breaks altogether. This is a false economy, based on the premise that one can keep going indefinitely – in fact, it leads to greater inefficiency and is harmful to both the worker and their work.

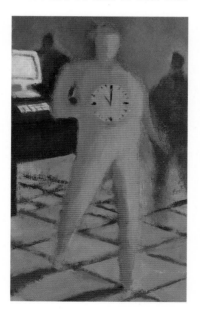

◀ BE AWARE OF YOUR BIOLOGICAL CLOCK THROUGHOUT THE WORKING DAY AND TRY TO TAKE A BREAK EVERY 90 MINUTES.

Gaining the meditative state: exercises

The first rule in approaching the meditative state is to learn to relax completely. When you stop working, the tension that has built up in your mind and body remains, and this must be diffused before you can benefit from rest.

A programme of exercises will loosen contracted muscles and make you feel refreshed, revitalized and physically relaxed. As well as unwinding the stresses in your body, exercise has the added benefit of releasing mental tension, so it can be a helpful prelude to every meditation session.

If strains and tensions are allowed to build up in the body, they may lead to a variety of aches and pains, as well as increasing mental strain and diminishing co-ordination and efficiency. A single session of exercises

for relaxation will instantly refresh and calm you. Loosening your muscles will also make you aware of areas of tension in your body, so that you can give some attention to the causes: improving your posture and the way you sit at your desk, or changing the shoes you wear when you are constantly on your feet.

Relaxation reduces not only muscular tension, but also rates of respiration and digestion, blood pressure and heart rate. It also increases the efficiency of the internal organs and the immune system.

▶ RELAX IN A POSITION THAT IS COMFORTABLE FOR YOU.

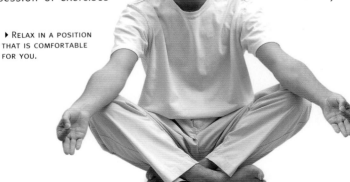

While it is vital to relieve tension when you feel it building up into aching or stiffness, it is better to avoid such a build-up by incorporating relaxation exercises into your daily routine. Use them to stretch stiff muscles when you get up in the morning, or during a mid-morning or afternoon break from work. At bedtime, taking a few minutes to release tension in your neck, back and shoulders will aid sound, relaxing sleep. Training your body to relax fully will calm your mind and prepare it for the meditative state.

STANDING RELAXATION EXERCISES FOR NECK, BACK AND SHOULDERS

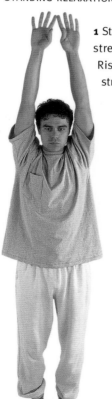

1 Stand upright with your arms stretched above your head. Rise up on your toes and stretch further still.

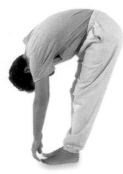

2 Drop forward, keeping your knees relaxed, and let your arms, head and shoulders hang heavy and loose for a while.

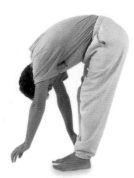

3 Shake your head and arms vigorously, then slowly return to a standing position. Repeat the exercise two or three times.

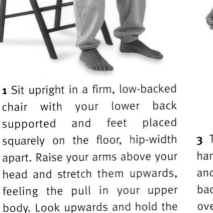

2 Drop forward, allowing your head and arms to relax completely. Return to the starting position and repeat the exercise, staying aware of the changing tensions in the muscles.

1 Sit upright in a firm, low-backed chair with your lower back supported and feet placed squarely on the floor, hip-width apart. Raise your arms above your head and stretch them upwards, feeling the pull in your upper body. Look upwards and hold the stretch for 20–30 seconds.

3 To stretch the back, link your hands together behind the chair, and lift your arms slightly. Lean back gradually, arching your back over the chair, hold for 10 seconds, then repeat.

The three "Ss" of meditation

When you begin to meditate, there are three things that you can focus on to make the process easier and more fluid. These will help you to "close off" the outside world and concentrate on the rich vastness of the inner world.

STILLNESS

Being able to sit relaxed and completely still is very important: it will enable you to drift into the state of awareness where your inner world can be reached and enjoyed. If you start to fidget or become aware that you are not comfortable, the stream of concentration will be broken. The ideal is to maintain stillness throughout the meditation.

SILENCE

Many people use personal stereos to try and block out the noise around them, but this can be very counterproductive: it is much better to meditate during a quiet time of day and learn to create inner silence. This will encourage your mind to see images and hear sounds coming from your inner self. The more you allow images and feelings to surface, the less you will be distracted. A teacher once said that when you can meditate on a busy railway platform, you will know you can really meditate.

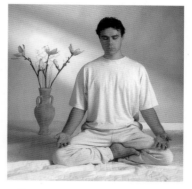

▲ MEDITATION IS THE BEST GATEWAY TO INNER WISDOM; FIND TIME EVERY DAY TO INCREASE YOUR ABILITY.

SENSITIVITY

When you begin any new meditation technique, it is important to listen, watch and perceive whatever images, symbols, sounds and other sensations appear in your mind. These may be vague and fleeting at first, but by noticing and focusing on them, you will aid the whole process. You will become more still and quiet, and your overall awareness will become sharper – in meditation and, eventually, in the rest of your life.

Breathing and meditation

The power of proper breathing should not be underestimated – it oxygenates the blood, aiding thought processes and boosting physical energy. It also assists the flow of toxins out of the bloodstream, thus reducing the effects of stress.

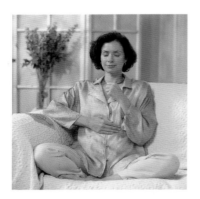

▲ COUNT EACH BREATH FROM ONE TO TEN.

In meditation, your breath provides an ever-present and easily accessible focus on which to concentrate – you are always breathing. Many schools of meditation advocate using the breath in various ways, such as imagining that the breath originates at certain points in the body. The areas usually focused on are the "hara" just below the navel and the "tan tien", the heart in the centre of the chest. The crown of the head, the base of the spine and the soles of the feet may all be included in the awareness.

There are many ways of concentrating the mind in order to distract the inner "voice" that chatters incessantly, worrying and becoming obsessive about problems or people:

• Slowly count your breaths, from one to ten.

• Notice the physical changes at the nostrils and the abdomen, as your breath moves in and out.

• Notice the inner stillness as you change from exhalation to inhalation, from inhalation to exhalation.

• Conjure up an image that evokes a feeling of joy and serenity. This could be a beautiful natural scene with mountains or ocean waves, the sun's rays or a child. Breathe the image into your heart.

◀ IMAGINE EACH BREATH ORIGINATES AT THE HEART.

CHAKRA-BALANCING MEDITATION

The following exercise is a powerful way of activating and balancing personal energies, thus improving your overall health and wellbeing.

1 Sit comfortably, with your spine straight and relaxed. Breathe from your lower abdominal area and focus your attention on the first chakra, at the base of your spine. Imagine that you are breathing in and out of this point, and sense the external energies brought in by your breath.

2 Bring your attention to your second chakra, above the genitals, and repeat the process.

3 Continue the exercise through all the chakras, until you reach the crown chakra. You may find that with some of the chakras, the energies are a bit stagnant and a little extra time and attention is needed to bring them into focus.

4 Now review each chakra in turn, from bottom to top, and imagine you are unblocking the natural energy flow in each and redressing the balance between them.

5 Be aware that the base chakra connects you to the earth and the crown chakra to cosmic energies; sense the integration between your physical and spiritual energies with that of the whole universe.

◀ FOCUS ON THE CHAKRAS INDIVIDUALLY AND BREATHE IN AND OUT AT THE POINT OF EACH ONE.

Postures for meditation

Meditation is a personal experience, but one that you need not practise in private. You can meditate almost anywhere – on the bus, in the park, or sitting at your desk – but it is important to find a position that feels comfortable for you.

When choosing a position in which to meditate, remember that you should feel relaxed without drifting off to sleep. In addition, you should be able to remain still for the period of meditation without experiencing any numbness or cramp in your limbs, as this would be distracting and counterproductive. Experiment with the following suggestions until you discover which position feels best for you.

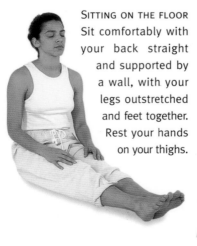

SITTING ON YOUR HEELS
This posture is a good one for your back, as it keeps the spine straight. Your feet should be relaxed, with the toes pointing backwards. Rest your hands lightly on your lap. Put a cushion underneath your feet if you wish.

SITTING ON THE FLOOR
Sit comfortably with your back straight and supported by a wall, with your legs outstretched and feet together. Rest your hands on your thighs.

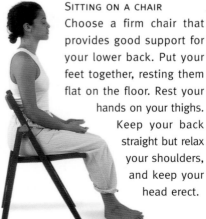

SITTING ON A CHAIR
Choose a firm chair that provides good support for your lower back. Put your feet together, resting them flat on the floor. Rest your hands on your thighs. Keep your back straight but relax your shoulders, and keep your head erect.

The Lotus Position

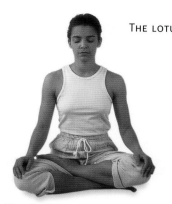 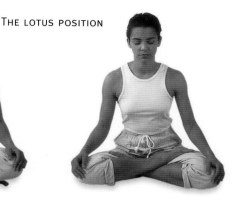

1 The half-lotus is the simpler version: bend one leg so that the foot rests under the opposite inner thigh. Place the second foot on top of the thigh of the first leg. Keep the spine upright, and rest the hands lightly on the knees.

2 To achieve the full lotus position, one leg should be bent with the foot resting on top of your other thigh; then bend your other leg so that the foot crosses over the first leg on to the opposite thigh.

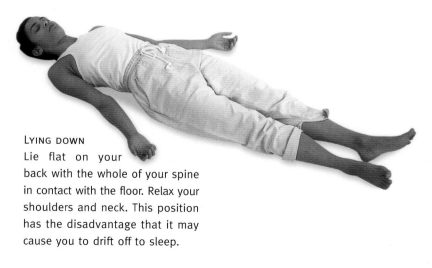

Lying Down
Lie flat on your back with the whole of your spine in contact with the floor. Relax your shoulders and neck. This position has the disadvantage that it may cause you to drift off to sleep.

Using sounds

Many adherents of transcendental meditation and religious groups talk of using a sound to assist with meditation. The repetition of a phrase, a word or a sound creates the alpha state by an almost hypnotic focus upon the sound.

An effortless sound, repeated with the natural rhythm of breathing, can have the same soothing, mentally liberating effect as the constant natural sound of running water, rustling leaves or a beating heart. The single sound, or mantra as it is known, is used to blot out the chatter of intrusive thoughts, allowing the mind to find repose.

Speaking or chanting a mantra as a stream of endless sound is a very ancient method of heightening an individual's awareness by concentrating the senses. The simple gentle sound "om" or "aum" is sometimes known as the first mantra, which is literally an instrument of thought. From the ancient Hindu language, the curving Sanskrit symbol for this primordial word represents the states of consciousness: waking, dreaming, deep dreamless sleep and the transcendental state.

The Hare Krishna movement is well known for its chant, which is repeated over and over again,

and can lead its members to become "high" – again the effects of endorphin release. However, the sound need not be a special word or incantation; something simple and meaningful will be just as effective. Any word that appeals to you will do, repeated with the outflow of breath – silently in the mind, or spoken out loud.

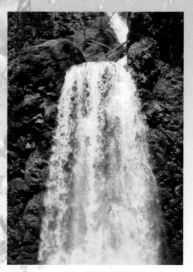

▲ The constant, yet variable sound of running water can be especially soothing and therapeutic.

Using touch

You can use your sense of touch in a soothing way to induce a state of meditation when you are under stress. Young children do this when they take a smooth ribbon or blanket end to hold and manipulate whenever they feel tense.

For centuries in the Middle East, people have benefited from the soothing sense of touch by using strings of worry beads: these are passed rhythmically through the fingers during times of stress and difficulty, in order to focus the mind and calm anxiety. The beads' uniform size, gentle round shapes, smooth surfaces and rhythmic, orderly clicking as they pass along their string all assist the state of mind.

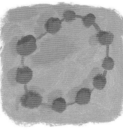

◀ FEEDING WORRY BEADS THROUGH YOUR FINGERS CAN HELP TO FOCUS AND CALM THE MIND.

such as a favourite velvet or silk scarf, which you can feed slowly from one hand to the other as you concentrate on clearing your mind.

You can use one or two smooth, rounded stones or crystals in the same way, passing them from one hand to the other, and concentrating on their temperature, shape and surface.

Alternatively, choose an object with a soothing and tactile quality that particularly appeals to you,

▶ THE SMOOTH FEEL OF A SILK SCARF BETWEEN YOUR HANDS MAY HELP TO LULL YOU INTO THE MEDITATIVE STATE.

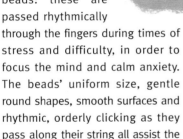

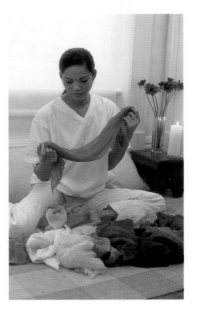

Using colours

Some colours are associated with relaxation. Summoning up and concentrating on these can be a helpful way to clear the mind of tension. They can be an ideal entry into the quiet of a meditation session.

Sit with your eyes closed, and be aware of the first colour that comes into your mind: it may be any colour of the rainbow – though red and purple are common. Slowly let the colour change to blue or green, allowing it to fill the whole of your mind's eye and replace all other colours; pink hues are also beneficial. A feeling of relaxation will grow as the new colour builds in your mind. When it is complete, you will experience pleasant feelings of inner peace and stillness.

BREATHING IN COLOUR
You can help the colour to build by associating it with your breathing. Establish a comfortable rhythm of breathing, and focus on it until your mind is clear. Allow the colour to fill your mind's eye; then, as you breathe in, imagine the colour filling your body, from the soles of your feet right up to the top of your head.

▶ TRY TO BECOME AWARE OF THE WONDERFUL COLOURS OF THE NATURAL WORLD, SUCH AS IN THIS FIELD OF BRIGHTLY COLOURED TULIPS.

COLOUR VISUALIZATION EXERCISE
Shut your eyes and breathe calmly and regularly, focusing on your breathing. As you inhale, imagine that you are sitting on a soft lawn in a peaceful garden. Sense the cool freshness of the green surrounding you. As you exhale, imagine the silken magenta of a rose. Breathe in again and let the cleansing green fill your mind. Repeat this exercise once or twice, then sit quietly for a few moments.

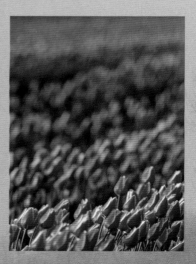

COLOUR PROPERTIES

Colours are associated with various qualities, so choose a colour to suit your current needs. Its complementary colour is shown in brackets. Often meditators visualize moving from their chosen colour to its complement – a way of creating change. Or they may move from one colour to another to gain these qualities.

- Red: vitality, energy, strength and will power (turquoise)
- Orange: happiness and laughter (blue)
- Yellow: intellect and objectivity (violet)
- Green: cleansing and harmony (magenta)

- Turquoise: strengthens the immune system, counteracts disease (red)
- Blue: peace and relaxation, restful sleep (orange)
- Violet: beauty, dignity, self-respect (yellow)
- Magenta: release of obsessional thoughts and memories (green)

The numbers game

This is a simple meditation that uses a blackboard – real or imaginary. It is a good "game" to use with children, to give them an experience of meditation. Practised after bath-time, it is an ideal way to relax in the evening.

The game is presented as if you are leading a group of children, but it can be easily used by an adult. It is an excellent way to clear the mind through concentration, imagination and patterns, all of which are wonderful ways of gaining a real experience of deep meditation.

1 Ask the participants to sit or lie down in a relaxed position. Once they have found a really comfortable position, tell them to remember it, and then ask them to sit up. Tell them they are going to return to their relaxed positions in just a few moments.

2 With chalk on the blackboard, draw a diagram of numbers, three lines by three columns, making sure that there are no mathematical links, like this:

3	1	5
8	6	9
4	7	2

▶ EVEN CHILDREN CAN ENJOY AND BENEFIT FROM MEDITATION EXERCISES.

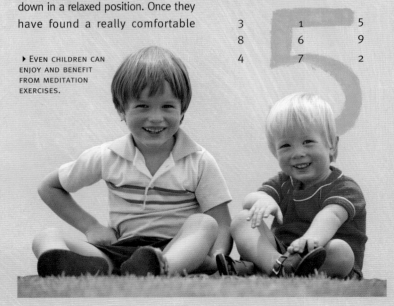

3 Give the children one minute — be sure that they see you are timing it — to memorize this pattern in lines and columns. They will be working with this later in their mind's eye (the imaginary screen on the inside of the forehead).

4 Ask them to return to their relaxed position, with their eyes closed. Tell them to concentrate on the numbers and, if anything else comes into their mind, to recognize it and push it away (repeat this often during the session).

5 Rub out lines or columns of numbers, telling the children what you are doing and asking them to do the same in their mind's own diagram — do this slowly. Keep the pace of your speech slow, too. Give them time to adjust, and tell them what is left as a check, for example, "That leaves just four numbers." Continue until they reach the last number, and say "Really concentrate on that number." Then take a long pause.

6 Rub out the last number, saying "Now concentrate on what is left." Let them remain in silence until you notice a restlessness — this is often after three or more minutes.

7 Wake them gently, by speaking in a soft voice becoming louder with an instruction to "Sit up." Ask them what the last number was and for their reactions.

The haven

Once you have managed to achieve a state of complete physical relaxation and calm, allow your mind to enter a place that is special to you. Whether real or imaginary, you will be able to rest and feel good about yourself in this place.

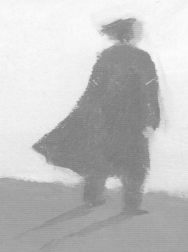

▲ CLOSE YOUR EYES AND ALLOW YOUR MIND TO DRIFT OFF TO YOUR FAVOURITE REFUGE FOR PEACE AND RELAXATION.

Where is this special place? It may be lying in bed, in a warm bath, or a place that you visited when you were a child, in a quiet corner of a wood, or a secret room in a ruined castle, where you found yourself suddenly away from all other people. Perhaps it is a windswept beach, where pieces of driftwood wash up on the sand. Whether a real or an imaginary place, it is somewhere you really can relax, safe and secure.

Go to your special place . . . feel what made it appeal to you . . . what makes it special still . . . It belongs only to you, so you can think and do whatever you like here . . . In this safe, secure place no one and nothing can ever bother you. Allow yourself to realize that this is a haven, a unique haven of tranquillity and safety, where you will always feel able to relax completely . . .

Now you can allow your mind to drift . . . drift. Notice what kind of light shines through the

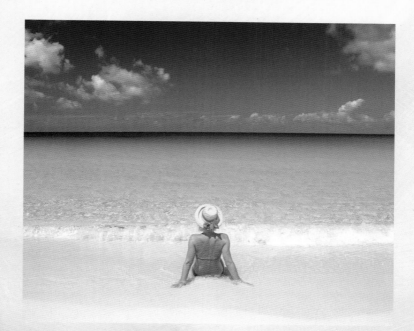

branches or the drifting clouds or in through the window . . . Is it bright or hazy or dim? . . . Does the temperature feel soothingly warm or refreshingly cool? . . . What sounds do you hear? Distant voices, or perhaps birds singing . . . Be aware of the colours that surround you . . . the shapes . . . and textures . . . the familiar objects that make that place special. You can just be there . . . whether sitting, lying or reclining, enjoying the sounds . . . the smells . . . the atmosphere . . .

▲ CONJURE UP A TIME AND PLACE, REAL OR IMAGINARY, TO ADOPT AS YOUR SPECIAL MEDITATIVE PLACE.

No one is asking anything of you here . . . no one expects anything of you . . . you do not need to do anything . . . you have no need to be anywhere . . . except here in this peaceful place, where everything is perfectly calm and you can truly let yourself . . . relax. Breathe in the quiet solitude and feel completely at one with your tranquil private place.

A guided visit to a country house

This meditation takes you on a tour of a beautiful, old, country estate. Imagine that you are visiting a sprawling stately home, on a warm summer's afternoon. Begin by standing at the top of the wide staircase that leads down into the entrance hall.

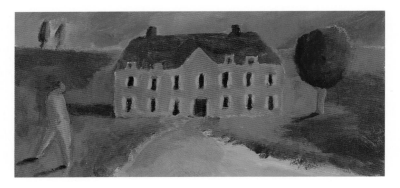

▲ PICTURE YOURSELF IN THE GROUNDS OF A STUNNING STATELY HOME.

As you look down across the entrance hall, you can just glimpse a gravel drive through the open doors opposite, and sunlight on the gravel. There is no one around to bother you as you stand poised to descend the staircase . . .

You slowly begin to ease down the steps, and now you are moving down the last ten steps to the hallway, relaxing more as each foot reaches the next step:

10 Taking one step down, relax and let go . . .

9 Taking the next step down, feel at ease . . .

8 Becoming even more relaxed . . .

let go even more . . .

7 Drifting deeper . . . and deeper . . . and even deeper down still . . .

6 Becoming calmer . . . and calmer . . . even calmer still . . .

5 Continuing to relax . . .

4 Relaxing further, let go even more . . .

3 Sinking deeper, drifting further into this welcoming, relaxed state . . .

2 Enjoy these good feelings, feelings of inner peace . . .

1 Nearly all the way down, feeling very good . . . feeling beautifully relaxed . . . and **0**.

You are wandering across that hallway now, towards the open doors and the gardens beyond, soaking up the atmosphere of peace and permanence in this lovely old building. You wander out through the doors and down the stone steps . . . and find yourself standing on a wide gravel drive that leads from the lush green lawns . . . and the shrubs and trees, towards the entrance gates. Notice the different shades of green and brown against a clear, blue sky . . . You can feel the sun's warmth on your head and shoulders on this beautiful afternoon . . . There are flowerbeds with splashes of colour happily bobbing in the gentle breeze. And there's nobody else about . . . no one needing anything, no one wanting anything and

▾ WALK STEADILY DOWN THE PATH, AWARE OF ALL THE COLOURS, SCENTS AND SOUNDS.

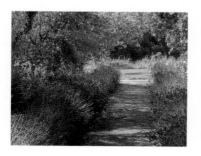

nobody expecting anything from you . . . You can enjoy the serenity and solitude of this pleasant garden that has existed for centuries.

Further down the driveway, you notice an ornamental fish pond. You wander down, with nothing disturbing the stillness of the afternoon but the crunch of the gravel as it moves beneath your feet, and the occasional bird song from far away . . . You are wandering down towards the fish pond, soaking up the atmosphere of the myriad flowers and butterflies.

Eventually . . . eventually you find yourself standing close to the edge of the fish pond, looking down into the clear, cool, shallow water, just gazing at the fish . . . large ornamental goldfish of red and gold, black and silver, swimming so easily . . . gliding so effortlessly among the pondweed, in and out of shadows and around the lily pads. Sometimes they seem almost to disappear behind the weed and shadows . . . but always they reappear, their scales catching the sunlight: red, gold, silver, black . . .

And as you stare at the fish, your mind becomes even more deeply relaxed . . .

a guided visit to a country house **607**

The well

This continues from the previous visualization of the country house. It is intended to take you to even deeper levels of meditation. Alternatively, you can use it just on its own to focus the mind, using the clarity and depth of the water.

As you watch the fish, you notice that the centre of the pond is very, very deep. It could be the top of a disused well . . .

You take from your pocket a silver coin and, with great care, toss the coin so that it lands over the very centre of the pond . . . then watch as it swivels down through the water. The ripples drift out to the edges of the pond, but you just watch the coin as it drifts and sinks, deeper and deeper through that cool, clear water, twisting and turning . . . Sometimes it seems to disappear as it turns on edge; at other times a face of the coin catches the sunlight and flashes through the water . . . sinking, drifting deeper and deeper, twisting and turning as it makes its way down.

Finally, it comes to rest at the bottom of the well, lying on a cushion of soft mud, a silver coin in the still, clean water . . .

And you feel as still and undisturbed as the coin . . . as still and cool and motionless as the water, enjoying the feeling of inner peace and utter tranquillity.

▼ WATCH THE SPREADING RIPPLES AS THE COIN LANDS IN THE CENTRE OF THE POND.

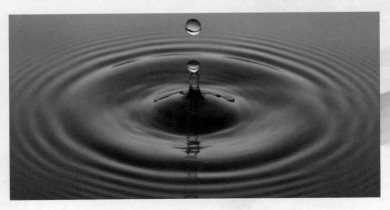

A mountain

Once you can reach a state of complete relaxation, you can use this time to focus your attention in various ways. You may meditate on an image to gain insights and self-knowledge. The mountain is a potent symbol for overcoming obstacles.

The mountain has existed for thousands of years . . . it stands tall . . . still . . . silent . . . and regal. Pushing up against the bright blue sky, nestled in-between the white, white clouds that drift past, its ancient ragged peak endures . . . for years . . . and centuries . . . and millennia. Nothing can shake the stillness of the mountain, its underlying rock made to last forever, its trees towering into the mist, their ever-changing cycles of life . . . beginning, ending, beginning again . . . Animals live among the trees and munch the plants tucked in the crevices . . . deer dwell here . . . birds nest up on the high rocks near the cliffs . . . and at the top of the mountain, at the very highest point, the air is crystal clear, imbued with the purest, invigorating oxygen . . . At the very highest point, the world stretches out before you, a vast tapestry of towns and lakes and continents . . . and as the sun sinks into the horizon, the infinite and uncountable stars glisten in a sky that stretches on forever . . . and forever . . . and forever.

▼ A MOUNTAIN MEDITATION HELPS YOU TO PUT PROBLEMS INTO PERSPECTIVE.

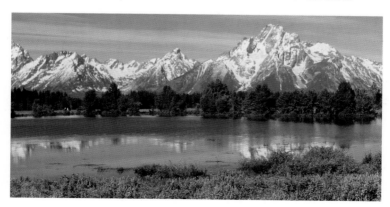

A flower

In this meditation, place a real flower in front of you. Use your chosen technique to obtain inner quiet. Now open your eyes and focus on the flower, a symbol of growth and rebirth. If you find thoughts or words developing, let them flow naturally.

Consider a single flower, in full bloom, the colour in the petals, the connection to the stalk, how each petal is formed, and the differences and similarities there. How natural and beautiful it is, the shading and subtle changes caused by the light . . . This flower is at its peak of perfection . . . soon the petals will open and then fall . . . a seed pod will develop there . . . the seeds will scatter . . . some will find earth in which to rest, and in the natural cycle of things will stay dormant . . . until the time is right . . . The light and temperature trigger new growth . . . a tiny shoot will develop and grow, emerging from the soil . . . larger leaves will unfold, then a stalk carrying a tiny green bud will emerge, and as this swells

◀ THE NATURAL CYCLE OF BIRTH, GROWTH, DEATH AND REBIRTH.

through the casing, the flower bud will appear . . . and form into another flower just like this one, and light and shade will allow its true beauty to be enjoyed again . . . Natural beauty . . . colour . . . light . . . shade . . . perpetual change . . . the seasons . . . death . . . decay . . . rebirth . . . growth . . . perfection . . . the natural cycle of living things.

▶ FOCUS YOUR MIND UPON A BEAUTIFUL, EXOTIC FLOWER IN FULL BLOOM.

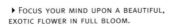

A clock ticking

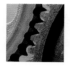

The hands of a clock record the passage of time: time never stands still, but our perception of it can change. Past – present – future, the clock registers the moments of life moving forward. Focusing on the image of a clock can be very therapeutic.

The clock ticks . . . the hands move . . . so slowly . . . always moving . . . seconds tick away . . . The one just past is over . . . a new second takes its place . . . it too is replaced . . . as time moves on. Each moment lasts for just a second . . . The clock may stop . . . time never stops . . . it moves on . . . and on . . . The moment that is over is out of reach . . . the moment to come has not yet arrived, but . . . this moment . . . is all MINE . . . this moment I can use exactly as I wish . . . I focus on this moment . . . I influence this moment . . . I can use this moment . . . and no other NOW!

Measurement . . . movement . . . monitoring . . . invention . . . mechanism . . . complexity . . . regularity . . . cogs . . . gears . . . chains . . . weights . . . pendulum . . . interaction . . . perpetual motion . . . never still . . . always moving . . . on and on . . . into the next moment . . . into infinity . . . for ever.

▼ YOU ARE ONLY ABLE TO INFLUENCE THE PRESENT MOMENT, SO TRY TO STAY FOCUSED ON THE HERE AND NOW.

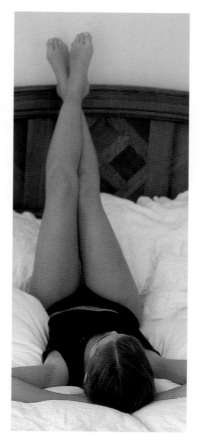

A bird

This meditation is effective when you feel cares weighing you down, curtailing your freedom. It is even more effective when done outside in the fresh air. If you have the chance to watch a real bird, follow its flight as far as you can.

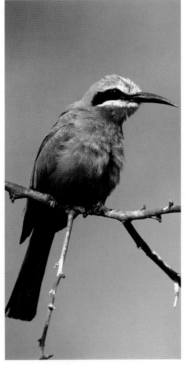

◀ Picture a colourful bird perched on top of a tall tree.

it sang . . . soaring upwards and upwards . . . coasting through the serene blue sky . . . skimming the feather-light clouds so effortlessly. It doesn't have a care in the world . . . all its attention is concentrated on flying . . . swooping . . . swerving in and out of the clouds so gracefully . . . For the moment, it forgets about finding food for its mate and its chicks . . . for the moment, it is free to play . . . to glide . . . to sail through the huge swathe of azure, lost in the pure joy of flying . . . lost in the happiness of being alive . . .

A bird perches at the top of a tall tree . . . it sings . . . sings a song to its mate . . . sings a song to its chicks . . . Suddenly, it flutters its wings and takes off. Flying, it finds itself high above the tree in which

▲ Follow the flight and movements of a bird as far as your eye can see.

A picture

This can be a way of bringing the outside world into your meditation, or coming to an understanding of another person's point of view of the world. Let your mind do the work for you, and you can be sure it will stimulate new and exciting insights.

Select a picture with an evocative scene. It might be a religious, historical or allegorical scene, or simply an image of a landscape that appeals to you, but it should be representative of the outside world in some form. Try not to choose something too harsh and dark in its subject matter, so you feel at ease.

Now allow your mind to gain a meditative state whilst focusing on the image in front of you. Let the colours wash over you and allow your mind to wander as if you were actually able to traverse the canvas and enter the scene in the picture.

Every picture tells a story. It might be the story as seen by the artist or photographer, or it might seek to tell a tale as seen by the subjects of the image – as told in their expressions and responses to the scene around them. The viewer of the picture might reach a totally different interpretation to the former two. All versions are completely valid, and this meditation should allow your thoughts to rest upon all the different possibilities of the picture: the total scene, a single aspect of it, or the making of it as envisaged by its original creator.

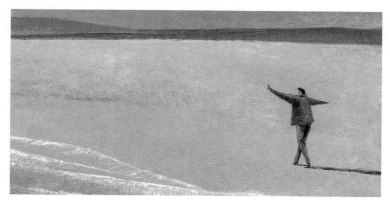

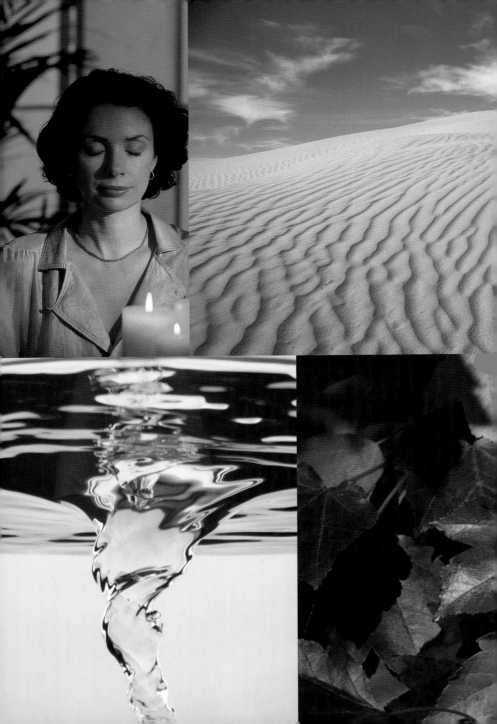

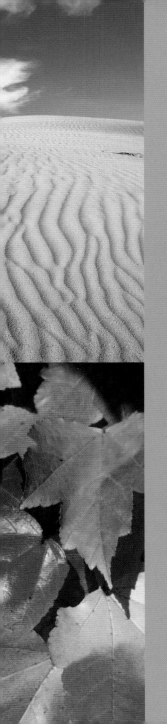

HEALING
MEDITATIONS

Now you have mastered the techniques for gaining the meditative state, you are ready to tackle specific problems in your life. Following the healing meditations given in this section, draw on your knowledge of postures, colour properties, chakras, affirmations and visualizations to focus the mind on a variety of tasks, whether this is to energize or relax the body, cleanse the mind or complete a challenge, forget the past or take exciting decisions about the future.

Don't try to learn everything by heart in one go. You may find it easier to record the exercises on tape, so that you can concentrate on gaining the images, or focusing attention, without worrying about forgetting a passage or having to refer to the appropriate page.

For cleansing the mind

Meditating lets you focus on yourself with greater clarity. It allows you to sift through all your scattered energies, and release thoughts and desires you no longer need. Try this exercise to cleanse your psyche with healing rays of colour.

1 Close your eyes and imagine that you are sitting in a green meadow. A cool, crystal-clear stream runs nearby, with abundant fragrant flowers all around. It is a fine, bright day with a gentle breeze; the sky is blue, with a scattering of soft, white clouds.

2 Choose a colour that you need (see Colour Properties) for your personal healing and well-being.

3 Choose one of the clouds above you and fill it with the colour until it starts to shimmer with its sparkling light.

4 Let the cloud float over you. Allow it to release a coloured shower that envelops you with a sweet, sparkling mist, like stars cascading in all directions.

5 The mist settles on your skin and is gently absorbed, until it has completely saturated your system with its healing vibration.

6 Allow the hue to run through your bloodstream for 3–4 minutes,

giving your body a therapeutic colour wash.

7 Let the pores of your skin open so that the coloured vapour can escape, taking any toxins with it. When the vapour runs clear, close your pores again.

8 Sit quietly with your cleared, healed body and mind for a few minutes. Take three deep breaths, releasing each gently, then open your eyes.

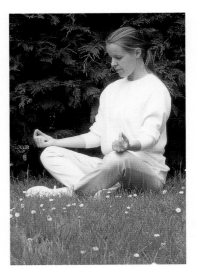

▶ MEDITATE OUT OF DOORS TO CONNECT TO YOUR HIGHER SPIRITUAL DIMENSION.

For maintaining stamina

In this meditation, you will use the enlivening colour gold to recharge your body and mind, letting its warmth restore your physical energy and lift your spirits. It is perfect for use in the midst of an active period, to help restore or maintain stamina.

1 Recline in a comfortable position and take a deep breath in. When you inhale, imagine yourself lying on a floating sunbed on the ocean or in a swimming pool, gently moving with the waves of the water.

2 Look up at the sky – it is pale blue, with an arch of pure gold, high up. Focus on this shimmering band of sun-gold.

3 After a few moments, allow the arch to vibrate gently, so that cascades of its sparkling golden crystals float gently towards you.

4 As they lightly touch your body, the crystals turn to golden dew drops that are absorbed into your skin.

5 Feel the internal warmth deep within you, as the golden hue surges through you, warming your body and soul and creating a wonderful glow.

6 Take a deep breath and, as you exhale, slowly open your eyes. Feel the way in which your mind and body have been recharged and revitalized.

For personal development

Affirmations are a deceptively simple device that can be used by anyone, and they prove remarkably effective. Try using this method while in the meditative state, having previously planned and memorized the affirmations involved.

In using affirmations with meditation, you combine ease of communication with all parts of the mind and the effectiveness of repeated powerful phrases. The technique requires you to say to yourself, out loud, a positive statement about yourself as you wish to be. In order to make your affirmations effective, they should:

• be made in the present tense
• be positively phrased
• have an emotional reward.

If you notice what happens if you are asked not to think of elephants, you will realize why negatives (the words "no", "not", "never" and so on) have the opposite effect to that intended. Yours is the most influential voice in your life, because you believe it! Be aware of any negative statements that you make regularly about yourself, either to others or to yourself – "I am shy", "I am lacking in confidence", "I cannot", "I get easily nervous when . . ." and so on. These are all self-limiting beliefs that you reinforce each time they slip into your conversation or mind. Now you will be able to use affirmations whenever you are meditating in order to change those beliefs: "I am strong", "I am able to do this", "I feel really confident when . . . "

▲ AFFIRMATIONS CHANGE THE WAY YOU THINK ABOUT YOURSELF AND THE WAY YOU ACT AND REACT.

For peak performance

 Visualization requires you to imagine yourself behaving, reacting and looking as you would wish to do in a given situation. This could be at an interview or a social gathering – any situation where peak performance is important to you.

In the same way that you can utilize your voice, so you can use your imagination. The imagination can stimulate emotions and can instil new attitudes in the mind. It can be a direct communication with your unconscious mind, and it can provide a powerful influence for improvements in your attitudes, behaviour patterns and overall confidence.

Imagine yourself at an important event. What will it mean for you? What will your reactions and those of people around you be? Most importantly, feel all the good feelings that will occur.

Imagination is like playing a video of the event in the mind's eye, from the beginning of the situation through to the perfect outcome. Get in touch with the feelings that will be there when you reach that outcome. Should any doubts or negative images creep into your "video", push them away and replace them with positive ones. Keep the scenario realistic, and base it upon real information from your past. Once you are happy with the images you are seeing, note the way you are standing and presenting yourself. Then allow yourself to view the scene from inside your imagined self. Now you can get in touch with the feelings and attitudes that will make the event successful. The best time to do this is when you are relaxed mentally and physically – during meditation. Teach yourself to expect new, positive outcomes. This can be combined with affirmations, to make the exercise doubly effective.

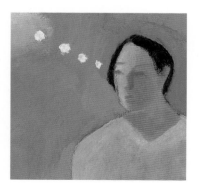

▶ REHEARSE THE FORTHCOMING EVENT IN YOUR MIND'S EYE SO THAT YOU ARE FULLY PREPARED.

For leaving troubles behind

This meditation, known as the "railway tunnel", is particularly helpful in leaving troubles behind, gaining perspective and focusing on the here and now. It can be very effective after the break-up of a relationship, loss of job or any major change.

Imagine yourself strolling along a straight flat path. It's a dull, cloudy, drizzly day. The path is leading between two high banks. There is damp grass beneath your feet, and you can see the cloudy sky above. You feel the weight of a heavy backpack on your shoulders, making your steps heavy and slow, and you seem to be looking at the ground in front of you as you trudge along the path, feeling damp and cold. You glance up and notice the entrance to an old railway tunnel: this must be a disused railway line. As you look, you can see a point of light at the other end of the tunnel, so it can't be too long. As you approach the entrance, the tunnel seems very dark, but that small circle of light at the far end is reassuring . . . At first it seems very dark, but the floor feels even and it is easy to walk along. As you do so, all those old doubts about yourself begin to surface; you are aware of your own failings, regrets and missed opportunities . . . Just

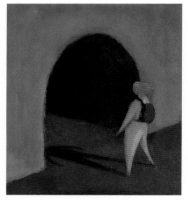

▲ IMAGINE YOURSELF ENTERING A DARK TUNNEL AND WALKING TOWARDS A CIRCLE OF LIGHT AT THE FAR END.

let them come gently to the surface of your mind. The backpack is getting a little lighter as these doubts and regrets surface, gently and easily . . .

You keep walking and notice a pool of light on the floor ahead . . . there must be an air shaft there. As you go through the pool of light, you suddenly remember a happy time, when someone really enjoyed your company . . . a time when you felt really good about being you. As you move into the darkness again, you feel lighter still; the backpack is emptying.

The circle of light at the end of the tunnel is growing, but here is another air shaft, with light penetrating the gloom. Again, as you pass through that light, another good memory of being appreciated for who you are, being praised or complimented, comes into your mind. Now you are back in the gloom, but it doesn't seem as intense as before. It is getting lighter and warmer with each step, and you experience more good memories of those who have loved you and happy events . . . As you near the end of the tunnel, you notice that the sun must be shining, and you feel so much lighter, as if you have lost that backpack altogether. A pleasant warmth begins to replace any traces of damp and cold that you felt before.

Eventually, you step out into the bright sunshine with a light tread, valuing yourself and the world much more. You realize you have so many opportunities awaiting you, and new chances to do things that make you feel good about yourself, building upon those positive events of the past. Your contribution is important – you are a valuable human being.

▾ WALK OUT OF THE TUNNEL INTO A BRIGHTER, LIGHTER WORLD.

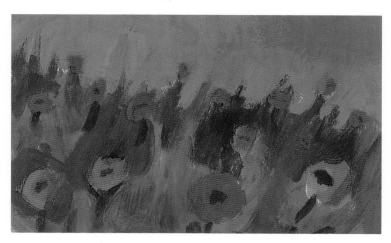

For relaxation

Having trained yourself to meditate, you can utilize your "triggers" – evocative words and images – to take you back into a state of relaxation. If you have imagined a certain place, for example, doing so again will give you the same positive feelings.

It may be that you are aware of certain physical symptoms during meditation, such as a tingling sensation in the hands or feet: this may be a useful trigger, too. Imagine that you feel those symptoms, and within seconds you will gain the sensations and feelings associated with meditation. This can be especially useful before an important meeting, or any occasion about which you may be feeling a little apprehensive. Use the trigger to gain the calm confidence you need and to put things into their proper perspective. With practice, your mind will accept the training and linkages you have created during meditation, and will respond to these same signals at any time, quickly and easily, giving you instant access to all the benefits that come with deep relaxation.

▼ MEDITATION IS EXCELLENT FOR RECHARGING THE BATTERIES AND REDISCOVERING VITALITY, ENERGY AND WELL-BEING.

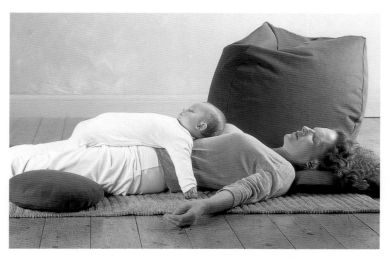

For confidence in meetings

The meditative state, affirmations and visualization can all create a valuable preparation for a future event. Athletes use the power of these "rehearsal techniques" in training, and you can use them to achieve optimum performance in any situation.

• I am quietly confident in meetings.
• I speak slowly, quietly and confidently so that others listen.
• My contribution is wanted and valued by others.
• I enjoy meetings, as they bring forth new ideas and renew my enthusiasm.

Imagine a meeting that is about to happen, and see yourself there, filling in all the details that you know, and the people too; imagine yourself looking confident and relaxed, concentrating on what is happening. Be aware of the acute interest you have in what is happening – complete, concentrated attention – and then imagine yourself speaking: hear yourself speaking quietly, slowly and calmly . . . Notice people listening to what you are saying; they wish you well and support you, as you are expressing a viewpoint or raising a question they may well have wanted to raise themselves. Take notice of how you are sitting or standing, how you lean slightly

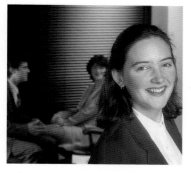

▲ IMAGINE YOURSELF AT AN IMPORTANT EVENT WHERE YOU FEEL AT EASE.

forward when speaking . . . that expression of calm confidence on your face. When this is clear in your mind, just like a film playing in your mind's eye, play it back and forth. When you are feeling comfortable with it, get into that imaginary you, "climb aboard" and be there in your mind, seeing things from that perspective. As you speak, get in touch with the attitudes that allow you to feel calm, in control, and quietly confident . . . It is like a rehearsal; the more you rehearse, the better your final performance will be.

For living for now

We cannot change the past, but we can learn from it and build up skills and useful insights from what we have experienced. The future is unknown – now is the only moment in which we can really make an impact.

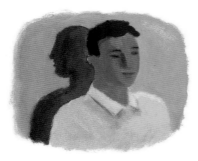

◀ THE PAST IS OVER, AND YOU CANNOT BE SURE ABOUT THE FUTURE, SO THE ONLY TIME YOU CAN TRULY AFFECT IS NOW.

• I have learned from the past.
• The future is an exciting range of opportunities.
• I am able to enjoy my acute awareness of this moment.
• I am living NOW.
• I enjoy laying good foundations now on which to build a better future.

Imagine standing on a pathway that stretches in front of you and trails behind you, the way you have come . . . As you look around, you are aware that the area immediately around you – to the left, right and above – is brilliantly illuminated, and that sounds are amazingly clear. You are intensely aware of all that is happening around you, and your reactions to it. Look ahead again; you see the path in front, but it is dim in comparison with this area. As you check over your shoulder, you notice that the path behind is even less clear. A distant clock chimes, you take a step forward, and the bright, acute awareness travels with you . . . You notice the slightest of noises, movements or shifts of light, and take pleasure even in the sound of silence. You hear the same clock ticking, and with each tick take a small step forward, effortlessly, along the path . . . and illumination and awareness moves with you, in the here and now . . . At any fork in the path you can make decisions easily, because you are truly involved in the moment, rather than looking back at what might have been, or staring blindly into the future at what might happen. You enjoy an acute awareness of sound, hearing, feeling, taste and smell that is NOW.

For decision making

When a decision must be made, talking to an inner adviser can be helpful. Each of us has a higher self, made up of a conscience and an ideal self, towards which we strive. Meditation puts you in touch with your own inner wisdom.

First choose an adviser. You may wish to imagine sitting in front of a wise old person – someone you know, or an imaginary being. Some people choose to focus on an animal. Now imagine being with that adviser and asking a simple question about your problem, then wait . . . You may get a real insight straight away, or your adviser may use a symbolic present, or show you a scene to think about. They may even open up a possibility not yet considered. At first the answer may seem obscure, but at some

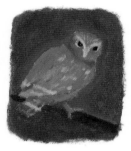

◀ DIFFERENT CULTURES HAVE ADOPTED PARTICULAR ANIMALS AS SYMBOLS OF WISDOM.

point the meaning will become obvious. We all have an inner adviser who is a source of wisdom – perhaps formed before birth, but who is constantly being brought up to date by our daily experience of the world and our reactions to it. The adviser is a valuable resource and can give you the confidence to make decisions, and move forward into your future.

▼ YOU MAY LIKE TO IMAGINE A FRIEND AS YOUR INNER ADVISER.

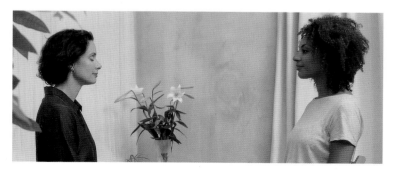

For improved health

The mind and body are so completely interlinked that if we keep physically fit, we will be mentally alert too. Likewise, if we utilize our mental capacities in a positive way, we can affect our physical health and performance for the better.

- I feel safe in the knowledge that my body is constantly renewing itself.
- It feels good to know that all damaged cells are replaced.
- My immune system is strong and fights off any infections easily.
- My mind and body are working in harmony to keep me healthy.

Imagine yourself lying or sitting comfortably. As you see yourself there, you notice a healing glow of coloured light surrounding your body, but not touching it. Let that colour become stronger, until it has a very clear, pure sheen, the colour of healing for you.

Now, as you watch, the healing light begins to flow into your crown. You can see it slowly draining into

▼ CONCENTRATE ON AREAS OF THE BODY THAT NEED HEALING, AND IMAGINE YOURSELF FREE OF ACHES, PAINS, ILLNESS AND TENSION.

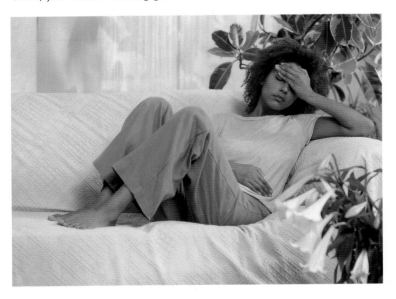

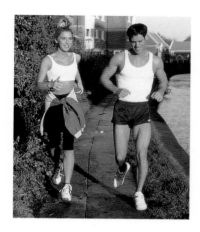

Now that the whole body is suffused with healing energy you notice the light concentrating in areas that need special attention. The warmth there seems more obvious as the light focuses upon repairing and replacing damaged tissue, and your own inner resources are focused in order to heal that area. Now you can allow the light to disperse again, and gradually return to your normal wakeful state.

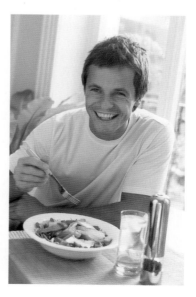

all parts of the head, face and ears, starting its journey down through the neck and shoulders, into the tops of the arms . . . It continues to flow down through the arms and chest, the healing colour penetrating all the muscles and organs . . . as you watch, you can also feel a healing warmth coming into your body . . . NOW . . . as it flows down into the stomach, the back, all the way down to the base of the spine. At the same time, it is reaching your fingertips too, and that warmth is in your body right now . . . It continues to flow down through the legs towards the knees, down into the calves and shins, the ankles, the feet . . . all the way into the toes . . .

For reducing stress

Stress features in everyone's life, and can even be a major motivator in some circumstances. Meditation can be a great help in coping with stress. Combined with visualization, it can change your whole response to the demands of modern living.

- I enjoy solving problems.
- I keep things in perspective.
- I am a calm, methodical and efficient worker.
- I love the feeling of having achieved so much in a day.
- I enjoy being calm when others around me are not.

Imagine yourself in a situation that has in the past caused stress. Picture the situation, and the other people involved . . . See yourself there . . . and notice a slight shimmer of light between yourself and those other people . . . a sort of bubble around you . . . a protective bubble that reflects any negative feelings back to them . . . leaving you able to get on with your tasks . . . your life, with an inner strength and calmness that surprises even you. The protective, invisible bubble surrounds you at all times. It will only allow those

▼ Your protective bubble will stay with you always, whatever you do.

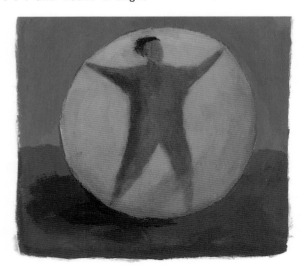

feelings that are positive and helpful to you to pass through for you to enjoy and build upon. Others may catch stress from each other . . . negativity, too, can be infectious . . . but you are protected . . . you continue to keep things in perspective . . . and to deal with things calmly and methodically. You are able to see the way forward clearly . . . solve problems . . . find ways around difficulties . . . by using your own inner resources and strengths, born of experience.

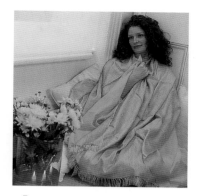

▲ TRY NOT TO LET WORRY DISTORT OR MAGNIFY YOUR PROBLEMS AND DIFFICULTIES.

Now see yourself talking to someone who has been causing tension in your life. Find yourself telling them that what they are doing is unhelpful in resolving the problem or difficulty. Find yourself able to let them know in such a way that they can accept this without offence . . . and find your own calmness and control . . . a strength that supports you. You can let someone know if too much is being expected, and explain why. See yourself in that situation . . . calmly explaining the areas of difficulty . . . being able to supply examples and information until they understand the position. Ask them to prioritize – or give new ways

that things can be dealt with. At all times you are surrounded by that protective bubble of light that keeps you calm and quietly confident. Next, imagine pushing out through that same protective bubble emotions that are unhelpful . . . past resentments . . . hurts . . . and embarrassments. Push them out through the bubble . . . where they can no longer limit or harm you. You are now better able to control the way you feel and react . . . The bubble stays with you and enables you to remain in control . . . keeping things in perspective . . . having the strength to change those things you can change . . . accept those things that you cannot . . . and move on.

For concentration

The pressures that are experienced when studying for an exam or learning a new skill can disrupt concentration, and so one's ability to absorb information. A visual image used during meditation can help re-energize your ability to learn.

- I enjoy moments of insight and understanding.
- I enjoy using my mind and expanding the boundaries of my knowledge.
- My memory forms links between the known and the new information.
- My learning ability improves with use.
- I concentrate so completely that nothing but an emergency can distract me.

Imagine a huge jigsaw puzzle spread out in front of you: it is a giant picture made up of many smaller images, and each image is a jigsaw puzzle in itself. Some images are nearly complete, others are only just starting to form, some even seem a confused jumble of unattached pieces. Focus your attention on one image, one part of the giant puzzle that is nearly complete but is still a little confusing.

A new piece comes into your hand and it fills a gap as it interlocks with all the surrounding pieces . . . The image suddenly becomes clear, and you can see it now. You have a wonderful feeling of achievement: that which was confusing is now fully understood. You feel as you do when a new piece of information interlocks with others and you understand the whole subject. This insight . . . the joy of understanding . . . is what makes learning so worthwhile.

Should you ever need to retrieve that piece of the puzzle, to answer a question of some kind, you know that all the interlocking pieces will arrive with it to give insight and understanding – you can select and use them as you wish. The memory is like a giant puzzle, and the moments of achievement when understanding and enlightenment occur are the joy of learning itself and an important part of life's beauty.

As you learn, so you enjoy total concentration as you study and gain information. Only an emergency could distract you. Learning is a continuous part of being alive.

For achieving goals

In all areas of life – personal relationships, social interactions and career – having a goal is important in focusing your attention and inner resources. A goal provides a sense of direction, and ultimately brings the joy of achievement.

Be aware of the different areas of your life: work, social, emotional and spiritual. Select one for this exercise . . . think about what you want to achieve and describe your goal on paper before beginning.

While in the meditative state, imagine that you have achieved this goal. Surround yourself with the things or people that indicate that you have achieved the goal. Be as specific as you can . . . be aware of all you see, hear, touch or sense . . . Be there . . . make it real . . . be specific about colours . . . temperatures . . . lighting. Be there and know how it feels to have achieved that goal . . . how it affects your mood.

Now, from where you are at that moment of achieving that goal . . . look back . . . as though along a pathway of time . . . to where you were . . . and notice the stages of change . . . of movement towards achieving the goal . . . the actions you have taken . . . the contacts that you have made . . . the people involved. Be aware of the smallest moments of change that have occurred, from the start of the journey to its fulfilment . . . Remain in touch with the feelings that will make it all worthwhile . . . feel more determined to take one step at a time . . . make just one change at a time . . . Become more determined to be successful in the achievement of your goal . . . Take the first step towards it, today.

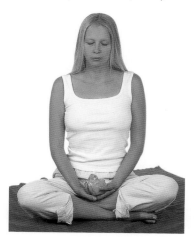

▸ VISUALIZE YOURSELF TAKING ONE STEP AT A TIME TOWARDS YOUR GOAL.

For increased creativity

Many adults long to be creative but underestimate their ability to be so. Self-expression takes many forms, and everyone is creative in one way or another. Use these exercises to discover your latent talents and build confidence.

- I enjoy my own creativity.
- I am blessed with having a vivid imagination.
- I love to express myself in creative ways.
- I enjoy my own imaginative responses to the world as I see, feel and experience it.

▼ AS CHILDREN WE ARE ALL NATURALLY CREATIVE AND THIS CREATIVITY REMAINS WITH US INTO ADULTHOOD. IT IS THERE WITHIN US JUST WAITING TO BE REKINDLED.

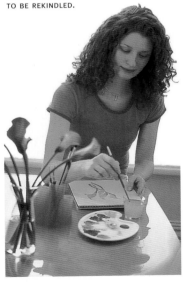

Imagine yourself in a wonderful room . . . a room surrounded by windows looking out on to countryside . . . In this room there are many small areas, and you can move freely around trying each of the areas to see how you feel . . . Here on the left is a large piece of paper with pens and pencils, in a small studio for drawing and sketching . . . Another area has an easel and paints set out for you, the artist, to take up . . . Another has clay for you to handle and form into shapes or pots . . . Another has a computer ready for you to create images in poetry or prose . . . Yet another has engineering tools for the inventor . . . Here is one with cameras and photographic equipment . . . Just spend a little time moving around and trying them all . . . these are some of the areas into which you may choose to channel your own creativity, and where no one else need judge or approve. Only your opinion matters, and the joy of translating the inner

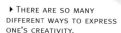

world of the imagination into a form or expression that suits you . . . Which feels most stimulating, most exciting, most comfortable?

Become aware that everyone has a creative ability – to tell stories, to create beauty, to capture a moment . . . Imagine yourself using one of the areas in this marvellous room, or finding another area not yet described . . . in order to create your response to the world around you, or your inner world. Be aware of the feeling of having time and energy to channel into this creative activity . . . the ability to utilize your innate creativity . . . and the joy that comes when something tangible forms in front of you.

Sometimes we drive smoothly and happily along a road, we come to traffic lights on red and have to pause. The creative flow can be like that too, but the lights turn to amber and then green and off we go, just as you will when a temporary block dissolves . . . Enjoy your creative and imaginative power, and translate it into the world around you. You can do it, for your own sake . . . free of the need to please anyone else but yourself.

▼ INSPIRATION CAN COME IN MANY
DIFFERENT FORMS: NATURAL OR ARTIFICIAL;
REAL OR IMAGINARY.

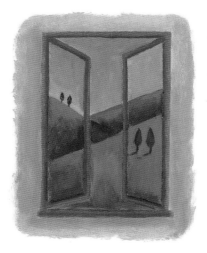

Index

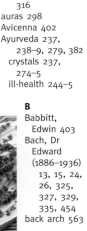
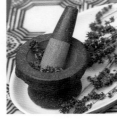

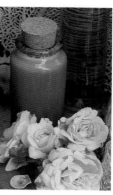

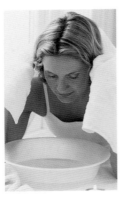

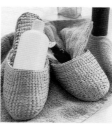

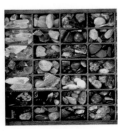

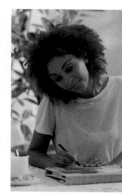

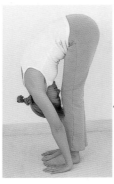

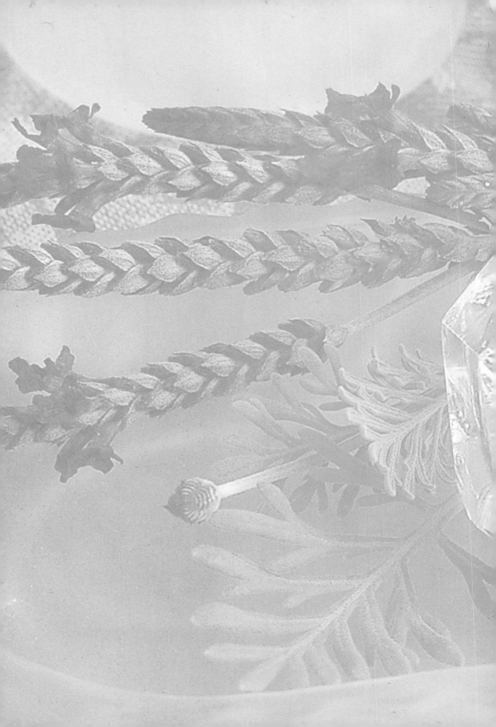